Geriatrics

Guest Editor

WILLIAM D. FORTNEY, DVM

VETERINARY CLINICS OF NORTH AMERICA: SMALL ANIMAL PRACTICE

www.vetsmall.theclinics.com

July 2012 • Volume 42 • Number 4

SAUNDERS an imprint of ELSEVIER, Inc.

W.B. SAUNDERS COMPANY
A Division of Elsevier Inc.

1600 John F. Kennedy Blvd. • Suite 1800 • Philadelphia, PA 19103-2899

http://www.vetsmall.theclinics.com

VETERINARY CLINICS OF NORTH AMERICA: SMALL ANIMAL PRACTICE Volume 42, Number 4
July 2012 ISSN 0195-5616, ISBN-13: 978-1-4557-3958-5

Editor: John Vassallo; j.vassallo@elsevier.com
Developmental Editor: Teia Stone

Veterinary Clinics of North America: Small Animal Practice (ISSN 0195-5616) is published bimonthly (For Post Office use only: volume 42 issue 1 of 6) by Elsevier Inc., 360 Park Avenue South, New York, NY 10010-1710. Months of issue are January, March, May, July, September, and November. Business and Editorial Offices: 1600 John F. Kennedy Blvd., Ste. 1800, Philadelphia, PA 19103-2899. Customer Service Office: 3251 Riverport Lane, Maryland Heights, MO 63043. Periodicals postage paid at New York, NY and additional mailing offices. Subscription prices are $283.00 per year (domestic individuals), $455.00 per year (domestic institutions), $138.00 per year (domestic students/residents), $375.00 per year (Canadian individuals), $559.00 per year (Canadian institutions), $416.00 per year (international individuals), $559.00 per year (international institutions), and $201.00 per year (international and Canadian students/residents). To receive student/resident rate, orders must be accompanied by name of affiliated institution, date of term, and the signature of program/residency coordinator on institution letterhead. Orders will be billed at individual rate until proof of status is received. Foreign air speed delivery is included in all *Clinics* subscription prices. All prices are subject to change without notice. **POSTMASTER:** Send address changes to *Veterinary Clinics of North America: Small Animal Practice,* Elsevier Health Sciences Division, Subscription Customer Service, 3251 Riverport Lane, Maryland Heights, MO 63043. Customer Service (orders, claims, online, change of address): Elsevier Periodicals Customer Service, Elsevier Health Sciences Division, Subscription Customer Service, 3251 Riverport Lane, Maryland Heights, MO 63043. Tel: 1-800-654-2452 (U.S. and Canada); 314-447-8871 (outside U.S. andCanada). Fax: 314-447-8029. E-mail: journalscustomerservice-usa@elsevier.com (for print support); journalsonlinesupport-usa@elsevier.com (for online support).

Reprints. For copies of 100 or more of articles in this publication, please contact the Commercial Reprints Department, Elsevier Inc., 360 Park Avenue South, New York, NY 10010-1710. Tel.: 212-633-3812; Fax: 212-462-1935; E-mail: reprints@elsevier.com.

Veterinary Clinics of North America: Small Animal Practice is also published in Japanese by Inter Zoo Publishing Co., Ltd., Aoyama Crystal-Bldg 5F, 3-5-12 Kitaaoyama, Minato-ku, Tokyo 107-0061, Japan.

Veterinary Clinics of North America: Small Animal Practice is covered in *Current Contents/Agriculture, Biology and Environmental Sciences, Science Citation Index, ASCA, MEDLINE/PubMed (Index Medicus), Excerpta Medica,* and *BIOSIS.*

Printed in the United States of America.

Contributors

GUEST EDITOR

WILLIAM D. FORTNEY, DVM
Assistant Professor, Department of Pathobiology and Diagnostic Medicine, Kansas State University, College of Veterinary Medicine, Manhattan, Kansas

AUTHORS

JOSEPH A. ARAUJO, BSc
CanCog Technologies Inc; InterVivo Solutions Inc; and Department of Pharmacology and Toxicology, University of Toronto, Toronto, Ontario, Canada

COURTNEY L. BAETGE, DVM
Diplomate, American College of Veterinary Anesthesiologists; College Station, Texas

JOSEPH W. BARTGES, DVM, PhD
Diplomate, American College of Veterinary Internal Medicine; Diplomate, American College of Veterinary Nutrition; Professor of Medicine and Nutrition, The Acree Endowed Chair of Small Animal Research, Department of Small Animal Clinical Sciences, College of Veterinary Medicine, The University of Tennessee, Knoxville, Tennessee

WILLIAM D. FORTNEY, DVM
Assistant Professor, Department of Pathobiology and Diagnostic Medicine, Kansas State University, College of Veterinary Medicine, Manhattan, Kansas

STEVEN M. FOX, MS, DVM, MBA, PhD
Independent Consultant, Fox Third Bearing Inc, Clive, Iowa; Adjunct Professor, University of Illinois, Urbana, Illinois; Adjunct Professor, University of Tennessee, Knoxville, Tennessee; and Adjunct Professor, Massey University, Palmerston North, New Zealand

STEVEN E. HOLMSTROM, DVM
Diplomate, American Veterinary Dental College; Animal Dental Clinic, San Carlos, California

J. RANDY KIDD, DVM, PhD
Retired Holistic Practitioner and Owner, Coyote Consulting LLD, McLouth, Kansas

BUTCH KUKANICH, DVM, PhD
Diplomate, American College of Veterinary Clinical Pharmacology; Associate Professor, Department of Anatomy and Physiology, College of Veterinary Medicine, Kansas State University, Manhattan, Kansas

D.P. LAFLAMME, DVM, PhD
Diplomate, American College of Veterinary Nutrition; Nestlé Purina PetCare Research, St Louis, Missouri

GARY M. LANDSBERG, DVM
Diplomate, American College of Veterinary Behaviorists; Diplomate, European College of Animal Welfare and Behavioural Medicine (Behaviour); North Toronto Animal Clinic, Thornhill; and CanCog Technologies Inc, Toronto, Ontario, Canada

NORA S. MATTHEWS, DVM
Diplomate, American College of Veterinary Anesthesiologists; Professor, Department of Small Animal Clinical Sciences, College of Veterinary Medicine and Biomedical Sciences, Texas A&M University, College Station, Texas

FRED L. METZGER, DVM
Diplomate, American Board of Veterinary Practitioners (Canine/Feline); Director, Metzger Animal Hospital, State College, Pennsylvania

JEFF NICHOL, DVM
Veterinary Emergency and Specialty Center of New Mexico, Albuquerque, New Mexico

ALAN H. REBAR, DVM, PhD
Diplomate, American College of Veterinary Pathologists; Senior Associate Vice President for Research, Executive Director, Discovery Park, Purdue University, West Lafayette, Indiana

ASHLEY B. SAUNDERS, DVM
Diplomate, American College of Veterinary Internal Medicine (Cardiology); Assistant Professor, Department of Small Animal Clinical Sciences, College of Veterinary Medicine and Biomedical Sciences, Texas A&M University, College Station, Texas

J. CATHARINE SCOTT-MONCRIEFF, MA, MS, Vet MB, MRCVS
Diplomate, American College Veterinary Internal Medicine; Diplomate, European College Veterinary Internal Medicine; Professor of Internal Medicine, Department of Veterinary Clinical Sciences, College of Veterinary Medicine, Purdue University, West Lafayette, Indiana

MICHAEL D. WILLARD, DVM, MS
Diplomate, American College of Veterinary Internal Medicine; Professor of Veterinary Clinical Sciences, Department of Small Animal Clinical Sciences, College of Veterinary Medicine and Biomedical Sciences, Texas A&M University, College Station, Texas

Contents

> Routine monitoring of clinicopathologic data is a critical component in the management of older patients because blood and urine testing allows the veterinarian to monitor trends in laboratory parameters, which may be the early indicators of disease. Laboratory profiling often provides an objective and sensitive indicator of developing disease before obvious clinical signs or physical examination abnormalities are observed. The primary key to the power of this evaluation is that the data are collected year after year during wellness checks and are examined serially. Chronic renal failure, chronic active hepatitis, canine hyperadrenocorticism, diabetes mellitus, and feline hyperthyroidism were reviewed and expected laboratory findings are summarized.

> Geriatric dogs and cats are an important group of patients in veterinary medicine. Healthy geriatric patients have similar physiology and presumably pharmacology as healthy adult animals. Geriatric patients with subclinical organ dysfunction are overtly healthy but have some organ dysfunction that may alter the clinical pharmacology of some drugs. Geriatric patients with an overt disease are expected to have altered drug pharmacology for some drugs based on the underlying disease. Diseases including cardiovascular, renal, hepatic, osteoarthritis, neurologic, and neoplastic are expected in the geriatric population and discussed, including the effects of the underlying disease and potential drug-drug interactions.

> The number of geriatric veterinary patients presented for anesthesia appears to be increasing. This article summarizes physiologic changes that occur in geriatric patients that are relevant to anesthesia. Proper patient preparation and vigilant monitoring are the best defense against anesthetic problems in the geriatric animal. The authors also discuss particular anesthetic problems as they relate to geriatric patients and seek to present solutions to these problems.

The American Veterinary Medical Association reported 81.7 million cats and 72.1 million dogs in the United States, with more than 10% over 11 years of age. Disorders of the cardiovascular system are one of the most commonly encountered disease entities in the aging pet population. This article reviews the diseases affecting older cats and dogs including how to make the diagnosis and when to treat while keeping in mind the unique aspects of comorbid conditions and polypharmacy situations encountered while managing pets with cardiovascular disease.

Chronic kidney disease (CKD) occurs commonly in older dogs and cats. Advances in diagnostics, staging, and treatment are associated with increased quality and quantity of life. Dietary modification has been shown to increase survival and quality of life and involves more than protein restriction as diets modified for use with CKD are lower in phosphorous and sodium, potassium and B-vitamin replete, and alkalinizing, and they contain n3-fatty acids. Additionally, recognition and management of CKD-associated diseases such as systemic arterial hypertension, proteinuria, and anemia benefit patients. This article summarizes staging and management of CKD in dogs and cats.

Lymphomas, carcinomas, leiomyomas, and stromal tumors are the most common tumors found in the canine and feline gastrointestinal tract. Endoscopic and surgical biopsies are often the mainstays of diagnosis, although ultrasound is playing an increasingly greater role. Small cell lymphocytic lymphoma of the feline intestines poses a special diagnostic dilemma and may require immunohistochemistry as well as polymerase chain reaction to distinguish it from lymphocytic-plasmacytic enteritis. This article will focus on the more common neoplastic problems of the esophagus and gastrointestinal tract (GIT) of geriatric dogs and cats.

The effects of age, concurrent illness, and administered medications complicate diagnosis of thyroid dysfunction in geriatric patients. Interpretation of thyroid hormone testing should take these factors into account. The most common thyroid disorder in dogs is acquired hypothyroidism. Therapeutic monitoring should be utilized for monitoring treatment of canine hypothyroidism. The most common thyroid disorder in cats is benign hyperthyroidism. Diagnosis is most often complicated by the presence of concurrent illness. Treatment should be individualized based on individual case characteristics and presence of concurrent illness. Some older cats have a palpable goiter months to years before development of clinical signs of hyperthyroidism.

Osteoarthritis and cancer are the inevitable consequences of aging and significantly contribute to the cause of death in cats and dogs. Managing the pain associated with these disease states is the veterinarian's mandate. Many treatment modalities and agents are available for patient management; however, it is only with an understanding of disease neurobiology and a mechanism-based approach to problem diagnosis that the clinician can offer patients an optimal quality of life based on evidence-based best medicine. When treating pain, knowledge is still our best weapon.

Brain aging is a degenerative process manifest by impairment of cognitive function; although not all pets are affected at the same level, once cognitive decline begins it is generally a progressive disorder. Diagnosis of cognitive dysfunction syndrome (CDS) is based on recognition of behavioral signs and exclusion of other medical causes that might mimic CDS or complicate its diagnosis. Drugs, diets, and supplements are now available that might slow CDS progression by various mechanisms including reducing oxidative stress and inflammation or improving mitochondrial and neuronal function. Moreover, available therapeutics may provide some level of improvement in cognitive and clinical signs of CDS.

Veterinarians need to be prepared to provide nutritional advice for healthy pets as well as for pets that are ill. Before instituting a dietary change in any patient, especially an older dog or cat, a nutritional evaluation should be completed. This should include an evaluation of the patient, the current diet, and feeding management. Diets should be appropriate to the unique needs of the individual patient. Many diseases in senior pets are "diet-sensitive" meaning that diet can play a role in managing the effects of the disease. Common examples discussed include cognitive dysfunction of aging, osteoarthritis, and obesity.

THE CLINICS ARE NOW AVAILABLE ONLINE!

Access your subscription at:
www.theclinics.com

Preface

Geriatrics

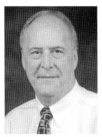

William D. Fortney, DVM
Guest Editor

Geriatric medicine is a major growth area in the veterinary profession. Advanced diagnostics and equipment, once reserved for universities and specialty referral centers, are currently accessible to these progressive primary care veterinarians. Those hospitals can now provide their older patients with the high-quality health care that even the "average" pet owner expects. Enhanced senior diets, improved dental care, pain management plans, safer preanesthetic protocols, new drugs, advanced surgery techniques, cancer chemotherapy protocol, drug-monitoring schedules, and the use of multimodal management strategies have changed the senior health care landscape.

What is commonplace today was just an idea in the mid 1980s when I began lecturing in the area. Momentum was painfully slow as the concept began to take shape . . . one practice at a time. I would like to recognize some of the leaders responsible for where senior care is today: foremost is my mentor Dr Jacob (Jake) Mosier for all his help; Drs Johnny Hoskins and Richard (Bill) Goldston for taking the discipline to the next level; Dr Fred Metzger for his unceasing passion for senior care programs; and Dr Gary Landsberg for all of the older pets he has helped during his career.

This Geriatrics edition represents a "topic-based" approach to many of the age-related problems commonly seen in older dogs and cats. Each author was selected based on their expertise and ability to convey practical knowledge to the reader. Their efforts exceeded my expectations. But without Mr John Vassallo's leadership, editorial genius, and patience with me, this issue would not have been possible. My sincere hope is that every veterinarian and veterinary technician reading this issue will share my enthusiasm and passion for older dogs and cats.

Vet Clin Small Anim 42 (2012) xi–xii
http://dx.doi.org/10.1016/j.cvsm.2012.05.002
0195-5616/12/$ – see front matter © 2012 Elsevier Inc. All rights reserved.

vetsmall.theclinics.com

Last, a special thanks to my amazing wife of 42 years, Sheila, who has devotedly helped me deal with the consequences of my recent stroke. She spent countless hours re-teaching me the alphabet and elementary level reading, writing, and arithmetic.

William D. Fortney, DVM
Department of Pathobiology and Diagnostic Medicine
Kansas State University
College of Veterinary Medicine
Manhattan, KS 66506, USA

E-mail address:
wfortney@vet.k-state.edu

Clinical Pathology Interpretation in Geriatric Veterinary Patients

Fred L. Metzger, DVM[a],*, Alan H. Rebar, DVM, PhD[b]

KEYWORDS

- Geriatric dogs • Geriatric cats • Laboratory trending • Hematology

KEY POINTS

- Routine monitoring of clinicopathologic data is a critical component in the management of older patients.
- Serial data evaluations on an individual animal can prove to be a highly objective effective means of characterizing developing disease.
- The complete blood count provides a broad overview of the general health status of the patient.
- The minimum canine geriatric database includes the CBC, biochemical profile (with electrolytes), complete urinalysis.
- The minimum senior feline database includes the CBC, biochemical profile (with electrolytes), complete urinalysis, total T_4.
- Important geriatric conditions in dogs cats include chronic renal disease, hepatobilliary disease endocrine metabolic disorders.

INTRODUCTION

Early disease recognition can help improve the quality of life for all dogs and cats, but especially for older dogs and cats and their owners. Complete diagnostic efforts, including laboratory profiling, are critical because geriatric pets frequently have abnormalities in multiple body systems and often receive long-term medications for chronic diseases or conditions related to aging.

Veterinarians should evaluate serial hematologic and biochemical data on an individual patient when performing yearly wellness testing and when following the progression or regression of a disease once recognized. Serial data evaluations on an individual animal can prove to be a highly objective and effective means of characterizing

---

The authors have nothing to disclose.
[a] Metzger Animal Hospital, 1044 Benner Pike, State College, PA 16801, USA; [b] Discovery Park, Purdue University, West Lafayette, IN, USA
* Corresponding author.
E-mail address: FLMDVM@aol.com

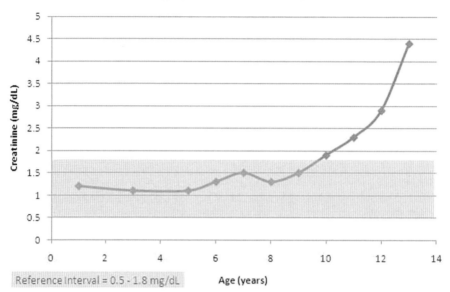

Fig. 1. Yearly creatinine measurements for a geriatric poodle.

developing disease in the clinically normal patient or of objectively determining if therapy is working appropriately with ill patients.

This article presents a brief review of important hematologic and biochemical testing parameters and concludes with a synopsis of laboratory findings for several common geriatric diseases, including chronic renal disease, canine chronic hepatitis, canine hyperadrenocorticism (Cushing disease), diabetes mellitus (DM), and feline hyperthyroidism.

TRENDING DATA DURING HEALTH

Serial laboratory data are especially critical in the interpretation of laboratory profiles in geriatric patients because laboratory data are much more objective and sensitive than clinical presenting signs or physical examination findings.

Fig. 1 represents yearly creatinine measurements for a geriatric poodle. Not until year 11 is there a clear increase out of the reference interval. However, in as early as years 7 through 10, the trend toward increasing creatinine values is observed. This type of trend should prompt further investigation to more critically evaluate the kidney (graphic examination of concentrating ability with retrospective serial specific gravity review, diagnostic imaging of the kidney, urine protein:creatinine ratio measurement, etc) and institute therapy earlier.

THE GERIATRIC SCREENING PANEL

The minimum canine geriatric database includes the complete blood count (CBC), biochemical profile (with electrolytes), and complete urinalysis. The minimum senior feline database includes the CBC, biochemical profile (with electrolytes), complete urinalysis, and total T_4.[1]

OTHER COMMONLY PERFORMED GERIATRIC TESTS

Primary senior profiling may reveal abnormalities that require further investigation. More specific geriatric laboratory tests include urinary tract protein evaluation (microalbuminuria, urine protein:creatinine ratio), hepatic function tests (bile acids and ammonia tolerance), endocrine assays (serum fructosamine, free T_4, canine thyroid-stimulating hormone, insulin, ionized calcium, parathyroid-like peptide, parathyroid hormone assay, urine cortisol:creatinine ratio, adrenocorticotropic hormone stimulation, dexamethasone suppression, 17-hydroxyprogesterone), and cardiac markers (N-terminal prohormone of brain natriuretic peptide [NT pro-BNP]) among others.

This article will focus only on the minimum geriatric database (hemogram, biochemical profile, urinalysis and total T_4) and recommends that the reader pursue additional readings suggested at the end more comprehensive information.

INTERPRETING THE GERIATRIC HEMOGRAM (CBC)

The CBC provides a broad overview of the general health status of the patient. The peripheral blood serves as the transport medium between the bone marrow and the tissues; consequently, the CBC provides a snapshot of the hematopoietic system at a specific point in time. The peripheral blood film examination is especially important in geriatric patients because erythrocyte, leukocyte, and thrombocyte changes are common in older patients and may give clues to occult underlying diseases.

Evaluating the Red Blood Cells

Red blood cell (RBC) data include the hematocrit, RBC count, hemoglobin concentration, absolute reticulocyte count, and indices such as mean cell volume, mean cell hemoglobin concentration, and red cell distribution width.

If RBC mass is reduced, the animal is anemic. The degree of anemia should be further considered in conjunction with plasma protein concentrations. If protein concentrations are elevated, then the animal may be dehydrated, and the anemia may be more severe than RBC mass measurements indicate. Anemia is a common syndrome detected in senior patients and prompt recognition allows earlier detection of underlying causes.

Peripheral blood film evaluation may provide important information if red cell abnormalities such as poikilocytes are identified (abnormally shaped red cells); the specific type of poikilocyte often proves to be a good indication of specific types of developing disease.

Regenerative or nonregenerative anemia?

Reticulocytosis is the hallmark and best single indicator of intensified erythropoiesis, allowing classification of anemias into regenerative or nonregenerative types based on bone marrow responsiveness.[2] The absolute reticulocyte count is the most objective measure of current bone marrow responsiveness in cases of anemia. If the bone marrow responds with an increase in RBC production of appropriate magnitude, the anemia is regenerative (responsive). Common types of regenerative anemia include blood loss anemia (secondary to any of a number of causes including bleeding neoplasm) immune-mediated hemolytic anemia, fragmentation anemia (microangiopathic hemolysis), and occasionally Heinz body hemolytic anemia due to oxidative injury.

The finding of a bone marrow response and a significant reticulocytosis in the absence of anemia may be an important early indicator of underlying disease.[3] In some circumstances where RBC life span is decreased and the bone marrow has the

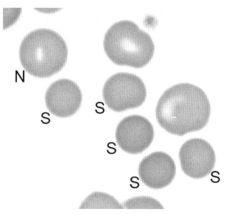

Fig. 2. Spherocytes (S) are spherical erythrocytes that have lost their normal biconcave shape resulting in more intense staining than normal erythrocytes (N). They have no central zone of pallor and they appear smaller than normal erythrocytes.

capability of responding, compensation may occur with an underlying finding of reticulocytosis without anemia. When this is observed, investigation into developing liver, splenic, renal, and immune-mediated disease and other conditions resulting in this type of response is warranted.[3]

Nonregenerative anemias (and in particular the anemia associated with inflammation and chronic disease) are the most frequently encountered anemias in geriatric patients because of the increased incidence of chronic renal failure, chronic hepatitis/hepatopathy, neoplasia, and endocrinopathies.

Important poikilocytes in senior patients

Spherocytes are spherical erythrocytes that have lost their normal biconcave shape, resulting in more intense staining than normal erythrocytes. They have no central zone of pallor and they appear smaller than normal erythrocytes (**Fig. 2**). Spherocytes are commonly seen with many of the immune-mediated hemolytic anemias encountered in veterinary medicine. Caution must be used when attempting to identify spherocytes in feline erythrocytes because feline erythrocytes are much less biconcave in shape than red cells of dogs and therefore normally have significantly less central pallor.[4]

Acanthocytes are abnormally shaped erythrocytes, having 2 to 10, blunt, finger-like projections of varying sizes on their surface (**Fig. 3**). Acanthocytosis is most commonly associated with liver disease where lipid metabolism is altered and lipid loading of red cell membranes occurs. Chronic hepatitis/hepatopathy and hepatic hemangiosarcoma in dogs and hepatic lipidosis in cats are relatively frequent causes.[4]

Evaluating the White Blood Cells

Leukogram data include total and differential white blood cell (WBC) counts and a description of WBC morphology from the peripheral blood film. Differential cell counts should always be expressed and interpreted in absolute numbers, not percentages. All leukocyte compartments—neutrophils and their precursors, lymphocytes, monocytes, eosinophils, and basophils—must be evaluated. Neutrophilic left shifts, persistent eosinophilia, and monocytosis are the best indicators of inflammation.[5] Left

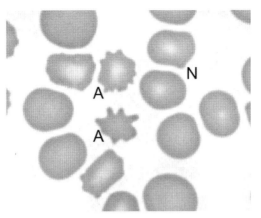

Fig. 3. Acanthocytes (A) are abnormally shaped erythrocytes having 2 to 10, blunt, finger-like projections of varying sizes on their surface.

shifts (increased numbers of immature [band] neutrophils in circulation) indicate increased turnover and tissue use of neutrophils. Eosinophilias are commonly associated with inflammatory diseases involving parasitic infestations and hypersensitivity responses. Monocytosis is seen in peripheral blood when there is a demand for phagocytosis.

Inflammatory leukograms may be present in senior patients for many reasons including inflammatory processes associated with underlying conditions such as DM, hyperadrenocorticism, and neoplasia, among others. Persistent peripheral eosinophilia indicates a systemic allergic or hypersensitivity reaction and may be associated with feline asthma, systemic parasitic disease, and certain cancers. Some neoplasms, such as lymphoma, mast cell tumor, and solid tumors, are associated with eosinophilia caused by tumor cell elaboration of interleukin 5 and other cytokines.[6] Persistent marked neutrophilia with no obvious underlying inflammatory process must be investigated for potential underlying chronic myelogenous leukemia, even when atypical neutrophil forms are not observed in the peripheral blood.

Lymphocyte evaluation is especially important in senior patients because stress leukograms may indicate undetected underlying disease including hyperadrenocorticism. When "atypical" lymphocytes or marked lymphocytosis with "normal" appearing lymphocytes are identified, investigation into potential underlying lymphoproliferative disease is warranted. Review by a veterinary clinical pathologist recommended and possible immunophenotyping or polymerase chain reaction clonality testing may be warranted.

Evaluating the Platelets

An assessment of platelet numbers is an important part of every CBC. As with RBCs, the principal issue is whether platelet numbers are normal, increased (thrombocytosis), or reduced (thrombocytopenia).

Transient or intermittent thrombocytosis may be associated with conditions such as the following: blood loss, fractures, gastrointestinal disorders, drug therapy, and nonhematologic neoplasias.[7] Persistently high platelet counts (sometimes >1 million/μL) may be the result of platelet leukemia (essential thrombocythemia) and should be thoroughly investigated. Essential thrombocythemias may have both platelets and blasts in circulation. Other hematologic abnormalities (severe nonregenerative anemia, panleukopenia, etc) may also be present as a result of bone marrow replacement by neoplastic platelet precursors.

Thrombocytopenia is of great clinical significance in any patient. Platelet evaluation in geriatric veterinary patients is especially important because thrombocytopenia has been reported in approximately 13% of dogs that have neoplasia, particularly lymphoma, multiple myeloma, myelogenous leukemia, and hemangiosarcoma.[8]

Platelet counts below 40,000/μL can lead to overt bleeding; however, one should always keep in mind that automated platelet counts may be inaccurate because variable platelet size and/or platelet clumping can result in falsely low counts, particularly in cats. Suspected thrombocytopenia should always be confirmed by looking at a peripheral blood film before pursuing further diagnostics.

True thrombocytopenia can result from 4 mechanisms: sequestration of platelets in the spleen, increased peripheral use of platelets, peripheral destruction of platelets, or decreased platelet production.[5]

Sequestration thrombocytopenia is sometimes seen in cases of hypersplenism in humans but is rare in animals. Platelet counts are usually moderately reduced.

Consumption thrombocytopenia (increased peripheral use) is seen in association with severe inflammatory disease and is often a feature of disseminated intravascular coagulopathy. Again, peripheral platelet counts are moderately decreased. Bone marrow aspirates contain adequate numbers of megakaryocytes (platelet precursors). In dogs with disseminated intravascular coagulopathy, red cell fragments (schistocytes) are often seen on blood films.

Destruction thrombocytopenia is caused by antibodies directed against circulating platelets. Platelet counts can be quite low (<50,000/μL). Megakaryocytes are often present in increased numbers in the bone marrow. Destructive thrombocytopenias are often responsive to therapy with glucocorticoids or other immunosuppressive therapeutic agents.

Production thrombocytopenia is characterized by decreased numbers of bone marrow megakaryocytes. Peripheral counts may be quite low (often 50,000/μL or less). The cause is often obscure, but this condition may result from immune-mediated marrow disease (antibodies directed against bone marrow platelet precursors) and may also respond to immunosuppressive therapy.

INTERPRETING THE GERIATRIC BIOCHEMISTRY PROFILE

It is beyond the scope of this chapter to discuss every laboratory finding for geriatric patients. Important geriatric conditions in dogs and cats include chronic renal disease, hepatobilliary disease, and endocrine and metabolic disorders (Cushing disease, DM, canine hypothyroidism, and feline hyperthyroidism). Accordingly, here we will limit our comments to a discussion of the laboratory findings in several of these important conditions. For more detailed discussions of laboratory profiling in general, readers should consult the references listed at the end of the article.

EXPECTED CLINICOPATHOLOGIC PATTERNS WITH COMMON GERIATRIC CONDITIONS
Chronic Renal Disease

Chronic renal disease (CRD) is the most frequently encountered urinary system disease in geriatric dogs and especially cats. Laboratory profile abnormalities commonly associated with CRD include anemia, azotemia, hyperphosphatemia, hyperkalemia or hypokalemia, metabolic acidosis, and isosthenuria.[9] More severe changes are commonly seen with chronic renal failure (CRF).

Hemogram

Anemia is a frequent finding with CRF patients. Underlying mechanisms include decreased renal erythropoietin production, decreased erythrocyte survival, and possible uremia-induced gastrointestinal ulceration with blood loss.[10] The anemia associated with CRF is typically mild to moderate and usually nonregenerative. If bleeding associated with anemia is a prominent finding, some evidence of regeneration may be observed.

Biochemical profile

Blood urea nitrogen (BUN) and creatinine (Cr) Azotemia is defined as increased circulating levels of nitrogenous wastes and is characterized by elevated BUN and Cr levels. Elevated BUN and Cr are typical in CRF.

BUN and Cr are indicators of glomerular filtration (GFR) rate but do not elevate in renal disease until more than three-fourths of the nephrons are nonfunctional. Since BUN can be increased following a high protein diet or bleeding into the gastrointestinal tract, Cr is the superior measure of GFR. BUN and Cr must be interpreted in light of urine specific gravity. If BUN and Cr are elevated and urine specific gravity is greater than 1.030 in dogs and 1.035 in cats, then azotemia is most likely prerenal (resulting from hemoconcentration). If urine specific gravity is isosthenuric (between 1.008 and 1.012, essentially the specific gravity of plasma), then primary renal disease is suspected. It is important to note that the occasional feline patient may concentrate urine to greater than 1.040 and still have renal disease.[9]

Phosphorus Like BUN and Cr, phosphorus is also cleared via glomerular filtration. In general, elevations in phosphorous levels correlate with Cr elevations.

Phosphorus levels should be closely monitored during treatment for CRF because chronic hyperphosphatemia may result in renal secondary hyperparathyroidism and soft tissue mineralization.[11]

Potassium Potassium is predominantly an intracellular ion so serum potassium levels do not necessarily reflect total body potassium. Both hyperkalemia (increased serum potassium) and hypokalemia (decreased serum potassium) can be seen in CRF.

Hyperkalemia is seen in renal failure in association with metabolic acidosis caused by circulating uremic acids (sulfates and phosphates). In acidosis, hydrogen ions move into tissue cells in exchange for potassium ions, which migrate from within cells into blood.

Hypokalemia occurs when total body stores of potassium are depleted due to decreased renal tubular absorption and increased renal excretion. This is particularly an issue with CRD in feline patients. When this occurs, serum potassium levels may be low even in the face of acidosis.[12]

Total T_4

Decreased total T_4 levels may be seen as a result of nonthyroidal illness in CKD patients. Total T_4 should always be evaluated in any feline geriatric CRD or CRF patient because hyperthyroidism may occur simultaneously with CRD.

Urinalysis

Urinalysis is critical to making the diagnosis of CRD but findings may be somewhat variable depending on the underlying cause of the CRD. The most consistent finding is isothenuria (urine specific gravity between 1.008 and 1.012, the specific gravity of plasma). Casts may or may not be present. In true end-stage renal disease, casts are rare to occasional and are usually granular or waxy in characterization. If the underlying cause is pyelonephritis, white cell casts may be seen. In this circumstance white cells and red cells may also be present in the urine. Proteinuria is variable, again, dependent upon underlying cause of the CRD.

Canine Chronic Hepatitis

Canine chronic hepatitis (CCH) is a group of necrotizing inflammatory diseases of the liver with variable etiology and clinical history. CCH usually affects middle-age to older dogs and includes idiopathic chronic hepatitis, copper-associated hepatitis, and chronic hepatitis in Doberman pinschers among others.[13] Chronic hepatitis may result in hepatic cirrhosis and fibrosis if the underlying disease progresses to end-stage liver disease. Biochemical profiling is useful in defining the presence and to some degree the extent of liver and biliary tree involvement; however, liver biopsy is generally necessary to fully and accurately characterize these disorders.

Hemogram

Hemogram findings are variable depending upon underlying disease. Most cases of chronic liver disease are characterized by a mild to moderate nonregenerative anemia. An inflammatory leukogram is a common accompaniment. Acanthocytes may be present if lipid metabolism is altered.

Biochemical profile

Alanine aminotransferase (ALT) ALT is a cytoplasmic enzyme found primarily in hepatocytes of dogs and cats. Whenever there is hepatocyte injury in dogs and cats, ALT will leak into the blood in increased amounts. In general, peak elevations are reached in about 48 hours after injury. The circulating half-life of ALT is about 48 to 96 hours in dogs (much shorter in cats), so that continual or rising elevations indicate ongoing injury. A 2-fold increase in ALT caused by a single episode of hepatic injury can be expected to resolve in 48 to 72 hours.[5] In this respect, ALT is an indicator of acute hepatocellular injury.

It is important to note that ALT is not a liver function test; rather, it is best regarded as an indicator of the number of hepatocytes undergoing injury or damage at the same time. The more hepatocytes affected, the greater are the serum ALT levels. This indicates nothing about the reversibility of the lesion.

In the active phases of liver disease, large numbers of hepatocytes may be damaged and ALT levels may be quite high, elevating to 10 times the upper end of the reference interval or higher.[13] As disease progresses to the more chronic phase, ALT levels tend to decline as injured hepatocytes are lost. In end-stage liver disease with cirrhosis, ALT levels may even be within reference interval limits as a result of decreased hepatic mass.

Serum alkaline phosphatase (SAP) SAP is a membrane-bound enzyme found at the bile canalicular surface of hepatocytes. SAP production is induced whenever cholestasis occurs. Unfortunately, in the dog, SAP is not found only in biliary system. Isoenzymes of SAP can also be found in bone, placenta, kidney, and gastrointestinal tract and there is even an additional isoenzyme specifically induced by high circulating levels of glucocorticoids (as is seen with Cushing disease) and other stimuli.[12] The degree of elevation of SAP is therefore extremely important to interpretation in dogs. Elevations of 2 to 3 times above the upper end of the reference interval are regarded as nonspecific in dogs. Four-fold or greater elevations in dogs are regarded as indicative of either cholestasis or elevations of the steroid-induced isoenzyme of SAP.[5] These are differentiated by looking for secondary indicators of cholestasis (urine, serum bilirubin) and the presence of lymphopenia (as a result of high levels of circulating glucocorticoids) in the CBC.

In most cases of CCH, SAP gradually elevates over time because the cholestasis resulting from scarring of the liver is progressive. Levels may frequently reach greater than 5 times the upper end of the reference interval. Keep in mind that elevations in SAP do not necessarily occur in concert with elevations of ALT; often, hepatocellular injury has subsided and ALT levels have returned to normal by the time significant elevations in SAP are seen.

Gamma-glutamyl transferase (GGT) GGT is a membrane-bound enzyme associated with bile duct epithelium. As such, it is a second primary indicator of cholestasis. It has been suggested that GGT may be more useful than SAP in dogs since it is not directly induced by glucocorticoids.[14] However, in practice, SAP and GGT tend to elevate together, even when steroid induction is the underlying cause of the SAP elevation. This is probably because high circulating levels of glucocorticoids induce a steroid hepatopathy with hepatocellular swelling and secondary intrahepatic cholestasis, which causes the GGT to rise as well.

Canine cases are seen in which GGT is elevated to a greater proportion than alkaline phosphatase (ALP). Such patients generally suffer from biliary obstruction and extrahepatic cholestasis.

Total protein and albumin Total protein and albumin may be regarded as liver function tests. All of the plasma proteins with the exception of the immunoglobulins are produced by the liver. Consequently, patients with decreased functional hepatic mass, such as those with advanced CCH, often present with hypoproteinemia with hypoalbuminemia and normal to increased globulins. These changes are usually only seen in chronic liver disease primarily because plasma proteins have a long circulating half-life (7–10 days) and the hypoalbuminemia/hypoproteinemia takes significant time to develop.

Serum and urine bilirubin Serum bilirubin and urine bilirubin are also often elevated in CCH, primarily as a consequence of cholestasis. Bilirubin is a normal breakdown product of hemoglobin. When aged red cells are removed from circulation by splenic and other tissue macrophages, the heme from hemoglobin gives rise to unconjugated bilirubin, which is transported by blood to the liver, where it is conjugated to bilirubin diglucuronide. Normally, the conjugated bilirubin then passes out of the body with the bile.

Whenever cholestasis occurs, levels of conjugated bilirubin in the blood elevate. Over time, as liver disease and cholestasis become chronic, circulating levels of unconjugated bilirubin elevate as well because of decreased hepatic function.

Conjugated bilirubin is water soluble and readily passes through the glomerulus of the kidney as a part of the glomerular filtrate. Additionally, the ability of canine renal tubules to reabsorb conjugated bilirubin is limited. As a consequence of these 2 facts, increased circulating levels of conjugated bilirubin quickly lead to bilirubinuria.[12] Bilirubinuria may be recognized before bilirubinemia is detected.

Urine bilirubin and serum bilirubin are generally less sensitive indicators of cholestasis than are SAP and GGT.

Bun Although BUN is generally used as an indicator of glomerular filtration, it is also an indicator of liver function. When protein enters the gastrointestinal tract, it is converted to ammonia, which readily diffuses across the intestinal lining and enters the portal circulation. The portal circulation carries the ammonia to the liver where it is converted to urea via urea cycle enzymes. When urea cycle activity is reduced as a result of decreased functional hepatic mass or congenital or acquired portosystemic shunt, circulating urea levels may be decreased and circulating ammonia levels may be increased. Both decreased functional hepatic mass and acquired portosystemic shunt may be seen with some cases of CCH. A common accompaniment of high circulating ammonia levels is the potential presence of ammonium biurate crystals in the urine.

Glucose Low fasting blood glucose levels can also indicate reduced functional hepatic mass. The liver is central to carbohydrate metabolism and is the principal site of glycogen storage. When the liver's capacity to store glycogen is impaired, hypoglycemia can result. Hypoglycemia in the face of liver disease is a poor prognostic sign.

Cholesterol and triglycerides The liver also plays a central role in lipid metabolism; liver disease can therefore profoundly affect circulating lipid levels. In general, liver disease, particularly when there is a significant cholestatic component, is associated with hypercholesterolemia and normal triglycerides. However, this pattern is hardly specific for liver disease and may be associated with conditions such as hypothyroidism, Cushing syndrome, DM, and others. Since the liver is the site of de novo cholesterol synthesis, end-stage liver disease with profoundly decreased functional hepatic mass can also present with hypocholesterolemia. This finding is less frequent but actually more specific for liver disease than is hypercholesterolemia.

Urinalysis
Findings most suggestive of liver disease are elevated urine bilirubin and the presence of ammonium biurate crystals. These were discussed in greater detail earlier.

Liver biopsy
As stated earlier, hepatic biopsy is critical to properly evaluate the canine chronic hepatopathies. Once profiling has established the presence of liver pathology, biopsy is warranted. Coagulation panels should be evaluated prior to biopsy as the majority of clotting proteins are produced by the liver and the potential for bleeding following biopsy should be assessed.

Canine Hyperadrenocorticism (Cushing Disease)

Canine hyperadrenocorticism (HAC) occurs when the adrenal gland produces excess adrenal hormones. The clinical signs and laboratory abnormalities are largely the result of excessive circulating levels of cortisol. The majority of cases are usually the result of a pituitary tumor (80%–85%) causing adrenal hyperplasia or a primary adrenal tumor (15%–20%).[13]

Most HAC patients are older dogs; clinical signs can be quite variable and include polyuria/polydipsia, bilateral alopecia, muscular weakness, and pendulous abdomen.

Hemogram
The most common hemogram change is the stress leukogram. (leukocytosis characterized by lymphopenia, mild mature neutrophilia, eosinopenia, and variable mild monocytosis) and occurs in approximately 80% of HAC patients.[14] The most common hemogram change is the stress leukogram. Steroid hormones stimulate red

cell production so high normal to mildly polycythemic red cell counts are not uncommon. Mild inappropriate nucleated red cell responses (5–10 nucleated RBCs/100 WBCs in the absence of polychromasia) and reticulocytosis with a normal HCT to mild erythrocytosis are also sometimes present.

Biochemical profile

Hepatic enzymes Elevated circulating corticosteroids induce production of a steroid-specific hepatic isoenzyme of SAP. As a consequence, it is estimated that approximately 80% of all canine Cushing patients have elevated levels of SAP.[15]

High levels of circulating glucocorticoids also cause hepatocellular swelling with vacuolar degeneration (steroid hepatopathy). Steroid hepatopathy is associated with mild to moderate elevations in ALT as well as elevations in GGT. GGT elevations are probably secondary to intrahepatic cholestasis.

Glucose Glucocorticoids are gluconeogenic, and Cushing syndrome is commonly associated with mild to moderate elevations in blood glucose. Values generally fall between the upper end of the reference interval (~120 mg/dL) and the renal threshold (180 mg/dL).

Total T_4

Approximately 70% of dogs with naturally occurring HAC have decreased basal thyroid levels most likely from chronic elevations in cortisol (nonthyroidal illness).[15] Cushing's patients may have decreased total T_4 concentrations from nonthyroidal illness. Confirmatory thyroid testing (free T_4, thyroid-stimulating hormone assay) is recommended to differentiate thyroidal from nonthyroidal causes.

Urinalysis

Glucocorticoids block anti-diuretic hormone (ADH) receptors in the kidney, thereby inducing polydipsia and polyuria. As a result, urine specific gravity is often 1.020 or less. If DM is present, glucosuria with or without ketonuria (ketoacidosis) may be present. Concurrent urinary tract infection is common in HAC patients; urine culture and sensitivity should be performed.[15]

Diabetes Mellitus

DM can have variable presentations in dogs and cats because of the disease subtypes commonly encountered. Various subtypes include insulin-dependent DM (frequently referred to as "type 1" and most common in dogs), non–insulin-dependent DM (also referred to as "type 2" or "insulin resistant" and most common in cats), and, finally, complicated DM (also referred to as diabetic ketoacidosis).[15]

It is important to note that cats frequently have stress-induced hyperglycemia, which can result in glucose concentrations greater than 300 mg/dL and can further complicate the diagnosis of diabetes in cats.

Hemogram

Hemogram findings are variable depending on the presence of other concurrent diseases (pancreatitis, Cushing disease, acromegaly, etc), but stress leukograms are common in systemically ill patients.

DM is the feline disease with the greatest correlation with the presence of Heinz bodies.[16] Cats with DM are frequently nonanemic, but the presence of several Heinz bodies can result in reduced RBC life span and most patients are not anemic.[17]

Biochemical profile

Hepatic enzymes Elevated ALT is common with diabetes because of hepatocellular injury due to fatty change. Swelling of fat-laden hepatocytes leads to secondary intrahepatic cholestasis and elevations in SAP and GGT. SAP elevations are less striking in cats than in dogs because of the very short half-life of SAP in cats. In cats, proportionally higher elevations in SAP than GGT are highly suggestive of hepatic lipidosis.

Glucose Fasting hyperglycemia is present and often profound with glucose values frequently greater than 400 mg/dL. In dogs, fasting levels of greater than 180 mg/dL are diagnostic. In cats, because of the existence of stress hyperglycemias of greater than 300 mg/dL, diagnosis is more difficult and requires demonstration of fasting elevations when the patient is in an unstressed state. Finding ketones in urine is also helpful. Serum fructosamine values may be very elevated and therefore helpful in making the diagnosis in cats.

Fructosamine Serum fructosamine concentrations are used on diabetic patients as a marker of mean blood glucose concentrations during the preceding 2 to 3 weeks. The higher the average blood glucose concentration over this time, the higher is the serum fructosamine concentration, and vice versa.

Results for fructosamine may be increased up to 150% by the presence of hemolysis, so careful blood collection technique and sample handling are required.

Normal (nondiabetic) serum fructosamine reference intervals[18]:

Canine: 260–378 μmol/L
Feline: 191–349 μmol/L

BUN and creatinine Azotemia occurs relatively frequently especially with severely dehydrated patients. This prerenal azotemia is characterized by a concentrated urine specific gravity in conjunction with elevations in BUN and Cr.

Potassium As mentioned previously, because potassium is primarily an intracellular ion, serum potassium levels do not necessarily reflect total body potassium. Either hyperkalemia or hypokalemia can be seen in diabetics, depending on the metabolic state of the patient at the time of sample collection.

Hyperkalemia occurs with insulin deficiency because insulin is required to move potassium into cells. Furthermore, hyperkalemia is a common feature of acidosis, because, in acidosis, hydrogen ions move into cells in exchange for potassium ions, which move into the extracellular space (plasma). Thus, as unregulated diabetics become ketoacidotic, their hyperkalemia is exacerbated.

In long-standing DM, there is osmotic diuresis as a result of glucosuria. The osmotic diuresis also causes increased excretion of potassium, which may eventually result in total body potassium depletion. Therefore, in unregulated diabetics, hypokalemia can actually occur in the face of ketoacidosis. This can be a life-threatening event and potassium supplementation is required. Serum potassium must also be closely monitored during the routine treatment of diabetics. Regardless of the state of total body potassium balance at the time, treatment with insulin drives potassium intracellularly, making potassium supplementation essential.[15]

Phosphorus Hyperphosphatemia is seen as an accompaniment to azotemia in diabetics. Furthermore, severe hypophosphatemia may develop as a serious complication to diabetic ketoacidosis patients and result in hemolytic anemia, which can be life-threatening.[18]

Urinalysis

Glucosuria and ketonuria are common occurrences in uncontrolled diabetics. Keto-nuria may be accompanied by a metabolic ketoacidosis (increased anion gap in the peripheral blood), which may be life-threatening. Concurrent urinary tract infection is possible secondary to glucosuria. In these instances, white cells and red cells may be present in increased numbers and bacteria may be seen. Urine culture and sensitivity should be performed.

Feline Hyperthyroidism

Feline hyperthyroidism is a multisystemic metabolic disease and is the most common endocrinopathy in older cats. Hyperfunctioning adenomatous hyperplasia of the thyroid gland results in a variety of clinical signs and laboratory abnormalities. Thyroid evaluation (total T_4) should always be performed when evaluating the laboratory profiles of geriatric felines.

Hemogram

Slight polycythemia is found in more than 50% of hyperthyroid cats and macrocytosis may cause an elevation in the mean cell volume.[19] Heinz bodies in the absence of hemolytic anemia may be seen.

Biochemical profile

Mild to marked increases in the serum activities of many liver enzymes, including ALT and ALP are the most common and striking biochemical abnormalities of feline hyperthyroidism.[20] Elevations in hepatic enzymes and T_4 concentrations are related, with liver enzyme abnormalities being more common in cats with severe hyperthy-roidism. Although how thyroid hormone excess stimulates the high ALT and SAP activity is not completely understood, it is clear that these high liver enzymes return to normal upon successful treatment of hyperthyroidism.[21]

Mild to moderate azotemia occurs occasionally in hyperthyroid cats. Renal function should be closely monitored because increased cardiac output associated with elevated thyroid hormone levels may mask reduced glomerular filtration.

Total T_4

The majority of hyperthyroid patients have elevated total T_4 concentrations, which confirm the diagnosis in cats with compatible clinical signs. Total T_4 may be within the normal reference interval in patients with concurrent hyperthyroidism and nonthyroi-dal illnesses (chronic renal failure, diabetes, etc). Confirmatory thyroid testing (free T_4, T_3 suppression test, thyroid radionucleotide imaging) is recommended in cats with signs compatible with hyperthyroidism but normal total T_4 levels.

Urinalysis

Urinalysis is usually unremarkable but patients should be monitored for evidence of decompensating renal function when treatment for hyperthyroidism is initiated.

SUMMARY

Routine monitoring of clinicopathologic data is a critical component in the manage-ment of older patients because blood and urine testing allows the veterinarian to monitor trends in laboratory parameters which may be the early indicators of disease. Laboratory profiling often provides an objective and sensitive indicator of developing disease before obvious clinical signs or physical examination abnormalities are observed. The primary key to the power of this evaluation is that the data is collected year after year during wellness checks and is examined serially.

Chronic renal failure, chronic active hepatitis, canine hyperadrenocorticism, diabetes mellitus and feline hyperthyroidism were reviewed and expected laboratory findings were summarized.

REFERENCES

1. Epstein M, Kuehn NF, Landsberg G, et al. AAHA Senior care guidelines for dogs and cats. J Am Anim Hosp Assoc 2005;41:81–91.
2. Fernandez F, Grindem C. Reticulocyte response. In: Feldman BF, Zinkl JG, Jain NC, editors. Schalm's veterinary hematology. 5th edition. Philadelphia: Lippincott Williams and Wilkins; 2000. p. 109–14.
3. DeNicola D, Russell J, Burger S, et al. Automated reticulocyte counts from anemic and nonanemic dogs. Proceedings from ECVCP annual meeting. Dublin (Ireland), 2011.
4. Reagan W, Saunders T, DeNicola D. Veterinary hematology atlas of common domestic species. Ames (IA): Iowa State University Press; 1998. p. 19.
5. Rebar A, Metzger F. CE advisor: interpreting the hemogram in dogs and cats. Vet Med 2001;96:1–12.
6. Fermand JP, Mitjavila MT, Le Couedic JP, et al. Role of granulocyte-macrophage colony-stimulating factor, interleukin-3 and interleukin-5 in the eosinophilia associated with T cell lymphoma. Br J Haematol 1993;83(3):359–64.
7. Hammer A. Thrombocytosis in dogs and cats: a retrospective study. Compar Hematol Int 1991;1:181.
8. Russell K, Grindem C. Secondary thrombocytopenia. In: Feldman BF, Zinkl JG, Jain NC, editors. Schalm's veterinary hematology. 5th edition. Philadelphia: Lippincott Williams and Wilkins; 2000. p. 492.
9. Polzin D, Osbourne C, Ross S. Chronic kidney disease. In: Ettinger S, Feldman E, editors. Textbook of veterinary internal medicine. 6th edition. St Louis (MO): Elsevier; 2005. p. 85–9.
10. Dibartola SP. Clinical approach and laboratory evaluation of renal disease. In: Ettinger SJ, Feldman EC, editors. Textbook of veterinary internal medicine. 7th edition. St Louis (MO): Elsevier Saunders, 2010. p. 1955–2020.
11. Bates JA. Phosphorus: a quick reference. Vet Clin North Am Small Anim Pract 2008;38(3):471–5.
12. Thrall MA. Liver profiling. In: Laboratory evaluation of bone marrow veterinary hematology and clinical chemistry. Philadelphia: Lippincott Williams and Wilkins; 2004. p. 336–8.
13. Johnson S, Sherding R. Diseases of the liver and biliary tract. In: Johnson S, Sherding R, editors. Saunders manual of small animal practice. 3rd edition. Philadelphia: Elsevier; 2006. p. 777.
14. Willard M, Tvedten H, Turnwald G. Gastrointestinal, pancreatic and hepatic disorders. In: Willard M, Tvedten H, Turnwald G, editors. Small animal clinical diagnosis by laboratory methods. 3rd edition. Philadelphia: WB Saunders; 1999. p. 200.
15. Feldman EC, Kersey R, Nelson RW. Canine hyperadrenocorticism (Cushing's syndrome). In: Nelson F, editor. Canine and feline endocrinology and reproduction. 3rd edition. Philadelphia: WB Saunders; 2004. p. 263. Chapter 6.
16. Werner L, Christopher M, Snipes S. Spurious leukocytosis and abnormal WBC histograms with Heinz bodies. Vet Clin Pathol 1997;26:20.
17. Christopher M. Relation of endogenous Heinz bodies to disease and anemia in cats: 120 cases. J Am Vet Med Assoc 1989;194:1089.

18. Nelson R. Diabetes mellitus. In: Ettinger S, Feldman E, editors. Textbook of veterinary internal medicine. 6th edition. St Louis (MO): Elsevier; 2005. p. 1582.
19. Broussard JD, Peterson ME, Fox PR. Changes in clinical and laboratory findings in cats with hyperthyroidism from 1983-1993. J Am Vet Med Assoc 1995;206:302–5.
20. Thoday KL, Mooney CT. Historical, clinical and laboratory features of 126 hyperthyroid cats. Vet Rec 1992;1:257–64.
21. Drobatz KJ, Ziemer L, Johnson VS, et al. Liver function in cats with hyperthyroidism before and after 131-I therapy. J Vet Intern Med 2007;2:1217–23.

Geriatric Veterinary Pharmacology

Butch KuKanich, DVM, PhD

KEYWORDS

- Physiology • Metabolism • Elimination • Pharmacokinetics • Pharmacodynamics

KEY POINTS

- The geriatric population can be subclassified as (1) healthy geriatric patients, (2) geriatric patients with subclinical organ dysfunction, or (3) geriatric patients with an overt disease condition.
- Healthy geriatric dogs and cats appear to be similar to healthy adult animals in relevant physiology and pharmacology.
- Some geriatric animals may have subclinical organ dysfunction or overt disease processes that may affect drug disposition and effects.

INTRODUCTION

Geriatric dogs and cats are an important demographic in the pet population. However, not all geriatric animals should be thought of as being the same. The geriatric population can be subclassified as (1) healthy geriatric patients, (2) geriatric patients with subclinical organ dysfunction, and (3) geriatric patients with an overt disease condition. Healthy geriatric animals are similar to adult animals, with only minor differences in organ function (see later). Geriatric patients with subclinical organ dysfunction are overtly healthy, but decreased function of 1 or more organs such as the heart, liver, or kidneys is present. Geriatric patients with an overt disease may or may not appear healthy but have a diagnosed disease such as heart disease (ie, chronic valvular disease), endocrine disease (ie, hypothyroidism, hyperthyroidism), renal disease (chronic renal failure), or neoplasia, among other conditions.

Data recently published on the most common causes of death can help guide the clinician in identifying the most common types of fatal diseases occurring in geriatric animals. The most common cause of death in adult dogs and cats is neoplasia.[1–3] However, differences within dog breeds occur with degenerative and metabolic diseases, accounting for the primary causes of death in small breed dogs and neoplasia predominating in large breed dogs.[3] Smaller dogs also live longer than large

Dr KuKanich has been a paid consultant for Aratana Therapeutics, Bayer Animal Health, Central Life Sciences, Nexcyon Pharmaceuticals, and Pfizer Animal Health.
Department of Anatomy and Physiology, College of Veterinary Medicine, Kansas State University, 228 Coles Hall, Manhattan, KS 66506, USA
E-mail address: kukanich@ksu.edu

dogs with weight being a significant predictor of life span.[4] Deaths due to urinary system diseases were the second most common cause of death in cats[1] compared with traumatic causes, accounting for the second most common cause of death in dogs.[3] Data also support the notion that dogs and cats are living longer. Although specific data on dogs in the published literature are lacking, data indicate cats are living longer when evaluated from 2005–2006 compared with just 6 years earlier, 1999–2000.[1]

PHYSIOLOGY APPLIED TO GERIATRIC PHARMACOLOGY

Clinical pharmacology involves 2 primary areas: pharmacokinetics and pharmacodynamics. Pharmacokinetics describes the absorption, distribution, metabolism, and elimination of a drug. For example, carprofen is well absorbed after oral administration, with active drug distributing to most areas of the body including the central nervous system, and is metabolized to inactive metabolites, and the inactive metabolites are eliminated in the feces (70%–80%) and urine (10%–20%).[5] Pharmacodynamics describes the pharmacologic effect of the drug on the body. As an example, carprofen primarily inhibits cyclooxygenase, decreasing prostaglandin production, resulting in analgesia.[5] The pharmacodynamics of the drug is the reason a drug is administered and typically the reason adverse effects occur, while the pharmacokinetics determine the dose, dosing interval, and route of administration. Therefore, both pharmacokinetic and pharmacodynamic changes can alter the desired effect in an animal, potentially increasing adverse effects or decreasing the drug's desired effect.

Some basic understanding of pharmacokinetic parameters is needed to properly assess dosing adjustments in veterinary patients. The plasma (terminal) half-life describes the terminal slope of the plasma profile and is the amount of time needed for drug concentrations to decrease by half (50%). The volume of distribution is the apparent volume a drug distributes to after administration. The volume of distribution does not have to actually represent a true volume in the animal as it is essentially determined similar to a simple dilution by dividing the dose by the plasma concentration. For example, the plasma concentration of a drug is 5 mg/L after a 10 mg/kg dose of drug is administered. The volume of distribution is determined by dividing the dose by the plasma concentration (10 mg/kg) ÷ (5 mg/L) = 2 L/kg. The plasma clearance is the volume (of the volume of distribution) completely cleared of drug per unit time. For example, the plasma clearance of fentanyl is 30 mL/min/kg; therefore, 30 mL of the volume of distribution is completely cleared of fentanyl every minute per kilogram of body weight. The plasma clearance is an estimate of total body clearance and therefore can include hepatic, renal, and other mechanisms of drug clearance depending on the specific drug.

GENERAL GUIDELINES FOR DOSE ADJUSTMENTS

Dose adjustments are sometimes needed due to decreased drug clearance from organ dysfunction, drug-drug interactions, or greater drug sensitivity. The most well recognized drug-drug metabolism interactions are included in **Table 1**. However, very little data are available in dogs and cats as to the proper adjustments that are needed in animals with organ dysfunction.

Some general guidelines can be used when treating a patient with organ dysfunction. The simplest adjustment is substitution of a drug with a similar pharmacologic effect but different route of elimination that is not affected by the organ dysfunction or drug-drug interaction. For example, if renal dysfunction is present, choose a drug

Table 1		
Drug-drug metabolism interactions most well described in dogs and cats		
Drug	**Affected Drug(s)**	**Consequence**
Phenobarbital	Multiple drugs	Increased drug metabolism
Ketoconazole	Multiple drugs	Decreased drug metabolism
Itraconazole	Multiple drugs	Decreased drug metabolism
Chloramphenicol (including ophthalmic ointments)	Multiple drugs	Decreased drug metabolism
Fluoroquinolones	Theophylline	Decreased theophylline metabolism

that is eliminated via hepatic mechanisms; therefore, the rate of drug elimination is not expected to be changed. Sotalol is a nonselective β-adrenergic antagonist eliminated primarily via renal mechanisms, and therefore its elimination is expected to be decreased in renal dysfunction and subsequent adverse effects and toxicity are more likely. However, propranolol is a nonselective β-adrenergic antagonist eliminated primarily by hepatic metabolism, and as a result renal failure is expected to have minor effects on the elimination of propranolol. Conversely, sotalol may be a better choice in an animal with moderate to severe liver disease in which a nonselective β-adrenergic antagonist is indicated.

Choosing a drug with a wide safety margin is another option to minimize drug adverse effects due to decreased drug elimination. For example, both amoxicillin/clavulanate and enrofloxacin have markedly decreased elimination in animals with renal dysfunction. Enrofloxacin has resulted in seizures in both dogs and cats and blindness has occurred in cats receiving "normal doses" of enrofloxacin when renal dysfunction is present. However, few adverse effects are observed with amoxicillin/clavulanate administered to animals with renal dysfunction (B. KuKanich, personal observation, 2011). Therefore, amoxicillin/clavulanate may be a better choice in some patients with renal dysfunction if the bacteria are susceptible and the drugs penetrate to the location of the infection.

Choosing a drug that can be monitored with therapeutic drug monitoring is another option in which dosages can be adjusted to maintain the plasma drug concentration within a therapeutic and nontoxic range. Unfortunately, there are only a few drugs in which therapeutic drug monitoring is readily available, including phenobarbital, bromide, digoxin, aminoglycosides, cyclosporine, and theophylline. Since most of the drugs, except aminoglycosides, are dosed chronically, they are expected to be at steady state plasma concentrations. Since the concentrations are at steady state, dose adjustments are proportional to the desired concentration. For example, phenobarbital therapeutic drug monitoring results in plasma concentrations of 40 μg/mL in a specific patient, but your desired concentration is 20 μg/mL. Therefore, if you decrease the dose by 50%, the plasma concentrations will decrease by 50% if no other changes occur and your new steady state concentration in that patient should decrease by 50% from 40 μg/mL to 20 μg/mL.

Clinically monitoring the drug effect can be performed to maintain efficacy but minimize adverse effects. For example, amlodipine is primarily eliminated via hepatic metabolism in humans and is likely similar for dogs and cats. If amlodipine therapy is needed in an animal with hepatic dysfunction, the dose can slowly be titrated up while monitoring blood pressure until the desired blood pressure is achieved. This is not only appropriate when dosages need to be adjusted but also in healthy patients in order to achieve the desired therapeutic effect and minimize potential adverse effects.

Similarly, methimazole could be slowly titrated to effect for a cat with liver dysfunction and the dose adjusted based on serial thyroid hormone monitoring.

CARDIOVASCULAR SYSTEM

Several studies have evaluated the cardiovascular status of healthy geriatric dogs compared with healthy adult dogs. Cardiac output is a key parameter is assessing cardiac function. Cardiac output is the amount of blood pumped from the heart per unit of time and is the product of heart rate and stroke volume. The stroke volume is the amount of blood ejected per heartbeat. In comparing adult dogs to geriatric dogs, the cardiac output has varied from decreased in geriatric dogs,[6] to no difference,[7] to increased[8] relative to adult dogs. Similarly, the stroke volume in healthy geriatric dogs has ranged from decreased[6,8] to no difference[7] compared with healthy adult dogs. Therefore, assumptions of decreased cardiac function in all healthy geriatric dogs appear to be inappropriate.

Similar to cardiac function, vascular function appears to be relatively similar in healthy geriatric dogs compared with healthy adult dogs. Arterial blood pressure is the product of cardiac output and systemic vascular resistance. Systemic vascular resistance is an assessment of vascular tone and the amount of resistance the heart has to pump against. Systemic vascular resistance in geriatric dogs ranges from no difference[6] to increased,[8] but mean arterial blood pressure was not different[6,8] compared with healthy adult dogs. Evaluation of the pulmonary vasculature in healthy geriatric beagles resulted in higher pulmonary vascular resistance compared with healthy adult beagles,[7] which may indicate there are regional differences in the vascular tone of geriatric animals, but further studies are needed to thoroughly describe any vascular differences in dogs. Hepatic and renal blood flow in healthy geriatric dogs will be discussed in detail in their respective sections but also appear similar in healthy geriatric dogs compared with healthy adult dogs.

Many different diseases affecting the heart can occur in dogs and cats resulting in decreased cardiac output. Decreased cardiac output due to underlying diseases can result in decreased renal or hepatic blood flow and can potentially affect the elimination of some drugs by both renal and hepatic clearance. For a discussion on renal clearance, see later.

Decreased hepatic blood flow can occur in animals on cardiac depressant drugs or with diseases decreasing cardiac output. Decreased hepatic blood flow will affect drugs with a high intrinsic hepatic clearance to a greater degree than will drugs with low intrinsic clearance (**Table 2**). Due to the large metabolism capacity drugs with a high intrinsic clearance, the rate-limiting step in metabolism is drug delivery to the liver by hepatic blood flow. Therefore, decreases in hepatic blood flow result in proportionally decreased clearance and subsequently an increased half-life if other factors are not changed. Although extensive data are not available in dogs and cats as to the intrinsic clearances of most drugs, the plasma clearance of drugs primarily eliminated by hepatic metabolism can be an indicator of the drug's intrinsic clearance. Hepatic blood flow in the average healthy cat is 27 to 29 mL/min/kg[9] and is similar in the average healthy dog with 28 mL/min/kg.[10] As a general rule of thumb, if a drug is eliminated via hepatic metabolism and plasma clearance is within 70% of hepatic blood flow (plasma clearance = $\geq$19 mL/min/kg) after intravenous drug administration, then the drug can be hypothesized to be a high intrinsic clearance drug and may have decreased clearance and in an increased half-life in a patient with decreased cardiac output. The decreased clearance/increased half-life should be proportional to decreased cardiac output and decreased hepatic blood flow. Some examples of drugs that likely have a high intrinsic hepatic clearance and may have prolonged

Table 2
The expected effects of low cardiac output and liver dysfunction on drugs that have low intrinsic hepatic clearance or high intrinsic hepatic clearance

	Low Cardiac Output Resulting in Decreased Hepatic Blood Flow	Mild to Moderate Liver Dysfunction	Moderate to Severe Liver Dysfunction
High intrinsic clearance	↓ Clearance, ↑ half-life	↑ Oral bioavailability, minimal effects on clearance/half-life	↓ Clearance, ↑ half-life, ↑ oral bioavailability
Low intrinsic clearance	Minimal effects	↓ Clearance, ↑ half-life proportional to severity of liver dysfunction	↓ Clearance, ↑ half-life

effects in conditions producing decreased cardiac output are morphine,[11] fentanyl,[12] buprenorphine,[13] and midazolam,[14] among others.

In contrast, the rate-limiting step in the metabolism of drugs with a low intrinsic clearance (<9 mL/min/kg) is the metabolizing capacity of the liver and is relatively independent of hepatic blood flow (see hepatic discussion later). The clearance of some drugs is between these classifications of low and high intrinsic clearance (ie, clearance 9–19 mL/min/kg) and are therefore only expected to be affected with moderate to severe hepatic impairment (see hepatic discussion) or severe decreases in cardiac output resulting in decreased clearance.

Drug-drug interactions are possible with numerous drugs used in the management of heart disease. Nonsteroidal anti-inflammatory drugs (NSAIDs) can decrease the effectiveness of angiotensin-converting enzyme (ACE) inhibitors and β-blockers in decreasing blood pressure.[15,16] Aspirin decreases the diuretic effect of furosemide in dogs, but it is unclear if other NSAIDs affect furosemide similarly.[17] Digoxin bioavailability can be decreased by aluminum hydroxide and increased by omeprazole.[18] Digoxin is a P-glycoprotein substrate and administration of P-glycoprotein inhibitors such as ketoconazole, itraconazole, cyclosporine, and quinidine may also increase the absorption of digoxin and potentially result in toxicity.

HEPATIC

The effects of hepatic impairment on drug disposition can involve several different processes. Reduced hepatic function can result in decreased elimination of some drugs (see later) or increased bioavailability of some oral drugs with both effects potentially increasing the risk adverse drug effects (see **Table 2**). Unfortunately, there are no readily available tests of hepatic function. Although bile acid testing is routinely used to assess hepatobiliary disease when clinical/pathologic changes are present, the sensitivity is relatively low (54%–74%) to routinely use them to assess hepatic function in an otherwise healthy animal.[19] Up to 46% of subclinical cases of hepatic dysfunction would be missed with bile acids testing.

The oral bioavailability of some drugs will be increased with hepatic dysfunction. The oral bioavailability of drugs is dependent on several factors. The drug has to remain intact through the harsh environments of the stomach and proximal small intestine in order to reach the areas of drug absorption in the intestines. The drug must be soluble within the gastrointestinal (GI) tract in order to be absorbed and must have enough lipid solubility (lipophilicity) to penetrate the mucous membranes in the intestines. Active transporters are also present in the intestines, which can either enhance drug absorption of low lipophilicity drugs or active transporters can decrease drug absorption by effluxing drug that is absorbed back into the intestinal lumen. If the drug is stable, soluble in the intestines, and absorbed intact through the intestinal mucosa, then it must pass metabolizing enzymes in the intestines and finally pass through the portal circulation and the metabolizing enzymes in the liver to reach the systemic circulation. Therefore, oral bioavailability depends not only on drug absorption but also on drug metabolism, known as first-pass metabolism. Some drugs are well absorbed after oral administration but are almost completely metabolized after absorption, but prior to reaching systemic circulation. For example, codeine is essentially completely absorbed after oral administration to dogs, but only 4% reaches systemic circulation as codeine due to hepatic metabolism.[20] Therefore, alterations in drug metabolism can markedly increase oral bioavailability of some drugs. The drugs most likely affected are high intrinsic hepatic clearance drugs. Examples include propranolol, carvedilol, opioids, and benzodiazepines, among others, that may have higher bioavailability when administered to an animal with hepatic dysfunction. Therefore, the dosages of high intrinsic clearance drugs administered orally may need to be lower to avoid toxicity. However, the doses of high intrinsic clearance drugs typically do not need to be changed if administered via other routes of administration if mild to moderate liver impairment is present as these routes of administration are not subject to first-pass hepatic metabolism.

Hepatic disease can also result in decreased drug clearance of some drugs but does not affect all drugs similarly. As stated in the cardiovascular section, high intrinsic hepatic clearance drugs are more likely affected by hepatic blood flow compared with liver activity, unless severe liver impairment is present. Drugs most likely to have decreased clearance caused by mild to moderate changes in liver function are the low intrinsic clearance drugs, in which case the clearance will decrease proportionally to the amount of liver dysfunction. Most NSAIDs, phenobarbital, and theophylline, among others, would need to have doses decreased to maintain similar plasma drug concentrations in an animal with hepatic impairment compared with a healthy geriatric animal regardless of the route of administration. Unfortunately, little data are available describing the actual dose adjustments that are needed.

RENAL

Renal clearance is the sum of glomerular filtration and renal tubular secretion minus renal tubular reabsorption. Glomerular filtration is dependent on renal blood flow, intact glomeruli, and plasma oncotic pressure. Healthy geriatric dogs appear to have similar renal function as assessed by glomerular filtration rate[21] to slightly decreased glomerular filtration rate.[22] Therefore, routine adjustments to drugs eliminated by renal mechanisms are not recommended for healthy geriatric dogs and cats with no indications of renal dysfunction. However, animals with renal dysfunction are expected to have decreased renal clearance of drugs eliminated via renal mechanisms and dose adjustments may be needed. Unfortunately, the effects of renal dysfunction on the magnitude of drug elimination have not been well described in dogs and cats, nor have methods of dose adjustment that are readily available to the practicing veterinarian. Dosing options for patients with renal dysfunction can include choosing a drug eliminated by hepatic mechanisms, choosing a drug with a large safety margin, and choosing a drug in which therapeutic drug monitoring is available.

It is important to consider potential drug adverse effects when choosing a drug for your patients. Drugs that cause renal toxicity should only be used when the benefits of treatment are greater than the potential adverse effects when renal dysfunction is present. NSAIDs, aminoglycosides, amphotericin B, cisplatin, ACE inhibitors in patients with renal hypotension, sulfonamides, and tetracyclines have the potential for nephrotoxicity and should be used cautiously in susceptible patients.

Another consideration with renal failure is the potential of electrolyte abnormalities including hyperkalemia in acute renal failure, but more common in geriatric animals is chronic renal failure and subsequent hypokalemia. Hypokalemic can be worsened with use of diuretics such as furosemide[23] and increases the risk of arrhythmias from digoxin in dogs.[24] Hypokalemia can also prolong the cardiac QT interval in dogs,[23] which can increase the risk of fatal arrhythmias.

Uremia has numerous deleterious effects including ulceration of mucous membranes of the GI tract.[25] Drugs such as NSAIDs and glucocorticoids will likely result in increased GI adverse effects such as bleeding, ulceration, and potentially perforation in uremic animals. NSAIDs may also result in decreased renal blood flow[26] and potentially worsening renal disease, but this has not been well defined in animals with naturally occurring disease. Glucocorticoids such as prednisone, prednisolone, and dexamethasone will also likely increase the risk of GI adverse effects in animals with renal disease and should only be used if the benefits outweigh the risks. Many animals with renal disease are also on gastric acid reduction therapy to decrease the GI adverse effects of renal disease. Histamine (H2) antagonists such as famotidine or proton pump inhibitors such as omeprazole are commonly recommended acid suppressors. Acid suppression is generally well tolerated but can result in decreased absorption of some drugs such as ketoconazole and itraconazole (not fluconazole) but can increase the absorption of digoxin.[18]

Hyperphosphatemia is commonly present in chronic kidney disease. Hyperphosphatemia can hasten the progression of chronic kidney disease due to elevations of the calcium-phosphate product, producing metastatic calcification. Management of hyperphosphatemia by reducing dietary phosphate absorption is best accomplished by administering phosphate binding agents such as aluminum hydroxide. Aluminum hydroxide is an antacid and may decrease the absorption of ketoconazole and itraconazole as do H2 antagonists and proton pump inhibitors. Aluminum also decreases the absorption of fluoroquinolones and tetracyclines and may decrease the absorption of digoxin.

NEOPLASIA

Recent studies have indicated neoplasia is a common cause of death in dogs and cats, and many pet owners are choosing to treat their animals with either palliative treatments or to induce remission. Regardless of the treatment goals, adverse effects and drug-drug interactions are still a concern for the well-being of the patient. Common adverse effects of antineoplastic treatment include anorexia, nausea, vomiting, diarrhea, and immunosuppression, and some specific agents can result in cardiac and renal adverse effects. The specific antineoplastics routinely used for canine and feline patients are beyond the scope of this article, but the GI adverse effects of neoplasia and antineoplastics will be discussed.

Anorexia, nausea, vomiting, and diarrhea can be the result of the neoplastic process or the drug therapy. Since antineoplastics often target rapidly growing cells, the GI tract and bone marrow progenitor cells are often killed in addition to the neoplastic tissue. Therefore, it is not surprising that GI adverse effects and myelosuppression are common in antineoplastic therapy.

Cyroheptadine can be administered for the symptomatic treatment of anorexia, probably due to anti-serotonin effects (5-HT$_2$ antagonist). Cyroheptadine may antagonize the effects of selective serotonin reuptake inhibitors (ie, fluoxetine), tricyclic antidepressants (ie, clomipramine), and tramadol,[27] resulting in decreased efficacy of these drugs. Benzodiazepines including diazepam and oxazepam have also been administered as appetite stimulants. Benzodiazepines as a drug class tend to be well tolerated, with sedation and behavioral changes being the primary adverse effects. However, diazepam has resulted in fatal hepatic toxicity in cats, typically within 2 weeks of treatment.[28] Benzodiazepines are also Drug Enforcement Agency (DEA) schedule IV (CIV) controlled substances and are subject to abuse and therefore should be dispensed cautiously.

Famotidine or omeprazole may also provide some beneficial effects for anorectic animals as both drugs suppress acid secretion and may provide benefit for gastritis.[29] Omeprazole is more effective at reducing GI acidity than famotidine in dogs,[30] which is consistent with their effects in humans. Famotidine and omeprazole are generally well tolerated, but adverse effects such as diarrhea and decreased absorption of some drugs including ketoconazole and itraconazole (not fluconazole), or increased the absorption of digoxin can occur.[18]

Anorexia may also be directly related to nausea and vomiting; therefore antiemetics may be beneficial in restoring an animal's appetite. Metoclopramide is often administered to animals orally or as an injection. Metoclopramide has fair antiemetic effects and is an upper GI tract prokinetic. The antiemetic effects are thought to be due to inhibition of dopamine receptors in the chemoreceptor trigger zone and may also be in part to its prokinetic effects if ileus is present. Adverse effects can include sedation or excitement, exacerbation of seizures, abdominal pain due to hypermotility, and GI perforation if a GI foreign body is present. Metoclopramide can also result in aldosterone release causing sodium and water retention and subsequent edema and worsening of congestive heart failure. Metoclopramide may also result in elevated prolactin and in humans has produced galactorrhea and gynecomastia.

Maropitant is a veterinary licensed antiemetic for dogs and is considered a high efficacy antiemetic. Maropitant is a neurokinin (NK-1) antagonist resulting in antiemetic effects at both the chemoreceptor trigger zone and emetic center. Maropitant significantly decreases vomiting due to central and GI vomiting including chemotherapy induced vomiting.[31] The most common adverse effects include pain on injection, sedation, and diarrhea. Studies from the sponsor also indicate maropitant causes prolongation of the QT interval due to blockade of cardiac potassium channels. The safety of maropitant has not been reported in patients with underlying cardiac disease, when administered with cardiac antiarrhythmic drugs, or when administered with doxorubicin. Drug-drug interactions have not been investigated, but maropitant elimination may be enhanced or reduced if administered with drugs that alter metabolism (see **Table 1**).

Ondansetron is a serotonin (5-HT^3) antagonist that is an effective antiemetic in dogs when administered intravenously.[32] However, its oral bioavailability is low and may not be effective when administered orally to dogs.[33]

OSTEOARTHRITIS

Osteoarthritis (OA) is a common condition in dogs and cats, with estimates of up to 20% of dogs greater than 1 year of age having OA.[34] OA is most commonly managed with NSAIDs, and as previously stated, NSAIDs may worsen renal dysfunction, may have drug-drug interactions with cardiovascular drugs including furosemide and ACE inhibitors, and may have decreased clearance with hepatic dysfunction. The efficacy of the different NSAIDs appears similar with no studies consistently identifying a specific NSAID that produces better effects than any other. Thorough reviews of NSAID use in veterinary medicine have been previously published.[35,36]

The most common adverse effects of NSAIDs are GI adverse effects ranging from vomiting and diarrhea to erosions, perforations, and even death in dogs and cats. The newer veterinary-approved NSAIDs have a lower frequency of GI adverse effects compared with older drugs such as phenylbutazone and aspirin, but no study has identified any of the newer drugs as having less GI adverse effects than another newer drug. Gastric adverse effects are worsened when NSAIDs are combined with glucocorticoids and this drug combination should be avoided. Similar to exogenous glucocorticoid administration, hyperadrenocorticism results in high concentration of circulating cortisol, which may increase the risk of NSAID GI adverse effects in these animals. Omeprazole and misoprostol may decrease the GI adverse effects of NSAIDs, but they have not been extensively evaluated in dogs and cats. As stated previously, animals with renal failure may already have GI injury and NSAIDs may worsen the GI lesions.

Renal toxicity is the second most common cause of NSAID adverse effects. NSAIDs alter renal hemodynamics resulting in regional hypoperfusion and subsequently may result in renal failure.[36] The greatest risk factors for renal adverse effects from NSAIDs are hypotension (ie, anesthesia, shock), hypovelmia, hyponatremia, high doses of NSAIDs, and concurrent administration of nephrotoxic drugs. Although not well documented in dogs and cats, preexisting renal disease may also increase the risk of renal adverse effects, but this may be drug and disease specific.

Hepatotoxicity due to NSAIDs can either be dose-dependent (ie, high doses/overdoses) or dose-independent (normal dose), often referred to as idiosyncratic toxicity.[36] Dogs may be more susceptible to hepatotoxicity compared with cats, but hepatotoxicity has been reported in cats as adverse drug events to the Food and Drug Administration. Idiosyncratic hepatotoxicity most commonly occurs in the first few weeks of drug administration and is often treatable with discontinuation of the NSAID and appropriate supportive care. Although Labrador retrievers are often cited as being more susceptible to idiosyncratic hepatotoxicity, they are more likely overrepresented due to their large size, breed popularity, and high prevalence of orthopedic disease and OA within the breed. Hepatotoxicity has been reported for all approved veterinary NSAIDs and there are currently no data suggesting any specific NSAID is more likely to cause hepatotoxicity than another.

IDIOPATHIC EPILEPSY AND SEIZURES

Idiopathic epilepsy and seizures are not uncommon in dogs with up to 2% of dogs presumptively diagnosed.[37] Phenobarbital and bromide salts are the most common drug therapies for epilepsy. Phenobarbital is a cytochrome P450 metabolizing enzyme inducer and as a result can increase the metabolism of certain, but not all, drugs resulting in decreased efficacy. Phenobarbital increases its own metabolism[38] and the metabolism of levetiracetam,[39] other barbiturates,[40] and some benzodiazepines,[41] among other drugs. Conversely, phenobarbital may increase the toxicity of some drugs, such as acetaminophen, but this has not been extensively investigated in dogs.

Bromide is available as potassium bromide and sodium bromide. Potassium bromide is more commonly used but should be avoided in patients prone to hyperkalemia including dogs with hyperadrenocorticism. Bromide is primarily eliminated by renal mechanisms and decreased elimination could occur in animals with renal dysfunction. Dietary chloride can affect the elimination of bromide with high-chloride diets increasing bromide elimination potentially resulting in decreased efficacy and therapeutic failure.[42] Conversely, low-chloride diets may decrease elimination resulting in bromide toxicity. Therefore, it is important to keep the diet consistent, including treats, in patients treated with bromide to avoid therapeutic failure or toxicity of bromide.

SUMMARY

Healthy geriatric dogs and cats appear to be similar to healthy adult animals in relevant physiology and pharmacology. However, some geriatric animals may have subclinical organ dysfunction or overt disease processes that may affect drug disposition and effects. Geriatric animals may be treated for several different disease conditions; therefore, the clinician has to be cognizant of potential drug-drug interactions. The effects of hepatic dysfunction on hepatic metabolized drugs can range from no effect, to increased oral bioavailability, to decreased clearance depending on the specific drug and degree of hepatic dysfunction. Renal dysfunction may decrease the rate of elimination of drugs eliminated by renal mechanisms. Drug-drug interactions and drug-diet interactions may increase drug adverse effects and toxicity but may also decrease drug effectiveness. Careful review of current dosing recommendations is encouraged, especially when treating patients with more than a single drug, to avoid drug-drug interactions.

REFERENCES

1. Egenvall A, Nødtvedt A, Häggström J, et al. Mortality of life-insured Swedish cats during 1999–2006: age, breed, sex, and diagnosis. J Vet Intern Med 2009;23: 1175–83.
2. Adams VJ, Evans KM, Sampson J, Wood JL. Methods and mortality results of a health survey of purebred dogs in the UK. J Small Anim Pract 2010;51:512–24.
3. Fleming JM, Creevy KE, Promislow DE. Mortality in north american dogs from 1984 to 2004: an investigation into age-, size-, and breed-related causes of death. J Vet Intern Med 2011;25:187–98.
4. Greer KA, Canterberry SC, Murphy KE. Statistical analysis regarding the effects of height and weight on life span of the domestic dog. Res Vet Sci 2007;82:208–14.
5. Rimadyl. Pfizer Animal Health. New York (NY). Available at: https://www.rimadyl.com/default.aspx. Accessed November 1, 2011.
6. Haidet GC, Parsons D. Reduced exercise capacity in senescent beagles: an evaluation of the periphery. Am J Physiol 1991;260:H173–82.
7. Mercier E, Mathieu M, Sandersen CF, et al. Evaluation of the influence of age on pulmonary arterial pressure by use of right ventricular catheterization, pulsed-wave Doppler echocardiography, and pulsed-wave tissue Doppler imaging in healthy Beagles. Am J Vet Res 2010;71:891–7.
8. Haidet GC. Effects of age on beta-adrenergic-mediated reflex responses to induced muscular contraction in beagles. Mech Ageing Dev 1993;68:89–104.
9. Galvin MJ, Lefer AM. Hepatic blood flow in acute myocardial ischemia. Experientia 1979;35:1602–4.
10. Skerjanec A, O'Brien DW, Tam TK. Hepatic blood flow measurements and indocyanine green kinetics in a chronic dog model. Pharm Res 1994;11:1511–5.
11. KuKanich B, Lascelles BD, Papich MG. Pharmacokinetics of morphine and plasma concentrations of morphine-6-glucuronide following morphine administration to dogs. J Vet Pharmacol Ther 2005;28:371–6.
12. KuKanich B, Hubin M. The pharmacokinetics of ketoconazole and its effects on the pharmacokinetics of midazolam and fentanyl in dogs. J Vet Pharmacol Ther 2010;33: 42–9.

13. Andaluz A, Moll X, Abellán R, et al. Pharmacokinetics of buprenorphine after intravenous administration of clinical doses to dogs. Vet J 2009;181:299–304.
14. Court MH, Greenblatt DJ. Pharmacokinetics and preliminary observations of behavioral changes following administration of midazolam to dogs. J Vet Pharmacol Ther 1992;15:343–50.
15. Webster J. Interactions of NSAIDs with diuretics and beta-blockers mechanisms and clinical implications. Drugs 1985;30:32–41.
16. Morgan T, Anderson A. The effect of nonsteroidal anti-inflammatory drugs on blood pressure in patients treated with different antihypertensive drugs. J Clin Hypertens (Greenwich) 2003;5:53–7.
17. Berg KJ, Loew D. Inhibition of furosemide-induced natriuresis by acetylsalicylic acid in dogs. Scand J Clin Lab Invest 1977;37:125–31.
18. Cohen AF, Kroon R, Schoemaker R, et al. Influence of gastric acidity on the bioavailability of digoxin. Ann Intern Med 1991;115:540–5.
19. Webster CRL. History, clinical signs, and physical findings in hepatobiliary disease. In: Ettinger SJ, Feldman EC, editors. Textbook of veterinary internal medicine. 7th edition. St Louis: Saunders Elsevier; 2010. p. 1612–28.
20. KuKanich B. Pharmacokinetics of acetaminophen, codeine, and the codeine metabolites morphine and codeine-6-glucuronide in healthy Greyhound dogs. J Vet Pharmacol Ther 2010;33:15–21.
21. Bexfield NH, Heiene R, Gerritsen RJ, et al. Glomerular filtration rate estimated by 3-sample plasma clearance of iohexol in 118 healthy dogs. J Vet Intern Med 2008; 22:66–73.
22. Miyagawa Y, Takemura N, Hirose H. Assessments of factors that affect glomerular filtration rate and indirect markers of renal function in dogs and cats. J Vet Med Sci 2010;72:1129–36.
23. Hanton G, Yvon A, Provost JP, et al. Quantitative relationship between plasma potassium levels and QT interval in beagle dogs. Lab Anim 2007;41:204–17.
24. Hall RJ, Gelbart A, Billingham M, et al. Effect of chronic potassium depletion on digitalis-induced inotropy and arrhythmias. Cardiovasc Res 1981;15:98–107.
25. Polzin DJ. Chronic kidney disease in small animals. Vet Clin North Am Small Anim Pract 2011;41:15–30.
26. Rodríguez F, Llinás MT, González JD, et al. Renal changes induced by a cyclooxygenase-2 inhibitor during normal and low sodium intake. Hypertension 2000; 36:276–81.
27. Oliva P, Aurilio C, Massimo F, et al. The antinociceptive effect of tramadol in the formalin test is mediated by the serotonergic component. Eur J Pharmacol 2002;445: 179–85.
28. Center SA, Elston TH, Rowland PH, et al. Fulminant hepatic failure associated with oral administration of diazepam in 11 cats. J Am Vet Med Assoc 1996;209:618–25.
29. Williamson KK, Willard MD, Payton ME, Davis MS. Efficacy of omeprazole versus high-dose famotidine for prevention of exercise-induced gastritis in racing Alaskan sled dogs. J Vet Intern Med 2010;24:285–8.
30. Tolbert K, Bissett S, King A, et al. Efficacy of oral famotidine and 2 omeprazole formulations for the control of intragastric pH in dogs. J Vet Intern Med 2011;25: 47–54.
31. Vail DM, Rodabaugh HS, Conder GA, et al. Efficacy of injectable maropitant (Cerenia) in a randomized clinical trial for prevention and treatment of cisplatin-induced emesis in dogs presented as veterinary patients. Vet Comp Oncol 2007;5:38–46.

32. Haga K, Inaba K, Shoji H, et al. The effects of orally administered Y-25130, a selective serotonin3-receptor antagonist, on chemotherapeutic agent-induced emesis. Jpn J Pharmacol 1993;63:377–83.

33. Saynor DA, Dixon CM. The metabolism of ondansetron. Eur J Cancer Clin Oncol 1989;25 Suppl 1:S75–7.

34. Johnston SA. Osteoarthritis. Joint anatomy, physiology, and pathobiology. Vet Clin North Am Small Anim Pract 1997;27:699–723.

35. Papich MG. An update on nonsteroidal anti-inflammatory drugs (NSAIDs) in small animals. Vet Clin North Am Small Anim Pract 2008;38:1243–66.

36. KuKanich B, Bidgood T, Knesl O. Clinical pharmacology of nonsteroidal anti-inflammatory drugs in dogs. Vet Anaesth Analg 2011, in press.

37. Podell M, Fenner WR, Powers JD. Seizure classification in dogs from a nonreferral-based population. J Am Vet Med Assoc 1995;206:1721.

38. Hojo T, Ohno R, Shimoda M, Kokue E. Enzyme and plasma protein induction by multiple oral administrations of phenobarbital at a therapeutic dosage regimen in dogs. J Vet Pharmacol Ther 2002;25:121–7.

39. Moore SA, Muñana KR, Papich MG, Nettifee-Osborne JA. The pharmacokinetics of levetiracetam in healthy dogs concurrently receiving phenobarbital. J Vet Pharmacol Ther 2011;34:31–4.

40. Sams RA, Muir WW. Effects of phenobarbital on thiopental pharmacokinetics in greyhounds. Am J Vet Res 1988;49:245–9.

41. Wagner SO, Sams RA, Podell M. Chronic phenobarbital therapy reduces plasma benzodiazepine concentrations after intravenous and rectal administration of diazepam in the dog. J Vet Pharmacol Ther 1998;21:335–41.

42. Trepanier LA, Babish JG. Effect of dietary chloride content on the elimination of bromide by dogs. Res Vet Sci 1995;58:252–5.

Anesthesia and Analgesia for Geriatric Veterinary Patients

Courtney L. Baetge, DVM[a], Nora S. Matthews, DVM[b,*]

KEYWORDS

- Geriatric • Anesthesia • Analgesia • Drug protocols • Physiology

KEY POINTS

- The number of geriatric veterinary patients presented for anesthesia appears to be increasing.
- Proper patient preparation and vigilant monitoring are the best defense against anesthetic problems in the geriatric animal.
- Monitoring should include pulse oximetry, end-tidal CO_2, blood pressure monitoring, electrocardiogram, and temperature.
- There is no "ideal" anesthetic combination for all geriatric animals.

INTRODUCTION

Although exact numbers are not available, the number of geriatric patients presented for anesthesia appears to be increasing. One study estimated that nearly one-fifth of all pet dogs are now over the age of 10 years,[1] and more than $1.5 billion is spent annually on these geriatric pets.[2] Another study reported that in 2002, 30% of the US pet population were expected to be geriatric.[3] These studies did not include cats, which have outnumbered dogs as pets in the United States; exact figures may not be available, but most practitioners would agree that geriatric cats are becoming more common in every practice! While age may not be a disease, the physiologic deterioration that normally occurs with age can cause significant complications during the anesthetic period.[1] Brodbelt and colleagues[4] estimated the risk of anesthetic death increased with age as much as 7 times for patients over the age of 12 years. Given the increasing number of geriatric dogs and cats and awareness of these risks, planning for the anesthetic period can help the practitioner avoid complications often seen in the older patient; these include hypotension, bradycardia,

None of the authors have any financial interests in any companies with interest in the matter or materials discussed in this article.

[a] 5057 Drake Road, College Station, TX 77845, USA; [b] Department of Small Animal Clinical Sciences, Texas A&M University, College Station, TX 77843–4474, USA

* Corresponding author.

E-mail address: nmatthews@cvm.tamu.edu

hypoxemia, and prolonged recovery.[5] Concurrent disease must also be considered and has been well discussed in other references.[6]

First, it is important to define "geriatric." Most references have reverted to using a percentage of life span for that particular breed (usually 75%–80%) versus a concrete number (eg, 8 years old).[7,8] This allows for the huge variability in breed life spans. For example, a 6-year-old Chihuahua is not considered geriatric while a 6-year-old great Dane might be.

PHYSIOLOGIC CHANGES ASSOCIATED WITH AGING
Cardiovascular

Clinically normal geriatric patients may have a reduced blood volume and baroreceptor activity as well as increased circulatory time and vagal tone. Thickened elastic fibers, increased wall collagen content, and wall calcification in the vasculature can decrease the patient's ability to autoregulate blood flow.[9] Functional reserve is also reduced due to myocardial fibrosis and ventricular free wall thickening.[10] These changes reduce efficiency, filling, and cardiac output. If the pacemaker cells are involved, heart rate and rhythm may be affected as well. To compensate, geriatric patients will increase stroke volume more than heart rate.[10]

An increase in heart disease is also seen in geriatric patients, most notably valvular incompetence and conduction abnormalities. Chronic valvular disease is extremely prevalent in the canine geriatric population; up to 58% of dogs older than 9 years show evidence of chronic valvular disease.[11] Common arrhythmias seen include heart block, bundle branch block, ventricular premature complexes, and atrial fibrillation.[9]

Pulmonary

The pulmonary system also shows widespread changes with age. Mechanically, the patient loses thoracic compliance, has atrophy of the intercostal muscles, and has decreased alveolar elasticity.[12] These changes cause a decline in the arterial oxygen concentration.[12] The response to decreased oxygen or increased carbon dioxide is also blunted, which creates a slower ventilatory response to respiratory depression or apnea.[9] These changes decrease the patient's respiratory functional reserve providing less time for intervention should respiratory complication arise.

Renal

The renal system shows dramatic structural changes that may not be evident clinically.[13] A 50% decrease in functional nephrons is not unusual in the aging animal.[2] The kidney also has decreased renal blood flow and a decreased glomerular filtration rate.[9] This can lead to a longer duration of action for drugs metabolized by the kidneys (eg, ketamine in cats).

In addition, older patients have difficulty retaining sodium and water and the renin–angiotensin system becomes less responsive.[12] This leaves the patient less able to tolerate hypovolemia, hemorrhage, and electrolyte and acid-base disturbances. Excreting excess water loads may also be difficult and overly vigorous fluid or electrolyte therapy can lead to pulmonary edema or heart failure.[10]

Hepatic

There are 2 factors that can cause a significant decrease in the rate of drug metabolism and excretion. First, geriatrics may have a decrease in liver mass of up to 50%, which leads to decreases in available hepatic enzymes.[10] Second, the age-related decrease in cardiac output decreases blood flow to the liver, thereby decreasing the delivery of drugs to the liver for metabolism and excretion. This can lead to prolonged effects of drugs and, thus, slower patient recovery. Products of the liver may also be decreased, such as coagulation factors, plasma proteins, and glucose.

Central Nervous System

Total requirement for anesthetics declines as cognitive and sensory functions diminish.[7] The exact cause of this apparent increased sensitivity to anesthetics is not known exactly, but theories include neuron loss, depletion of neurotransmitters, decreased receptor affinity, and/or changes in myelination.[10,12]

Body Composition and Metabolism

Aging can affect the body's overall composition and metabolism.[14] Geriatric patients tend to have less muscle mass and total body water but a larger percentage of fat, which changes the distribution of fat- or water-soluble drugs including inhalants.[12] Basal metabolic rate decreases and poor thermoregulation may lead to hypothermia, which can produce arrhythmias, decreased coagulation, decreased minimum alveolar concentration value, and increased risk of infection.[2]

PATIENT PREPARATION

Proper patient preparation and vigilant monitoring are the best defense against anesthetic problems in the geriatric animal. In one study, nearly 30% of geriatric animals were found to have undiagnosed, subclinical disease present and 10% had anesthesia canceled due to these disease processes.[15]

Proper preparation should begin with a complete history and thorough physical exam with careful auscultation of the heart; chest films and electrocardiogram should be performed if any murmur is ausculted. Blood work, including a complete blood count, serum chemistry profile with electrolytes, and urinalysis, should be completed prior to anesthesia. Knowledge of underlying disease processes allows anesthetic protocols to be properly adjusted to fit the individual patient. History should include all previously diagnosed diseases and especially current drug administration to avoid interactions. For example, any of the behavior-modifying drugs being used on geriatric animals can have serious to even deadly interactions with anesthetic or analgesic drugs. Antidepressants, such as mirtazapine, may be used as appetite stimulants but have neuroendocrine activity. Radiographs, ultrasound, or echocardiography may be indicated in some patients based on findings or history. Attempts should be made to correct any significant fluid or electrolyte abnormalities prior to anesthesia. A clotting profile is recommended prior to invasive surgical procedures. Intravenous catheters should be placed in all patients to allow fluid therapy as well as emergency drug administration. Preoxygenation will help to increase the fraction of oxygen in the lungs and arterial blood to help prevent hypoxemia during the induction period. Intubation is highly recommended in all anesthetized patients to protect the airway as well as facilitate positive pressure ventilation should it become necessary. Fluids should be provided judiciously during anesthesia to replace fluid losses as well as to counteract the vasodilatory and hypotensive effects of anesthetic agents. Using a burette system or syringe pump for smaller patients (or those requiring very small volumes) may help to prevent inadvertent overadministration of fluids.

PATIENT MONITORING

Monitoring should include pulse oximetry, end-tidal CO_2, blood pressure monitoring, electrocardiogram, and temperature (**Table 1**). Monitoring urine production (normal,

Table 1	
Monitoring geriatric patients	
Parameter	Range
Pulse oximetry	93–100%
End-tidal CO_2	35–45 mm Hg
Mean blood pressure	60–100 mm Hg
Heart rate	60–160 bpm
Temperature	95°–102°F

1–2 mL/kg/hr) may also help to ensure proper renal perfusion in patients where preexisting renal disease is a concern. Vigilant monitoring allows early intervention and correction of problems before permanent consequences occur. For example, early recognition of hypothermia allows treatment, which will help prevent the prolonged recoveries seen with a cold patient.

ANESTHETIC PROTOCOLS

There is no "ideal" anesthetic combination for all geriatric animals. The decision should be based on the needs of each individual animal and tailored to the individual's responses. However, in general, the doses for geriatrics may be reduced by as much as 50% to account for increased sensitivity and reduced distribution, metabolism, and excretion. Use of local and regional anesthetic techniques can aid in reducing the dose of other more depressant drugs being used.

Premedication and Analgesics

Acepromazine (Acepromazine Maleate; Vedco Inc., St Joseph, MO, USA) may be beneficial in the anxious, distressed patient but should be used cautiously due to its hypotensive effects and concern that it may decrease the seizure threshold. Effects of acepromazine are prolonged with poor hepatic function, so the dose should be very low (Table 2) in the geriatric patient. Benzodiazepines (diazepam [Valium; Hospira, Inc., Lake Forest, IL, USA] or midazolam [Versed; Hospira, Inc., Lake Forest, IL, USA]) may be a better choice since they produce less cardiac depression. Unlike younger animals, aging patients tend to show greater sedation with the benzodiazepines (Fig. 1) and longer action. Opioids are reversible and can be used alone or in combination with other sedatives to provide analgesia and as part of general anesthesia. The more potent opioids, such as morphine (Astramorph; AstraZeneca, Wilmington, DE, USA), fentanyl (fentanyl citrate; Baxter Healthcare Corp., Deerfield, IL, USA), and hydromorphone (Hydromorphone HCl; West-Ward, Eatontown, NJ, USA), can provide powerful analgesia but produce significant respiratory depression; assisted or controlled ventilation should be provided for patients on constant-rate infusion of opioids. The partial agonists (buprenorphine [Buprenex; Reckitt Benckiser Healthcare, Hull, England]) or agonist-antagonists (butorphanol [Torbugesic; Fort Dodge Animal Health, Ft Dodge, IA, USA]) can provide mild to moderate analgesia with less cardiopulmonary depression. Nonsteroidal anti-inflammatory drugs (NSAIDs) and α_2-adrenergic agonists (dexmedetomidine [Dexdomitor; Pfizer Animal Health, Exton, PA, USA]) are not generally recommended for most geriatric protocols or should be used with caution; α_2 drugs produce profound decreases in cardiac output except in very small doses. NSAIDs such as carprofen (Rimadyl, Pfizer Animal Health, Exton, PA, USA) or meloxicam (Metacam; Boehringer Ingelheim, St Joseph, MO, USA) should be used

Table 2
Geriatric anesthetic drugs

Drugs	Dose	Effects	Contraindications
Anticholinergics			
Atropine	0.01–0.02 mg/kg	Decrease secretions, increase heart rate	Tachycardia
Glycopyrrolate	0.005–0.01 mg/kg		
Sedatives			
Acepromazine	0.01–0.05 mg/kg (1 mg max)	Sedation	Hypovolemia, hypotension, liver dysfunction
Diazepam	0.2–0.4 mg/kg	Anxiolysis, muscle relaxation, combined with dissociative or opioid for sedation or induction	Severe liver dysfunction
Midazolam	0.1–0.3 mg/kg		
Analgesics			
Oxymorphone	0.05–0.1 mg/kg	Moderate to severe pain relief, decrease requirement of other anesthetics	Severe respiratory dysfunction
Hydromorphone	0.1–0.2 mg/kg		
Morphine	0.05–0.1 mg/kg		
Fentanyl	0.003–0.01 mg/kg		
Buprenorphine	0.005–0.02 mg/kg	Mild to moderate pain relief, mild sedation	Severe pain managed with pure mu opioid
Butorphanol	0.2–0.4 mg/kg		
Induction agents			
Propofol	4–6 mg/kg	Induction or maintenance CRI	Severe CV or CP dysfunction
Etomidate	0.5–1.5 mg/kg	Induction (usually in combination)	Adrenal corticosteroid suppression
Ketamine	2–5 mg/kg	Induction (usually in combination), sedation	Seizures, severe renal or hepatic disease
Inhalants			
Sevoflurane	2.5%–4%	Maintenance	Chamber or face mask induction can cause significant respiratory or CV depression
Isoflurane	1.5%–3%		

Abbreviations: CP, cardiopulmonary; CRI, constant rate infusion; CV, cardiovascular.

with good fluid support and monitoring renal function. Local anesthetics are a common adjunct for either infiltration at the site or regional blocks, which will help to lower the dosage of other drugs (ie, inhalants), thereby reducing the hypotension seen with higher concentrations.

Induction and Maintenance

Propofol (PropoFlo; Abbott Animal Health, Abbott Park, IL, USA) and etomidate (Amidate; Hospira, Inc., Lake Forest, IL, USA) are 2 common induction agents that are

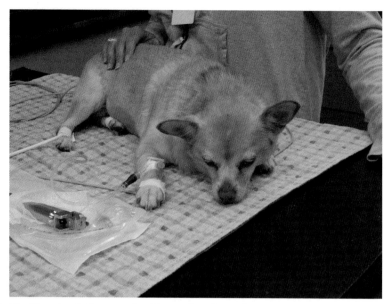

Fig. 1. Significant sedation seen in older patient from diazepam.

appropriate for geriatric patients. Propofol can cause moderate cardiopulmonary depression and apnea and so should be titrated slowly to effect and oxygen should be provided. However, the effects of propofol are very short; it is rapidly metabolized by hepatic and extrahepatic sites. Etomidate produces little cardiopulmonary depression, making it a good choice for patients with serious cardiac disease, but can cause rougher inductions with retching and twitching. Etomidate also produces transient adrenocortical suppression. Ketamine (KetaVed [Vedco Inc., St Joseph, MO, USA], Vetalar [Fort Dodge Animal Health, Ft Dodge, IA, USA], KetaFlo [Abbott Animal Health, Abbott Park, IL, USA]) is often used since it does not cause a decrease in heart rate or blood pressure due to sympathetic stimulation, but it can increase workload on patients with a decreased cardiac reserve. Ketamine also can cause seizures, muscle rigidity, or dysphoria, so it is often combined with a benzodiazepine. Maintenance with inhalants is recommended since they provide an oxygen-rich environment and quick recoveries. However, inhalants cause a dose-dependent cardiopulmonary depression; careful monitoring of blood pressure with adjustment in anesthetic depth and appropriate use of intravenous fluids will control this problem. The newer inhalants, isoflurane (IsoFlo [Abbott Animal Health, Abbott Park, IL, USA], Isothesia) and sevoflurane (SevoFlo; Abbott Animal Health, Abbott Park, IL, USA), require little metabolism so they are safer for patients with organ dysfunction. In geriatric patients, a combination of drugs to create balanced anesthesia is usually the most ideal solution. For example, premedications will decrease induction drug requirements, while infiltration of local anesthetics will reduce the need for intraoperative opioids; continuous-rate infusions can significantly decrease inhalant requirements.

Repeated Anesthetic Episodes in Geriatric Patients

With the increase in the number of patients undergoing radiation therapy, more geriatric patients are being anesthetized repeatedly. Our experience with daily

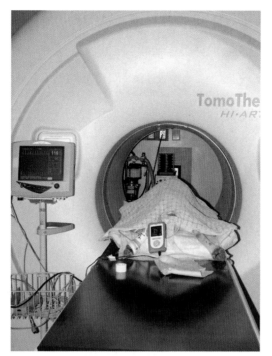

Fig. 2. Geriatric patient receiving radiation therapy.

anesthesia for TomoTherapy (**Fig. 2**) is that the patients (most of whom are quite geriatric and have cancer) are different from day to day in their response to the anesthetic protocol. We start with a basic anesthetic protocol (eg, glycopyrrolate and butorphanol premedication; propofol induction and maintenance on sevoflurane) and then modify it based on how the patient does under anesthesia. Very few patients complete 20 treatments without some modification to the initial anesthetic protocol; usually drug dosages have been decreased or dropped and supportive care measures (ie, dobutamine) increased. As for all geriatric patients, monitors are attached to the patient and reading are taken (**Fig. 3**) before the induction of anesthesia.

COMPLICATIONS
Hypotension

Hypotension is the most common concern in the geriatric patient. If the depth of anesthesia can be decreased, this may be sufficient to correct the problem. Substituting a less vasodilating drug may also be helpful; for example, providing a continuous-rate infusion of fentanyl may reduce the percentage of inhalant anesthetic needed. Administering a 5 to 10 mL/kg fluid bolus will help to rule out hypovolemia in a patient without significant cardiac disease; inotropic support may be needed if the patient cannot tolerate fluids. Dopamine and dobutamine are β-agonists, which increase cardiac contractility; however, this will increase the workload on the heart, so they should be titrated to the lowest possible rate.

Bradycardia

Depth of anesthesia should be assessed first. If possible, lighten the plane of anesthesia. An anticholinergic may be necessary to bring the heart rate back to

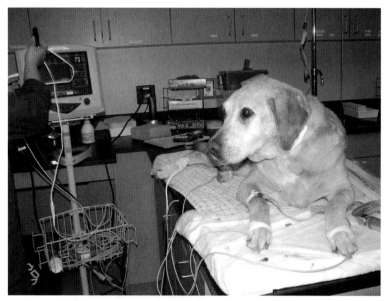

Fig. 3. Monitors attached prior to induction of anesthesia.

normal but should be used cautiously in geriatric patients since tachycardia will increase the workload and oxygen demand of the heart. Preoperative use of an anticholinergic such as glycopyrrolate (Robinul; Baxter Healthcare Corp., Deerfield, IL, USA) may prevent bradycardia without producing tachycardia, thereby avoiding increased workload. Hypothermia is also a common cause of bradycardia.[16] If the patient is severely hypothermic (<91°F), anticholinergic may not be effective at the time of administration but may create tachycardia once the patient is warmed. With profound hypothermia, immediate warming of the patient with forced warm air or water blankets is vital to avoid cardiac arrest.

Hypoxemia

The immediate action taken for the hypoxemic animal (ie, partial pressure of oxygen [PaO2] <80 mm Hg or saturation pressure of hemoglobin with oxygen [SpO2] <92%) should be to provide oxygen if not already being provided. Causes for hypoxemia can be broken into 3 causes: mechanical, ventilatory, or physiologic. First, rule out mechanical malfunction with the anesthetic machine, endotracheal tube, or oxygen supply. The endotracheal tube is easily kinked during positioning for surgery or imaging, especially in small patients. Next, confirm that the patient is ventilating adequately (by assessing CO_2 with a capnograph or blood gas sample if available). If necessary, provide assisted ventilation or place the patient on a ventilator. Due to the geriatric patient's decreased ventilatory drive and lack of reserves, this is often necessary. Positive pressure ventilation should be performed gently, not to exceed 15 to 20 cm H_2O, to prevent overinflation or barotrauma. Finally, auscult the chest to rule out bronchial intubation, pneumothorax, pulmonary edema, or atalectasis.

Insufficient Anesthetic Depth

It often takes a prolonged period to reach a stable anesthetic plane and is difficult to maintain in the geriatric patient. Pulmonary fibrosis ("old dog lung") and

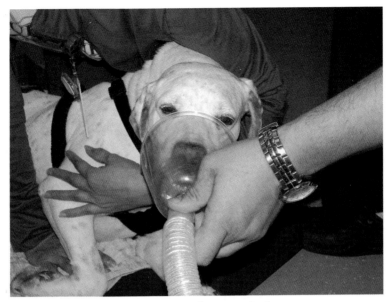

Fig. 4. Oxygen via face mask during recovery from anesthesia.

hypoventilation can cause lower levels of inhaled anesthetic to reach the brain and at a slower rate. Providing adequate premedication will aid in lowering the induction requirements as well as requirements for maintenance, thereby allowing for a smoother induction and anesthetic period. Assisting with ventilation is recommended to ensure oxygenation and provide a steady level of inhalant delivery. The addition of a continuous-rate infusion during anesthesia may also be helpful by providing more analgesia and relaxation, and decreasing needs for inhalant; however, as previously mentioned, the effect of an opioid continuous-rate infusion on ventilation must be taken into account.

Prolonged/Rough Recovery

Recovery can be a dangerous time for older patients. Monitoring and support MUST continue until the patient has regained full control of all physiologic functions; this may include the need for postextubation of oxygen given via facemask (**Fig. 4**). Doses of postoperative drugs should be reduced or carefully titrated to establish a good level of analgesia for each particular patient rather than giving them at fixed doses and intervals. If profound or prolonged depression occurs, reversing any reversible drugs may be necessary. Fluids should be continued throughout recovery to help maintain good perfusion and aid in excretion of metabolites. Older patients are prone to hypothermia, which will slow metabolism and recovery as well. The patient may be unable to increase his or her own temperature and external heat should be provided. Supportive care such as additional padding for arthritic patients and bladder expression will also help to keep the animal comfortable. Dysphoria is common with more senile patients. Once pain has been ruled out, very low doses of acepromazine may help to calm the distressed or dysphoric patient.

SEDATION VERSUS GENERAL ANESTHESIA?

It is often assumed that sedation would be safer in the geriatric patient, however, this maybe an incorrect assumption. General anesthesia can have many benefits over sedation such as control and protection of the airway, delivery of 100% oxygen, and inhalants that are not cumulative and do not require significant kidney or liver function and allow for quick control of depth of anesthesia. Careful evaluation of the patient, procedure, and risk:benefit ratio is necessary.

Unusual or Emerging Problems

Postoperative cognitive dysfunction (POCD) is an accepted problem in the human field. POCD is associated with normal consciousness but impairment of memory, concentration, language comprehension, and social integration.[17] Current thinking is that POCD may resolve within 3 months but may also be permanent, with no known treatment. It is not currently possible to say whether a similar problem exists for our patients, however, there may be anecdotal evidence that it exists. Since POCD is associated with age, it seems likely that, with the increase in geriatric patients, we might expect to see this problem.

Other sequelae that have been reported after anesthesia in geriatric patients include deafness.[18] This does not appear to be common, but the deafness has been permanent, and the cause is unknown.

SUMMARY

Geriatric patients are becoming a larger and larger portion of the pet population with owners willing to provide higher levels of care. This care will often necessitate anesthesia in old patients with significant underlying problems. The authors would like to emphasize that geriatric patients must be treated as *individuals*, and *each anesthetic episode* must also be treated individually; drug protocols and dosages should be carefully titrated based on the patient's response to prevent overdose or prolonged recovery. Although considerable care should be taken, with the right preparation and monitoring, the geriatric patient can be safely and comfortably anesthetized.

REFERENCES

1. Mosier JE. Caring for the aging dog in today's practice. Vet Med 1990;85:460–71.
2. Harvey RC, Paddleford RR. Management of geriatric patients. Vet Clin N Am Small Anim Pract 1999;29:683–99.
3. Carpenter R, Pettifer G, Tranquilli W. Anesthesia for geriatric patients. Vet Clin N Am Small Anim Pract 2005;35:571–80.
4. Brodbelt DC, Blissitt, KJ, Hammond RA, et al. The risk of death: the confidential enquiry into perioperative small animal fatalities. Vet Anaesth Analg 2008;35:365–73.
5. Baetge CL, Matthews NS. Geriatric anesthesia and analgesia. NAVC Clinician's Brief 2009;7:15–8.
6. Neiger-Aeschbacher G. Geriatric patients. In: Seymour C, Due-Novakovski, editors. BSAVA manual of canine and feline anaesthesia and analgesia. 2nd edition. Gloucester (UK): BSAVA; 2010. p. 303–9.
7. Paddleford RR. Anesthetic considerations for the geriatric patient. Vet Clin N Am Small Anim Pract 1989;19:13–31.
8. Dodman NH. Aging changes in the geriatric dog and their impact on anesthesia. Comp Contin Educ Pract Vet 1984;6:1106–13.

9. Ko JKH, Galloway DS. Anesthesia of the geriatric patient. In: Greene SA, editor. Veterinary anesthesia and pain management secrets. Philadelphia: Hanley & Belfus; 2002. p. 215–23.

10. Pettifer GR, Grubb TL. Neonatal and geriatric patients. In: Tranquilli WJ, Thurmon JC, Grimm KA, editors. Lumb & Jones' veterinary anesthesia and analgesia. 4th edition. Ames (IA): Blackwell; 2007. p. 986–91.

11. Maher ER, Rush JE. Cardiovascular changes in the geriatric dog. Comp Contin Educ 1990;12:921–31.

12. Mosley C, Grubb T. Anesthetic management of the geriatric patient small animal and exotics. Proceedings of the North American Veterinary Conference, vol. 20. Orlando (FL), January 7–11; 2006. p. 1323–6.

13. Polzin DJ. The effects of aging on the canine urinary tract. Vet Med 1990;85:472–82.

14. MacDougall DF, Barker J. An approach to canine geriatrics. Br Vet J 1984;140: 115–23.

15. Joubert KE. Pre-anesthetic screening of geriatric dogs. J S Afr Vet Assoc 2007;78: 31–5.

16. Harvey RC. Hypothermia. In: Greene SA, editor. Veterinary anesthesia and pain management secrets. Philadelphia: Hanley & Belfus; 2002. p. 149–52.

17. Grape S, Ravussin P, Rossi A, et al. Postoperative cognitive dysfunction. Trends Anaesth Crit Care 2012. DOI: http://dx.doi.org/10.1016/j.tacc.2012.02.002.

18. Stevens-Sparks C, Strain G. Post-anesthesia deafness in dogs and cats following dental and ear cleaning procedures. Vet Anaesth Analg 2010;37:347–51.

The Diagnosis and Management of Age-Related Veterinary Cardiovascular Disease

Ashley B. Saunders, DVM

KEYWORDS

- Cardiomyopathy • Geriatric • Hypertension • Pericardial • Senior
- Valvular disease

KEY POINTS

- Disorders of the cardiovascular system are one of the most commonly diagnosed disease entities in the aging pet population.
- Comorbid conditions and polypharmacy situations are frequently encountered while managing pets with cardiovascular disease.
- Blood pressure measurement is recommended as routine screening for cats older than 9 years of age in which systemic hypertension can complicate renal disease or hyperthyroidism.
- Myxomatous degeneration of the mitral valve accounts for approximately 75% of acquired heart disease in small to medium-sized dogs, in which progression of disease is variable consisting of a long preclinical period and with many dogs never progressing to heart failure.
- Successful management of heart disease often requires multimodal therapy with the goal of maintaining quality of life for patient and owner.

INTRODUCTION

At last count, the American Veterinary Medical Association reported 81.7 million cats and 72.1 million dogs in the United States with more than 10% over 11 years of age.[1] Disorders of the cardiovascular system are one of the most commonly encountered disease entities in the aging pet population.[2,3]

Guidelines developed by the American Association of Feline Practitioners categorize cats as mature at 7 years old and senior by 11 years.[4] Systemic hypertension and cardiomyopathies are of particular importance in the aging cat.[3] Dogs age at different rates depending on breed, and small breeds typically have longer life spans than giant

The author has nothing to disclose.
Department of Small Animal Clinical Sciences, College of Veterinary Medicine and Biomedical Sciences, Texas A&M University, 4474 TAMU, College Station, TX 77843-4474, USA
E-mail address: asaunders@cvm.tamu.edu

Vet Clin Small Anim 42 (2012) 655–668
http://dx.doi.org/10.1016/j.cvsm.2012.04.005
0195-5616/12/$ – see front matter © 2012 Elsevier Inc. All rights reserved.

breeds. Whereas a small breed dog may be considered senior around 9 years of age, a giant breed may have reached that stage by 6.[2] Alternatively, dogs and cats can be considered senior once they reach the last 25% of their predicted life span.[3] Valvular heart disease, dilated cardiomyopathy, pericardial disease, arrhythmias, and systemic hypertension are of particular importance in the aging dog.[3,5]

THE PATHOLOGY OF AGING

The cardiovascular system undergoes intrinsic physiologic changes during the natural aging process. In dogs, these changes include a reduced response to β-adrenergic stimulation, an increase in myocardial and vascular stiffness, and prolongation of the action potential duration as well as normal myocyte contraction and relaxation times.[6,7] With exercise, the cardiovascular system is not able to compensate to maintain cardiac output in older dogs.[8] Coronary arteriosclerosis and both valvular and myocardial fibrosis are common findings in dogs older than 12 years.[9,10] Myxomatous degeneration of the mitral valve, the most common acquired cardiac disease in dogs, is characterized by lengthening and thickening of the valve leaflets and a loss of connective tissues that is associated with age.[11] Degenerative changes of the atrioventricular node and terminal narrowing of the small arteries have been identified histopathologically in aging dogs and may contribute to arrhythmias and conduction abnormalities.[12,13]

Cardiac biomarker concentrations appear to be correlated with age. Cardiac troponin I, a marker of myocardial damage, can be detected in older, apparently healthy dogs and cats, suggesting that age is associated with myocardial changes.[14–16] In one study, concentrations of N-terminal pro-B-type natriuretic peptide (NT-proBNP), a marker produced by myocardial distension and neurohormonal stimulation,[17] were higher in apparently healthy Doberman pinschers older than 8 years using a specific NT-proBNP assay.[18] NT-proBNP is also correlated with age in healthy, older cats ranging from 9.9 to 12.3 years of age.[19] Elevations in NT-proBNP concentrations in healthy individuals may be related to renal dysfunction and changes in myocardial diastolic function.[20,21]

The development of acquired cardiovascular disease can be complicated by age-related physiologic changes in older animals. Other organ systems including the kidneys, liver, and thyroid are susceptible to age-related decreases in function and blood flow. Renal disease, canine hypothyroidism, feline hyperthyroidism, hyperadrenocorticism, arthritis, and dental disease create comorbid conditions that affect therapeutic planning, anesthesia protocols, and heart disease management.[22–24] Nutritional needs and energy requirements change with age and heart disease.[25–28] Drug absorption, metabolism, and distribution are altered in geriatric patients often related to changes in cardiac output, gastric absorption, renal blood flow, and hepatic metabolism.[29] It is not uncommon for geriatric patients to be receiving multiple medications that, when coupled with age-related organ system dysfunction, can result in drug toxicity.[29,30]

CLINICAL PRESENTATION

Most cardiac diseases diagnosed in the mature to older dog and cat are acquired and progressive. In many cases, they can exist without progressing to the point of causing clinical signs. For example, degenerative mitral valve disease can result in mitral regurgitation and a characteristic murmur but not advance to cardiomegaly or heart failure.[31] Although clinical signs of heart disease may be related to the particular disease, more often than not, they are nonspecific. Commonly reported are cough, tachypnea, dyspnea, lethargy, syncope, reduced appetite or anorexia, and ascites/abdominal distension. Coughing is a common complaint by small breed dog owners that can be caused by both cardiac and respiratory diseases. Even when a heart murmur is present, a history of a chronic cough in the absence of breathing difficulty in a dog with a good appetite and activity level would suggest respiratory disease or mainstem bronchial compression as a more likely cause of the coughing than congestive heart failure.

Inquiring about appetite, activity level, and behavior can assess quality of life issues. Exercise intolerance, lethargy, change in appetite, and weight loss can be vague and mistakenly attributed to aging. A detailed history would include not only information related to potential heart disease but also details regarding currently administered medications and other organ systems for evidence of concurrent disease.

Auscultatory abnormalities suggestive of heart disease include a murmur, gallop, and arrhythmia. Less common are split heart sounds and clicks. In dogs, the location and timing of a murmur can be very useful in combination with signalment for determining the type of heart disease present. For example, dogs with valvular heart disease typically have a left apical, systolic murmur indicative of mitral regurgitation. In one study of apparently healthy cats, the incidence of heart murmurs and heart disease increased with age.[32] Murmurs in cats with cardiomyopathy are typically located in the parasternal region.[33,34] Multiple studies in apparently healthy cats and cats with cardiomyopathy have demonstrated how insensitive cardiac auscultation is at detecting heart disease.[32–37] Cats with preclinical heart disease may have no auscultable abnormalities on physical examination highlighting the importance of echocardiography for diagnosing heart disease in cats. Additionally, anesthesia and fluid administration can precipitate heart failure in cats with preclinical heart disease.[38] To complicate matters, cats can have a heart murmur or gallop for a variety of reasons that are not exclusive to heart disease including anemia, hyperthyroidism, systemic hypertension, and physiologic dynamic outflow tract obstruction.[34,37,39] Auscultation alone cannot differentiate cats with and without heart disease.

Abnormal pulse quality, pulse deficits, abdominal distention, jugular venous distention, pale or cyanotic mucus membranes, increased lung sounds, tachypnea, dyspnea, and crackles are all indicators of heart disease. Muffled heart and lung sounds suggest the presence of pleural and pericardial effusion.

DIAGNOSIS

The objective of performing diagnostic tests is to identify the type of cardiac disease, determine if heart failure is present, monitor therapy, and detect abnormalities that when properly addressed will help maintain quality of life. In most cases, multiple tests are indicated (**Table 1**).

Thoracic Radiographs

Normal findings in apparently healthy, older cats include a more horizontal position of the heart toward the sternum and undulation of the thoracic aorta that is also identified in cats with systemic hypertension.[40,41] The vertebral heart scale system developed by Buchanan provides reference values for heart size in dogs and cats that are useful for detecting cardiomegaly and monitoring disease progression within a patient.[42,43]

Thoracic radiographs provide information regarding the size of the heart and pulmonary vasculature. Pulmonary arterial and venous enlargement is indicative of pulmonary

Table 1
Diagnostic tests recommendations for common cardiovascular diseases in aging cats and dogs

	Radiography	Echocardiography	Electrocardiography	Blood Pressure	Clinical Pathology
Cat					
Cardiomyopathy	+	++	+	+	Biochemistry panel, urinalysis, thyroid
Systemic hypertension	+	+		++	Biochemistry panel, urinalysis, thyroid
Pericardial disease	+	++	+		Biochemistry panel
Arrhythmias	+	+	++	+	Biochemistry panel, thyroid
Dog					
Valvular disease	++	++	+	+	Biochemistry panel
Dilated cardiomyopathy	++	++	++	+	Biochemistry panel, thyroid
Arrhythmogenic right ventricular cardiomyopathy	+	++	++	+	Biochemistry panel
Systemic hypertension				++	Biochemistry panel, urinalysis
Pericardial disease	+	++	+		Biochemistry panel
Arrhythmias			++		Biochemistry panel

+ indicates tests useful for making the diagnosis of each disease (with ++ being most useful).

hypertension and congestive heart failure, respectively. A distinct advantage of radiographs is visualization of the lungs for identifying heart failure. Left-sided heart failure typically presents as pulmonary edema in the dog and a combination of pulmonary edema and/or pleural or pericardial effusion in cats. Mainstem bronchial compression secondary to atrial enlargement can be identified in coughing dogs. A globoid cardiac silhouette is indicative of pericardial effusion.

Limitations include inability to assess cardiac function, the amount of valvular regurgitation, identify intracardiac masses, or determine type of feline cardiomyopathy. If a cat has clinical signs, physical exam findings, or radiographic evidence suggestive of heart disease, an echocardiogram is essential for diagnosing the specific type of cardiomyopathy, which can influence therapeutic decision-making.[34,37]

Echocardiography

In many instances, echocardiography is the test of choice for diagnosing cardiac disease. Information gained that is unique to echocardiography includes:

- Valve anatomy for abnormal thickening, prolapse, and chordal rupture
- Severity of valve regurgitation
- Atrial and ventricular size
- Systolic and diastolic ventricular function
- Type of cardiomyopathy
- Presence and severity of pulmonary hypertension
- Presence and severity of pericardial and pleural effusion
- Location of cardiac neoplasia.

Limitations include availability, operator experience, and cost associated with performing echocardiography.

Electrocardiography and Holter Monitoring

An electrocardiogram is indicated in patients with arrhythmias, when an arrhythmia is suspected based on a history of weakness or collapse, in canine breeds predisposed to developing arrhythmias (boxer, Doberman pinscher), as a preanesthetic workup, when monitoring antiarrhythmic therapy, and in patients with metabolic or endocrine diseases. Twenty-four–hour Holter monitor recordings are recommended to identify the presence of arrhythmias and to evaluate the frequency and severity of arrhythmias in predisposed breeds.[44,45]

Even though chamber enlargement criteria have been established based on specific changes in the components of normal complexes, an electrocardiogram is an insensitive means of assessing heart size.

Blood Pressure

Both hypertension and hypotension can be problematic in aging patients. Systemic hypertension is often secondary to other diseases and causes increased cardiac work. Hypotension in a patient with heart disease may indicate a decrease in cardiac output secondary to reduced ventricular function, arrhythmias, or overdiuresis. Many heart failure medications including angiotensin-converting enzyme inhibitors and pimobendan have vasodilatory effects that can alter blood pressure.[46,47] For optimal results in clinical cases, use an indirect oscillometric or Doppler device with the appropriate cuff size and position and allow for an acclimation period prior to taking measurements.[48]

Table 2
Age at diagnosis for common cardiovascular diseases in aging cats and dogs

	Mean Age at Diagnosis	Comments
Cat		
Cardiomyopathy	5.6–6.8 y[38,57]	Hypertrophic most common
Systemic hypertension	14.8 y[56]	Often associated with concurrent renal disease or hyperthyroidism
Pericardial disease	6.3 y[80]	Pericardial effusion is most often associated with heart failure
Arrhythmias	Atrial fibrillation 10.2 y[88] Atrioventricular block 14 y[89]	Uncommon
Dog		
Valvular disease	90% of Cavalier King Charles spaniels >10 y[73]	Predominantly small and medium-size breeds
Dilated cardiomyopathy	Median 5–7.5 y[93,94]	Predominantly large and giant breeds
Arrhythmogenic right ventricular cardiomyopathy	9.1 y[66]	Associated with arrhythmias in boxers
Systemic hypertension	9.6 y[51]	Often associated with concurrent renal or endocrine disease
Pericardial disease	Idiopathic 6 y Hemangiosarcoma 10.1 y[77]	
Arrhythmias	Atrioventricular block 11.1 y[81] Sick sinus syndrome 10.5 y[85]	

Clinical Pathology

Tests are selected to provide information regarding organ system function and for therapeutic monitoring. Complete blood count, biochemistries, electrolytes, heartworm antigen test, and urinalysis including urine protein:creatinine ratio are used to assess general health. Concurrent endocrine disorders require additional testing. Currently available cardiac specific biomarkers, including atrial natriuretic peptide, brain natriuretic peptide, and cardiac troponin I, are being evaluated for detection of preclinical disease, to differentiate cardiac and noncardiac causes of respiratory distress, to guide therapy, and as prognostic indicators.[49,50] Elevations in biomarker concentrations are detected in dogs and cats with heart disease, and specific values are unique to each biomarker and the assay being used.

DISEASES

In the following section, species-specific differences in cardiovascular disease in cats and dogs and distinct findings associated with aging will be addressed (**Table 2**).

Systemic Hypertension

Systemic hypertension can be a primary disease or, more often, it is secondary to another disease or condition.[51] Secondary conditions like renal and endocrine disease are typically more prevalent in older cats and dogs. Reported normal blood pressure values vary depending on age, sex, and breed. In general, persistent values greater than 150 mm Hg place a patient at risk for target organ damage to the kidneys, eyes, brain, and heart.[48] Clinical findings in cats and dogs include the presence of a murmur, gallop, and, in some cases, left ventricular hypertrophy and aortic valve insufficiency.[51,52]

Blood pressure measurement is recommended as routine screening for cats older than 9 years in which systemic hypertension is most often secondary to renal disease or hyperthyroidism.[53,54] Blood pressure measurement is recommended as routine screening for dogs older than 10 years in which systemic hypertension is associated with kidney disease, hyperadrenocorticism, diabetes mellitus, and pheochromocytoma.[48,55] Additional clinical pathologic testing is typically required to diagnose concurrent disease. Damage to target organs presents as hemorrhage, detachment, or edema of the retinas and seizures.[56] Therapy is recommended to avoid or limit damage related to sustained high pressures and consists of antihypertensive therapy with an angiotensin-converting enzyme inhibitor, calcium channel blocker (amlodipine), or both in addition to identifying and treating any concurrent disease.[48,53]

Cardiomyopathy

Cardiomyopathies are diseases of myocardial structure and function and are classified based on specific morphologic characteristics and abnormalities of systolic and diastolic function. The incidence of a specific type of cardiomyopathy differs between dogs and cats.

Cats

Hypertrophic cardiomyopathy is the most common cardiomyopathy diagnosed in cats.[57,58] Left ventricular hypertrophy characteristic of hypertrophic cardiomyopathy should be differentiated from left ventricular hypertrophy secondary to systemic hypertension and hyperthyroidism.[59] While the presence of a murmur, gallop, arrhythmia, or cardiomegaly on thoracic radiographs is suggestive of heart disease, many cats have disease without any detectable abnormalities and not all cats develop clinical signs. In multivariate analysis of cats with hypertrophic cardiomyopathy, age and left atrial size were negatively associated with survival.[38]

Important complications of the disease include:

- Congestive heart failure
- Arrhythmias
- Arterial thromboembolism.

Dogs

Dilated cardiomyopathy is characterized by enlargement and reduced systolic function of the ventricular chambers and typically affects large and giant breeds including the Doberman pinscher, Irish wolfhound, great Dane, and Newfoundland.[60,61] Cocker spaniels may be affected as well. Ventricular arrhythmias increase the risk of sudden death. A retrospective study suggested the use of an angiotensin-converting enzyme inhibitor may delay the onset of clinical signs in Doberman pinschers with preclinical disease.[62] Screening is recommended for at risk breeds using echocardiography and electrocardiography. Approximately 25% of Dobermans pinschers over the age of 10 years have clinical signs and many have concurrent hypothyroidism.[45,63]

Arrhythmogenic right ventricular cardiomyopathy is a familial disease in boxers characterized predominantly by ventricular arrhythmias and occasionally by myocardial failure.[64–66] In a recent study, boxers in the United Kingdom were more likely to have ventricular dilation and systolic dysfunction than what has been reported in North America.[67]

Therapeutic management is recommended for dogs with clinical signs, most often syncope, and ventricular arrhythmias with appropriate antiarrhythmic and heart failure therapy.

Important complications of the disease include:

- Congestive heart failure
- Arrhythmias
- Sudden death.

Valvular Disease

By far the most commonly acquired disease in dogs, myxomatous degeneration of the mitral valve accounts for approximately 75% of heart disease and affects mostly small- to medium-sized breeds, although large breeds have been reported.[68,69] The prevalence of valvular disease increases with age with the mitral valve being affected in most cases.[70–72] Prevalence in Cavalier King Charles Spaniels older than 10 years is greater than 90%.[73] Progression of disease is variable and typically takes years to progress to a severity that requires treatment.[9] Approximately 30% of dogs progress to heart failure.[31] In effect, many dogs will not develop clinical signs or require therapy. A heart murmur is a consistent finding and is characteristically systolic and left apical in origin. A classification system including 4 distinct stages (A–D) has recently been reported to assist with the diagnosis and treatment of valvular disease.[74] Stage A includes patients at risk for developing heart disease. Stage B includes patients with heart disease but without clinical signs and is further divided into normal heart size (B1) and heart enlargement (B2). Stages C and D include patients with heart failure that can be managed with standard heart failure therapy (Stage C) or are refractory to therapy and considered to have end-stage disease (Stage D).

Important complications of the disease are:

- Congestive heart failure
- Mainstem bronchial compression
- Pulmonary hypertension and right sided heart failure
- Arrhythmias
- Acute decompensation associated with chordae tendineae rupture
- Left atrial rupture.

Pericardial Disease

Dogs

In approximately 20% of dogs, there is no identifiable cause of pericardial effusion.[75] Potential causes in older dogs include neoplastic and cardiac. The most common neoplastic lesions are hemangiosarcoma of the right atrium and auricle, aortic body tumors (chemodectoma), and mesothelioma. Small volume pericardial effusion can be identified in dogs with right-sided heart failure or left atrial rupture. On average, the age at presentation with idiopathic effusions is less than with neoplastic effusions.[76,77] Clinical signs are often nonspecific lethargy and anorexia. Some dogs may present for abdominal distention. Pericardiocentesis is indicated in patients with evidence of hemodynamic compromise.

Cats

Pericardial effusion is uncommon in cats but can occur secondary to congestive heart failure.[78,79] Clinical findings are consistent with heart failure and include tachypnea, abnormal lung sounds, murmur, and gallop. Effusions are typically mild and may resolve with heart failure therapy.[80]

Arrhythmias

Dogs

Bradyarrhythmias including sick sinus syndrome and atrioventricular block can occur at any age but are more prevalent in older dogs.[81–83] Although advancing age is associated with a worse prognosis in humans with atrioventricular block, the same has not been found in dogs.[81,84] Clinical findings typically include lethargy, episodic weakness, and syncope.[82,83,85] The most commonly affected breeds are the miniature Schnauzer, Labrador retriever, cocker Spaniel, West Highland white terrier, and German shepherd. More than 50% of affected dogs have concurrent cardiac disease, often valvular disease.[82] Treatment for symptomatic dogs requires pacemaker implantation. In one review, clinical outcomes were good following pacemaker placement despite the prevalence of older patients and most owners were satisfied with the procedure.[82]

Cats

Arrhythmias in older cats are generally associated with cardiomyopathy and hyperthyroidism.[86,87] Abnormalities identified include atrial fibrillation, ventricular arrhythmias, prolonged QRS duration, and atrioventricular block.[86–89] Nearly all cats with atrial fibrillation had concurrent atrial enlargement.[88]

MANAGEMENT

Successful management of heart disease requires multimodal therapy (pharmacotherapy, centesis, device placement, nutritional management) with the goal of maintaining quality of life for patient and owner.

Medical management of heart failure consists of diuretic therapy and renin-angiotensin-aldosterone system blockade with angiotensin-converting enzyme inhibitors.[68,90] Pimobendan, an inodilator, has proven benefit in dogs with dilated cardiomyopathy and valvular disease.[91,92] Additional therapeutics including antiarrhythmic and anticoagulant medications may be required prophylactically or to manage complications and comorbid conditions, remembering that aging patients often have comorbid conditions and are receiving multiple medications. Changes in organ function for patients that have developed hemodynamically significant effusions secondary to congestive heart failure or pericardial disease, or centesis of the thorax, abdomen, or pericardial space can improve or resolve clinical signs. Nutritional support in heart disease should emphasize proper diets, sodium content, and the use of supplements (taurine, carnitine, fatty acids) when appropriate.

REFERENCES

1. American Veterinary Medical Association. U.S. pet ownership & demographics sourcebook, 2007 edition. Schaumberg (IL): American Veterinary Medical Association; 2007. p. 1–27.
2. Hoskins JD, McCurnin DM. Geriatric care in the late 1990s. Vet Clin North Am Small Anim Pract 1997;27:1273–84.
3. Epstein M, Kuehn NF, Landsberg G, et al. AAHA senior care guidelines for dogs and cats. J Am Anim Hosp Assoc 2005;41:81–91.

4. Hoyumpa Vogt A, Rodan I, Brown M, et al. AAFP AAHA feline life stage guidelines. J Fel Med Surg 2010;12:43–54.

5. Guglielmini C. Cardiovascular diseases in the ageing dog: diagnostic and therapeutic problems. Vet Res Comm 2003;27(Suppl 1):555–60.

6. Dai D, Wessells RJ, Bodmer R, et al. Cardiac aging. In: Wolf NS, editor. Comparative Biology of aging. London: Springer Dordrecht Heidelberg; 2010. p. 259–86.

7. Yin FC, Spurgeon HA, Greene HL, et al. Age-associated decrease in heart rate response to isoproterenol in dogs. Mech Ageing Dev 1979;10:17–25.

8. Yin FC, Weisfeldt, Milnor WR. Role of aortic input impedance in the decreased cardiovascular response to exercise with aging in dogs. J Clin Invest 1981;68:28–38.

9. Detweiler DK, Luginbuhl H, Buchanan JW, et al. The natural history of acquired cardiac disability of the dog. Ann N Y Acad Sci 1968;147:318–29.

10. Falk T, Jonsson L, Olsen LH, et al. Arteriosclerotic changes in the myocardium, lung, and kidney in dogs with chronic congestive heart failure and myxomatous mitral valve disease. Cardiovasc Pathol 2006;15:185–93.

11. Han RI, Black A, Culshaw G, et al. Structural and cellular changes in canine myxomatous mitral valve disease: an image analysis study. J Heart Valve Dis 2010;19:60–70.

12. Meierhenry EF, Liu SK. Atrioventricular bundle degeneration associated with sudden death in the dog. J Am Vet Med Assoc 1978;172:1418–22.

13. Sandusky GE, Kerr KM, Capen CC. Morphologic variations and aging in the atrioventricular conduction system of large breed dogs. Anat Rec 1979;193:883–902.

14. Oyama MA, Sisson DD. Cardiac troponin-I concentration in dogs with cardiac disease. J Vet Intern Med 2004;18:831–9.

15. Ljungvall I, Hoglund K, Tidholm A, et al. Cardiac troponin I is associated with severity of myxomatous mitral valve disease, age, and C- reactive protein in dogs. J Vet Intern Med 2010;24:153–9.

16. Serra M, Papakonstantinou S, Adamcova M, et al. Veterinary and toxicological applications for the detection of cardiac injury using cardiac troponin. Vet J 2010;185:50–7.

17. Clerico A, Giannoni A, Vittorini S, et al. Thirty years of the heart as an endocrine organ: physiological role and clinical utility of cardiac natriuretic hormones. Am J Physiol Heart Circ Physiol 2011;201:H12–20.

18. Wess G, Butz V, Mahling M, et al. Evaluation of N-terminal pro-B-type natriuretic peptide as a diagnostic marker of various stages of cardiomyopathy in Doberman Pinschers. Am J Vet Res 2011;72:642–9.

19. Lalor SM, Connolly DJ, Elliott J, et al. Plasma concentrations of natriuretic peptides in normal cats and normotensive and hypertensive cats with chronic kidney disease. J Vet Cardiol 2009;11:S71–9.

20. Sayama H, Nakamura Y, Kinoshita M. Why is the concentration of plasma brain natriuretic peptide in elderly inpatients greater than normal? Coron Artery Dis 1999;10:537–40.

21. Raymond I, Groenning BA, Hildebrandt PR, et al. The influence of age, sex and other variables on the plasma level of N-terminal pro-brain natriuretic peptide in a large sample of the general population. Heart 2003;89:745–51.

22. Lulich JP, Osborne CA, O'Brien TD, et al. Feline renal failure: questions, answers, questions. Comp Cont Educ Pract Vet 1992;14:127–52.

23. Syme HM. Cardiovascular and renal manifestations of hyperthyroidism. Vet Clin North Am Small Anim Pract 2007;37:723–43.

24. Scott-Moncrieff JCR. Clinical signs and concurrent diseases of hypothyroidism in dogs and cats. Vet Clin North Am Small Anim Pract 2007;37:709–22.

25. Harper EJ. Changing perspectives on aging and energy requirements: aging, body weight and body composition in humans, dogs and cats. J Nutr 1998;128:2627S–31S.

26. Laflamme DP. Nutrition for aging cats and dogs and the importance of body condition. Vet Clin North Am Small Anim Pract 2005;35:713–42.

27. Freeman LM, Rush JE, Cahalane AK, et al. Evaluation of dietary patterns in dogs with cardiac disease. J Am Vet Med Assoc 2003;223:1301–5.

28. Freeman LM, Rush JE, Markwell PJ. Effects of dietary modification in dogs with early chronic valvular disease. J Vet Intern Med 2006;20:1116–26.

29. Dowling P. Geriatric pharmacology. Vet Clin North Am Small Anim Pract 2005;35:557–69.

30. Fleg JL, Aronow WS, Frishman WH. Cardiovascular drug therapy in the elderly: benefits and challenges. Nat Rev Cardiol 2011;8:13–28.

31. Borgarelli M, Haggstrom J. Canine degenerative myxomatous mitral valve disease: natural history, clinical presentation and therapy. Vet Clin North Am Small Anim Pract 2010;40:651–63.

32. Drourr LT, Gordon SG, Roland RM, et al. Prevalence of heart murmurs and occult heart disease in apparently healthy adult cats. In: American College of Veterinary Internal Medicine 2010 Proceedings. Madison: Omnipress; 2010. p. 159.

33. Paige CF, Abbott JA, Elvinger F, et al. Prevalence of cardiomyopathy in apparently healthy cats. J Am Vet Med Assoc 2009;234:1398–403.

34. Dirven MJM, Cornelissen JMM, Barendse MAM, et al. Cause of heart murmurs in 57 apparently healthy cats. Tijdschr Diergeneeskd 2010;135:840–7.

35. Cote E, Manning AM, Emerson D, et al. Assessment of the prevalence of heart murmurs in overtly healthy cats. J Am Vet Med Assoc 2004;225:384–8.

36. Wagner T, Luis Fuentes V, Payne JR, et al. Comparison of auscultatory and echocardiographic findings in healthy adult cats. J Vet Cardiol 2010;12:171–82.

37. Nakamura RK, Rishniw M, King MK, et al. Prevalence of echocardiographic evidence of cardiac disease in apparently healthy cats with murmurs. J Fel Med Surg 2011;13:266–71.

38. Rush JE, Freeman LM, Fenollosa NK, et al. Population and survival characteristics of cats with hypertrophic cardiomyopathy: 260 cases (1990–1999). J Am Vet Med Assoc 2002;220:202–7.

39. Sisson DD, Ettinger SJ. The physical examination. In: Fox PR, Sisson DD, Moise NS, editors. Textbook of canine and feline cardiology. 2nd edition. Philadelphia: WB Saunders; 1999. p. 46–64.

40. Nelson OL, Reidesel E, Ware WA, et al. Echocardiographic and radiographic changes associated with systemic hypertension in cats. J Vet Intern Med 2002;16:418–25.

41. Moon ML, Keene BW, Lessard P, et al. Age related changes in the feline cardiac silhouette. Vet Radiol Ultrasound 1993;34:315–20.

42. Buchanan JW, Bucheler J. Vertebral scale system to measure canine heart size in radiographs. J Am Vet Med Assoc 1995;206:194–9.

43. Litster AL, Buchanan JW. Vertebral scale system to measure heart size in radiographs of cats. J Am Vet Med Assoc 2000;216:210–4.

44. Calvert CA, Jacobs G, Pickus CW, et al. Results of ambulatory electrocardiography in overtly healthy Doberman Pinschers with echocardiographic abnormalities. J Am Vet Med Assoc 2000;217:1328–32.

45. O'Grady MR, O'Sullivan ML. Dilated cardiomyopathy: an update. Vet Clin North Am Small Anim Pract 2004;34:1187–207.

46. Lefebvre HP, Brown SA, Chetboul V, et al. Angiotensin-converting enzyme inhibitors in veterinary medicine. Curr Pharm Des 2007;13:1347–61.

47. Haggstrom J, Hoglund K, Borgarelli M. An update on treatment and prognostic indicators in canine myxomatous mitral valve disease. J Sm Anim Pract 2009;50:25–33.
48. Brown S, Atkins C, Bagley A, et al. Guidelines for the identification, evaluation, and management of systemic hypertension in dogs and cats. J Vet Intern Med 2007;21: 542–58.
49. Boswood A. Editorial: the rise and fall of the cardiac biomarker. J Vet Intern Med 2004;18:797–9.
50. Boswood A, Dukes-McEwan J, Loureiro, et al. The diagnostic accuracy of different natriuretic peptides in the investigation of canine cardiac disease. J Sm Anim Pract 2008;49:26–32.
51. Misbach C, Gouni V, Tissier R, et al. Echocardiographic and tissue Doppler imaging alterations associated with spontaneous canine systemic hypertension. J Vet Intern Med 2011;25:1025–35.
52. Chetboul V, Lefebvre HP, Pinhas C, et al. Spontaneous feline hypertension: clinical and echocardiographic abnormalities, and survival rate. J Vet Intern Med 2003;17: 89–95.
53. Stepien RL. Feline systemic hypertension: diagnosis and management. J Fel Med Surg 2011;13:35–43.
54. Kobayashi DL, Peterson ME, Graves TK, et al. Hypertension in cats with chronic renal failure or hyperthyroidism. J Vet Intern Med 1990;4:58–62.
55. Wehner A, Hartmann K, Hirschberger J. Associations between proteinuria, systemic hypertension and glomerular filtration rate in dogs with renal and non-renal diseases. Vet Rec 2008;162:141–7.
56. Maggio F, DeFrancesco TC, Atkins CE, et al. Ocular lesions associated with systemic hypertension in cats: 69 cases (1985–1998). J Am Vet Med Assoc 2000;217:695–702.
57. Ferasin L, Sturgess CP, Cannon MJ, et al. Feline idiopathic cardiomyopathy: a retrospective study of 106 cats (1994–2001). J Feline Med Surg 2003;5:151–9.
58. Fox PR, Liu SK, Maron BJ. Echocardiographic assessment of spontaneously occurring feline hypertrophic cardiomyopathy: an animal model of human disease. Circulation 1995;92:2645–51.
59. Abbott JA. Feline hypertrophic cardiomyopathy: an update. Vet Clin North Am Small Anim Pract 2010;40:685–700.
60. Vollmar AC. The prevalence of cardiomyopathy in the Irish wolfhound: a clinical study of 500 dogs. J Am Anim Hosp Assoc 2000;36:125–32.
61. Tidholm A, Haagstrom J, Borgarelli M, et al. Canine idiopathic dilated cardiomyopathy. Part I: aetiology, clinical characteristics, epidemiology and pathology. Vet J 2001; 162:92–107.
62. O'Grady MR, O'Sullivan ML, Minors SL, et al. Efficacy of benazepril hydrochloride to delay the progression of occult dilated cardiomyopathy in Doberman pinschers. J Vet Intern Med 2009;23:977–83.
63. Calvert CA, Jacobs GJ, Medleau L, et al. Thyroid-stimulating hormone stimulation tests in cardiomyopathic Doberman pinschers: a retrospective study. J Vet Intern Med 1998;12:343–8.
64. Meurs KM, Spier AW, Miller MW, et al. Familial ventricular arrhythmias in boxers. J Vet Intern Med 1999;13:437–9.
65. Meurs KM. Boxer dog cardiomyopathy: an update. Vet Clin North Am Small Anim Pract 2004;34:1235–44.
66. Basso CB, Fox PR, Meurs KM, et al. Arrhythmogenic right ventricular cardiomyopathy causing sudden cardiac death in boxer dogs: new animal model of human disease. Circulation 2004;109:1180–5.

67. Palermo V, Stafford Johnson MJ, Sala E, et al. Cardiomyopathy in boxer dogs: a retrospective study of the clinical presentation, diagnostic findings and survival. J Vet Cardiol 2011;13:45–55.
68. Haggstrom J, Kvart C, Pedersen HD. Acquired valvular heart disease. In: Ettinger S, Feldmen E, editors. Textbook of veterinary internal medicine. Diseases of dogs and cats. 6th edition. Philadelphia: Elsevier Saunders; 2005. p. 1022–40.
69. Borgarelli M, Zini E, Dagnolo A, et al. Comparison of primary mitral valve disease in German Shepherd dogs and in small breeds. J Vet Cardiol 2004;6:27–34.
70. Jones TC, Zook BC. Aging changes in the vascular system of animals. Ann N Y Acad Sci 1965;127:671–84.
71. Detweiler DK, Patterson DF. The prevalence and types of cardiovascular disease in dogs. Ann N Y Acad Sci 1965;127:481–516.
72. Buchanan JW. Prevalence of cardiovascular disorders. In: Fox PR, Sisson DD, Moise NS, editors. Textbook of canine and feline cardiology. 2nd edition. Philadelphia: WB Saunders; 1999. p. 457–70.
73. Pedersen HD, Lorentzen K, Kristensen B. Echocardiographic mitral valve prolapse in cavalier King Charles spaniels: epidemiology and prognostic significance for regurgitation. Vet Record 1999:144;315–20.
74. Atkins C, Bonagura J, Ettinger S, et al. Guidelines for the diagnosis and treatment of canine chronic valvular heart disease. J Vet Intern Med 2009;26:1142–50.
75. Berg RJ, Wingfield W. Pericardial effusion in the dog: a review of 42 cases. J Am Anim Hosp Assoc 1983;20:721–30.
76. Dunning D, Monnet E, Orton C, et al. Analysis of prognostic indicators for dogs with pericardial effusion: 46 cases (1985–1996). J Am Vet Med Assoc 1998;212: 1279–80.
77. Aronsohn M. Cardiac hemangiosarcoma in the dog: a review of 38 cases. J Am Vet Med Assoc 1985;187:922–6.
78. Rush JE, Keene BW, Fox PR. Pericardial disease in the cat: a retrospective evaluation of 66 cases. J Am Anim Hosp Assoc 1990;26:39–46.
79. Hall DJ, Shofer F, Meier CK, et al. Pericardial effusion in cats: a retrospective study of clinical findings and outcome in 146 cats. J Vet Intern Med 2007,21:1002–7
80. Davidson BJ, Paling AC, Lahmers SL, et al. Disease association and clinical assessment of feline pericardial effusion. J Am Anim Hosp Assoc 2008;44:5–9.
81. Schrope DP, Kelch WJ. Signalment, clinical signs, and prognostic indicators associated with high-grade second- or third-degree atrioventricular block in dogs: 124 cases (January 1, 1997–December 31 1997). J Am Vet Med Assoc 2006;228: 1710–7.
82. Oyama MA, Sisson DD, Lehmkuhl LB. Practices and outcome of artificial cardiac pacing in 154 dogs. J Vet Intern Med 2001;15:229–39.
83. Wess G, Thomas WP, Berger DM, et al. Applications, complications, and outcomes of pacemaker implantation in 105 dogs (1997–2002). J Vet Intern Med 2006;20:877–84.
84. Johansson BW. Prognostic aspects of complete heart block. Acta Med Scand Suppl 1966;451:33–50.
85. Moneva-Jordan A, Corcoran BM, French A, et al. Sick sinus syndrome in nine West Highland white terriers. Vet Rec 2001;148:142–7.
86. Cote E. Feline arrhythmias: an update. Vet Clin North Am Small Anim Pract 2010;40: 643–50.
87. Petersen ME, Keene BW, Ferguson DC, et al. Electrocardiographic findings in 45 cats with hyperthyroidism. J Am Vet Med Assoc 1982;180:273–8.
88. Cote E, Harpster NK, Laste NJ, et al. Atrial fibrillation in cats: 50 cases (1979-2002). J Am Vet Med Assoc 2004;225:256–60.

89. Kellum HB, Stepien RL. Third-degree atrioventricular block in 21 cats (1997-2004). J Vet Intern Med 2006;20:97–103.
90. MacDonald K. Myocardial disease: feline. In: Ettinger S, Feldmen E, editors. Textbook of veterinary internal medicine. Diseases of dogs and cats. 7th edition. St Louis (MO): Saunders Elsevier; 2010. p. 1328–41.
91. O'Grady MR, Minors SL, O'Sullivan ML, et al. Effect of pimobendan on case fatality rate in Doberman Pinschers with congestive heart failure caused by dilated cardiomyopathy. J Vet Intern Med 2008;22:897–904.
92. Haggstrom J, Boswood A, O'Grady M, et al. Effect of pimobendan or benazepril hydrochloride on survival times in dogs with congestive heart failure caused by naturally occurring myxomatous mitral valve disease: the QUEST Study. J Vet Intern Med 2008;22:1124–35.
93. Borgarelli M, Santilli RA, Chiavegato D, et al. Prognostic indicators for dogs with dilated cardiomyopathy. J Vet Intern Med 2006;20:104–10.
94. Calvert CA, Pickus CW, Jacobs GJ, et al. Signalment, survival, and prognostic factors in Doberman pinschers with end-stage cardiomyopathy. J Vet Intern Med 1997;11:323–6.

Chronic Kidney Disease in Dogs and Cats

Joseph W. Bartges, DVM, PhD

KEYWORDS

- Chronic kidney disease • Geriatric • Nutrition • Treatment
- International Renal Interest Society

KEY POINTS

- Chronic kidney disease occurs commonly in dogs and cats.
- Chronic kidney disease is progressive; however, management utilizing dietary modification and pharmacologic agents may improve quality of life and survival.
- Management of dogs and cats with chronic kidney disease is directed at minimizing the excesses and deficiencies that occur.
- Specifically, management is directed at providing nutritional support, treating hypokalemia and metabolic acidosis, decreasing the degree of proteinuria, maintaining hydration, decreasing retention of wastes such as nitrogen containing compounds, avoiding other renal insults, improving anemia, minimizing renal secondary hyperparathyroidism and hyperphosphatemia, and decreasing blood pressure if systemic arterial hypertension is present.
- Serial monitoring of dogs and cats with chronic kidney disease is essential because of the progressive nature of the disease.

Chronic kidney disease (CKD) occurs commonly in older dogs and cats and is the most common renal disease occurring in elderly patients. It is defined as structural and/or functional impairment of one or both kidneys that has been present for more than approximately 3 months. In most patients, there is loss of function and structure with CKD; however, degree of functional impairment does not always mirror loss of structure. CKD implies irreversible loss of renal function and/or structure that remains stable for some period of time but is ultimately progressive. In some patients, CKD may be complicated by concurrent prerenal and/or postrenal problems that may worsen the condition, but if managed, they may improve the situation.

CKD is considered a disease of older animals, although it occurs at all ages. The estimated incidence of CKD in the general population of dogs and cats is 0.5% to

The author has nothing to disclose.
Department of Small Animal Clinical Sciences, College of Veterinary Medicine, The University of Tennessee, 2407 River Drive, Knoxville, TN 37996-4544, USA
E-mail address: jbartges@utk.edu

Vet Clin Small Anim 42 (2012) 669–692
http://dx.doi.org/10.1016/j.cvsm.2012.04.008
0195-5616/12/$ – see front matter
vetsmall.theclinics.com

1.5%.[1] At the University of Minnesota Veterinary Medical Center, more than 10% of dogs and 30% of cats over 15 years of age are diagnosed with CKD.[1] One retrospective study reported that 53% of cats with CKD were over 7 years old, but animals ranged in age from 9 months to 22 years.[2] In a study on age distribution of kidney disease in cats based on data submitted from 1980 to 1990 to the Veterinary Medical Data Base at Purdue University, 37% of cats with the diagnosis of "renal failure" were less than 10 years old, 31% of cats were between the ages of 10 and 15, and 32% of cats were older than 15 years.[3] Similarly, in a study of cats with CKD reported in 1988, the mean age was 12.6 years with a range of 1 to 26 years.[4] Mean age among 45 control cats in this study was 10.0 years. During 1990, the prevalence of kidney disease was reportedly 16 cases for every 1000 cats of all ages, 77 cases per 1000 cats over age 10 years, and 153 per 1000 among cats older than 15 years.[2] Maine coon, Abyssinian, Siamese, Russian blue, and Burmese cats were disproportionately reported as affected.

The kidneys are involved with whole body homeostasis; therefore, CKD affects many organ systems, is associated with many metabolic derangements, and affects general well-being. Glomerular filtration results in formation of urine in Bowman's space except for cells and protein-bound compounds; a small amount of albumin is filtered. Bulk reabsorption of the filtrate occurs in the proximal tubule with additional secretion or reabsorption of anionic and cationic compounds. The loop of Henle concentrates then dilutes the filtrate through selective reabsorption of water and sodium. The distal convoluted tubule and collecting ducts fine-tune the solute and moisture content of urine. In addition to these processes, the kidneys are intimately involved in metabolic regulation of acid-base status, have endocrine function (eg, erythropoietin and vitamin D), and have a role in blood pressure regulation (eg, renin production and adrenal secretion of aldosterone). Therefore, when renal function declines there is disruption of these normal processes resulting in retention of compounds that should be excreted (eg, phosphorous and creatinine) and loss of compounds that should be retained (eg, water and protein).

CLINICAL, BIOCHEMICAL, AND IMAGING FINDINGS WITH CKD

It is the retention or loss of compounds that results in clinical manifestations of CKD. Many, but not all, patients show clinical signs of chronic disease such as loss of body condition, BW, and muscle mass, and an unkempt appearance. Polyuria and polydipsia occur because of an inability of the kidneys to regulate water balance. Hyporexia/anorexia, vomiting, halitosis, and ulcerative stomatitis and gastroenteritis may be present (**Fig. 1**). With CKD, the kidneys often palpate small and irregular, and this is confirmed with abdominal radiography and ultrasonography. Occasionally, renomegaly is present with CKD when there is renal neoplasia, pyelonephritis, or ureteral obstruction present. Biochemically, azotemia with inappropriately dilute urine (urine specific gravity <1.030 in dogs and <1.035 in cats), metabolic acidosis, and hyperphosphatemia are present. Additionally, some patients may have hypokalemia (seen more commonly in cats than in dogs), nonregenerative anemia, hypoalbuminemia, dyslipidemia, and bacterial urinary tract infection. Arterial systemic hypertension occurs in 40% to 80% of patients.[1] Proteinuria may also occur and has been associated with a poorer prognosis and more rapid progression of CKD than in patients without proteinuria.[5,6]

TREATMENT OF CKD

Treatment of CKD is directed at correcting these imbalances and in slowing down progression; it is lifelong because CKD is irreversible. Additionally, treatment is

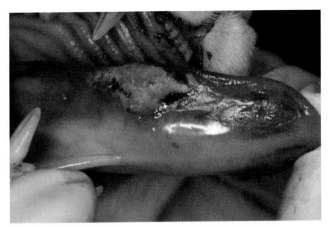

Fig. 1. Uremic stomatitis and glossitis in a 20-year-old, spayed female domestic shorthair cat with chronic kidney disease.

directed at ameliorating clinical signs of CKD and at correcting or controlling nonrenal disease that may affect a patient with CKD. We developed an acronym to assist in treating CKD based on excesses and deficiencies that occur: NEPHRONS.

N	nutrition
E	electrolytes
P	pH of blood (acid-base status); proteinuria
H	hydration
R	retention of wastes
O	other renal insults – avoid
N	neuroendocrine function – hyperparathyroidism, hypoproliferative anemia, and hypertension
S	serial monitoring – CKD is irreversible and progressive

Key Therapeutic Points

The kidneys are involved with homeostasis through filtration, reabsorption, secretion, and metabolism of compounds. A conservative medical treatment of CKD consists of supportive and symptomatic treatment designed to correct excesses and deficiencies that occur (NEPHRONS). Guidelines for managing dogs and cats with CKD have been established by the International Renal Insufficiency Society (http://www.IRIS-kidney.com). This staging system is designed for use with dogs and cats with CKD (**Table 1**).[7]

A diagnosis of CKD is made first and staging is accomplished by evaluating (1) 2 serum creatinine concentrations when patient is well hydrated, (2) 2 or 3 urine protein–to–urine creatinine ratios (UPCs), and (3) 2 to 3 indirect arterial blood pressure determinations.[1] CKD is staged by magnitude of renal dysfunction and further modified (substaged) by presence or absence of proteinuria and/or hypertension. Proteinuria ONLY refers to renal proteinuria and not prerenal (eg, hyperglobulinemia) or postrenal (eg, urinary tract infection, hematuria, etc), and is based on UPC.[8] Blood pressure determination should be performed several times with an nonsedated and calm patient that has acclimated to a quiet area using a standard protocol.[9]

Table 1
International Renal Interest Society (IRIS) System
Stage of CKD based on serum or plasma creatinine concentration

Stage	Plasma Ccreatinine, μmol/L, mg/dL Dogs	Cats	Comments
1	<125 <1.4	<140 <1.6	Nonazotemic Some other renal abnormality present such as inadequate concentrating ability without identifiable nonrenal cause; abnormal renal palpation and/or abnormal renal imaging findings; proteinuria of renal origin; abnormal renal biopsy results
2	125–179 1.4–2.0	140–249 1.6–2.8	Mild renal azotemia [lower end of the range lies within the reference range for many labs but the insensitivity of creatinine as a screening test means that animals with creatinine values close to the upper limit of normality often have excretory failure] Clinical signs usually mild or absent
3	180–439 2.1–5.0	250–439 2.9–5.0	Moderate renal azotemia Many systemic clinical signs may be present
4	>440 >5.0	>440 >5.0	Severe renal azotemia Many extrarenal clinical signs present

Substage of CKD based on presence or absence of proteinuria determined by a UPC

UPC Value

Dogs	Cats	Substage
<0.2	<0.2	Nonproteinuric
0.2–0.5	0.2–0.4	Borderline proteinuric
>0.5	>0.4	Proteinuric

Substage of CKD based on presence or absence of systemic arterial hypertension and risk of systemic arterial hypertension-related complications

Systolic Blood Pressure, mm Hg	Diastolic Blood Pressure, mm Hg	Adaptation When Breed-Specific Reference Range Is Available*	Substage
<150	<95	<10 mm Hg above reference range	AP0: Minimal Risk (N)
150–159	95–99	10–20 mm Hg above reference range	AP1: Low Risk (L)
160–179	100–119	20–40 mm Hg above reference range	AP2: Moderate Risk (M)
>180	>120	>40 mm Hg above reference range	AP3: High Risk (H)

Courtesy of Novartis Animal Health, Inc, Basel, Switzerland, sponsor of the International Renal Interest Society (IRIS), with permission.

Table 2
Body condition scoring systems

Descriptor	Description	5 point	9 point
CACHECTIC	Ribs are easily palpated with no fat cover; bony structures are prominent and easy to identify; muscle tone and mass often decreased; little to no subcutaneous fat; hair coat often poor; pronounced abdominal tuck	1	1
UNDERWEIGHT	Ribs are easily palpated with little fat cover; abdominal tuck present; bony structures are palpable but not prominent; hair coat may be poor; muscle tone and mass may be good or slightly decreased	2	3
IDEAL	Ribs are easily palpated, but fat cover is present; hourglass shape present and abdominal tuck is present, but not pronounced; bony prominences are palpable but not visible some subcutaneous fat, but no large accumulations; muscle tone and mass good; hair coat quality is good	3	5
OVERWEIGHT	Ribs are difficult to palpate due to overlying fat accumulation; hourglass shape is not prominent and abdominal tuck is absent; subcutaneous fat obvious with some areas of accumulation; muscle tone and mass good; hair coat quality may be decreased; cannot identify bony prominences	4	7
OBESE	Ribs are impossible to palpate due to overlying fat; hourglass shape is absent and animal may have a round appearance; subcutaneous fat is obvious and accumulations are present in the neck, tail-base, and abdominal regions; muscle tone and mass may be decreased; hair coat quality may be decreased	5	9

N Nutrition

The main goal of nutritional support of any patient with a chronic disease is maintenance of lean muscle mass and optimal body condition, and this is true of patients with CKD. A thorough physical examination is performed and a body condition score (BCS) and muscle condition score (MCS) are assigned.[10] There are 5- and 9-point BCS systems; either can be used.[11–13] Assigning a BCS (**Table 2**) provides more information than BW alone and estimates body fat content. The goal for most pets is a BCS of 2.5 to 3 of 5 or 4 to 5 of 9.

An MCS may also be assigned and is an assessment of muscle mass and tone.[10] Evaluation of muscle mass includes visual examination and palpation of muscles over temporal bones, scapulae, lumbar vertebrae, and pelvic bones. Muscle condition is an assessment of lean mass and loss of muscle mass may adversely affect strength, immune function, wound healing, and ability to compensate for chronic conditions such as CKD. A simple MCS has been suggested using a 0-to-3 scale where 0 = normal muscle mass and tone, 1 = slightly decreased muscle mass and tone,

Table 3
Activity and life stage factors used to estimate MERs after RERs are estimated

Life Stage	Canine Factor	Feline Factor
Gestation	1.0–3.0	1.6–2.0
Dogs: first ½–⅔	1.0–2.0	
Dogs: last ⅓	2.0–3.0	
Lactation	2.0–8.0	1.0–2.0
Growth	2.0–3.0	2.0–5.0
Adult intact	1.8	1.4
Adult neutered	1.6	1.2
Senior	1.4	1.1
Work: light	2.0	
Work: moderate	3.0	
Work: heavy	4.0–8.0	
Obese prone	1.4	1.0
Weight loss	1.0	0.8
Weight gain	1.2–1.4 ideal	0.8–1.0 ideal
Critical care (usually)	1.0	1.0

2 = moderately decreased muscle mass and tone, and 3 = markedly decreased muscle mass and tone.[14]

Daily caloric requirements are determined by estimating resting energy requirement (RER) using 1 of 2 equations[15]:

$$\text{Exponential}: 70\ BW_{kg}^{0.75}$$
$$\text{Linear}: 30(BW_{kg}) + 70$$

The exponential equation is more accurate because energy requirements relate to body weight (BW) in a parabolic fashion rather than a linear one. Once the RER is estimated, the result is multiplied by an activity or life stage factor (**Table 3**) to estimate the maintenance energy requirement (MER).[15] These equations give only estimates of daily energy requirements and energy intake should be adjusted based on response to estimated energy requirements and through serial monitoring of BW, BCS, and MCS.

Patients with CKD may exhibit some degree of anorexia depending on stage of CKD. Causes of anorexia and nausea include retention of uremic toxins, dehydration, biochemical alterations (azotemia, metabolic acidosis, electrolyte imbalances, and mineral imbalances), anemia, renal secondary hyperparathyroidism, and uremic gastroenteritis.[16] Gastric ulcers occur less commonly in dogs and cats than in human beings; however, many dogs and cats with CKD have gastric pathology including vascular changes and edema[17] and probable gastric hyperacidity associated with hypergastrinemia from decreased renal excretion.

Feed a highly palatable diet or increase the palatability of diet by adding water to dog food, using flavoring agents, and warming food to near body temperature.[18] Consuming diets that are more calorically dense than maintenance adult foods promotes adequate energy intake with less volume intake resulting in less gastric distention and nausea. Because dietary fat is more calorically dense than dietary protein and carbohydrates, diets formulated for patients with CKD are typically higher in fat compared with maintenance adult foods. Available diets contain 12% to 30% crude fat (dry matter basis).

Nausea and anorexia associated with chronic renal failure may also occur because of hypergastrinemia and gastric hyperacidity.[17] Dietary protein stimulates gastric acid secretion; therefore, dietary protein restriction may decrease gastric hyperacidity. Administration of histamine$_2$-receptor antagonists (famotidine: dogs and cats, 1.1 mg/kg po q 12–24 hours; ranitidine: dogs and cats, 1–2 mg/kg po q 8–12 hours)[19] or other antacids are beneficial in dogs and cats with CKD; many phosphate binders also bind gastric acid and act as antacids. Sucralfate (dogs, 0.5–2.0 g po q 6–12 hours; cats, 0.25–0.5 g po q 6–12 hours)[19] is an aluminum-containing compound that binds to exposed submucosal collagen in an acidic environment and may have cytoprotectant effects via prostaglandin E$_2$. It is used to treat active gastric ulcers, but may also act as an antacid and phosphate binder. Maropitant (dogs and cats: 2–8 mg/kg po q24h; although not recommended for more than 5 days)[19] is an anti-emetic that inhibits neurokinin-1; it is used for motion sickness but is effective with many other causes of vomiting including uremic gastroenteritis. Mirtazapine (dogs, 15–30 mg po q 24 hours; cats, 1.875–3.75 mg po q 48–72 hours)[19] is a noradrenergic and serotonergic antidepressant that stimulates appetite and has antiemetic properties. In cats with CKD, it should be administered every 48 hours.[20] Metoclopramide (dogs and cats, 0.1–0.5 mg/kg po q 6–24 hours),[19] an intestinal prokinetic agent that has central antiemetic effects via dopamine receptor antagonism, may also be used although it is less effective than serotonin receptor antagonists in uremic human beings.[21]

In patients that are unwilling or unable to eat, nutrition may be provided by feeding tubes including nasogastric, esophagostomy, and gastrostomy feeding tubes.[22–26] A study of 56 dogs with renal failure were managed with gastrostomy feeding tubes; 10 were low profile and 46 were standard mushroom-tipped tubes.[27] Gastrostomy tubes were used for 65 ± 91 days (range, 1–438 days). Eight dogs gained weight, 11 did not have a change in BW, and 17 lost weight; information was not available for 20 dogs. Mild stoma-site complications included discharge, swelling, erythema, and pain in 26 (46%) of dogs. Twenty-six gastrostomy tubes were replaced in 15 dogs; 11 were replaced because of patient removal, 6 were replaced because of tube wear, and 3 were replaced for other reasons. Three dogs were euthanatized because they removed their gastrostomy tubes, 2 were euthanatized because of evidence of tube migration, and 1 died of peritonitis. Based on this report, gastrostomy tubes appear to be safe and effective for improving nutritional status of dogs with renal failure. In another report, 96% of owners of dogs or cats managed with gastrostomy feeding tubes had a positive experience and would use a gastrostomy feeding tube again in their pet if necessary.[28]

In addition to providing calories (energy), there are specific nutrients that may alter progression of CKD in dogs and cats. With a decrease in numbers of functioning nephrons, pressure inside remaining nephrons increased; this is termed intraglomerular hypertension.[29,30] The intraglomerular hypertension increases the filtration rate in the remaining nephrons. The tradeoff of intraglomerular hypertension is damage to these nephrons over time. In dogs with induced CKD, feeding diets containing omega-3 fatty acids has been shown to decrease intraglomerular hypertension, maintain glomerular filtration rate, and increase survival.[31–34] In dogs fed omega-3 long chain fatty acids, renal function actually increased and remained above baseline over 20 months of the study. Glomerulosclerosis, tubulointerstitial fibrosis, and interstitial inflammatory cell infiltrates were less in dogs fed an omega-3 fatty acid–supplemented diet compared with dogs fed an omega-6 fatty acid–supplemented diet.[32] Omega-3 fatty acids reduce hypercholesterolemia, suppress inflammation and coagulation, lower blood pressure, and improve renal hemodynamics. An omega-6–to–omega-3 fatty acid ratio of 3:1 to 5:1 appears to be beneficial and is present in many renal failure diets.

B vitamins are water-soluble vitamins and may be decreased with CKD due to the polyuric state. B vitamin deficiency may be associated, in part, with hyporexia/anorexia, which occurs commonly with CKD. A recent study showed that B vitamin deficiency is not common in patients with CKD.[35] Nonetheless, diets formulated for CKD in dogs and cats are supplemented with B vitamins.

Oxidative stress may be an important component of CKD. Renal cells, particularly renal tubular cells, are among the most metabolically active cells. The kidneys maintain persistently high levels of mitochondrial oxidative phosphorylation and arterial blood flow, making them an environment in which reactive oxygen species formation occurs.[36] Important factors in generation of reactive oxygen species include angiotensin II, glomerular hypertension, hyperfiltration, tubular hypermetabolism, systemic arterial hypertension, anemia, regional hypoxia, and renal inflammation.[37,38] The result of reactive oxygen species formation may be glomerulosclerosis and interstitial fibrosis, thereby promoting progression of CKD. Renal oxidative stress may be decreased by treating systemic arterial hypertension, correcting anemia, providing omega-3 fatty acids, and treating with angiotensin-converting enzyme inhibitors.[37] In a study of cats with induced CKD, feeding a diet with vitamins C and E and beta-carotene for 4 weeks decreased evidence of oxidative stress as measured by serum levels of 8-hydroxy-2′-deoxyguanasine and comet assay parameters.[38]

Supplementation with omega-3 fatty acids and antioxidants has not been adequately evaluated in cats. A retrospective study on the effects of several renal diets did find that survival was greatest among cats fed the diet with the highest omega-3 fatty acid content.[39] The study, however, was retrospective and it is not possible to accurately assess effects of dietary omega-3 fatty acids from these data.

Recently, an extract of medicinal rhubarb (Rheum officinale) has become available for dogs and cats with CKD. Experimentally, it decreases renal fibrosis in an induced CKD model in rats.[40,41] One study of cats with CKD showed no benefit when administered alone or in combination with benazepril.[42]

E Electrolytes

The kidneys are involved with regulation of electrolyte balance. Electrolytes are filtered at the glomerulus, most of the filtered electrolytes are reabsorbed in the proximal convoluted tubule, and the remainder of the nephron reabsorbs or secretes electrolytes depending on status. A common electrolyte disturbance in cats and occasionally in dogs with CKD is hypokalemia,[43,44] which has been reported to occur in 20% to 30% of cats with stage 2 or 3 CKD.[2,4] Hypokalemia may occur because of hyporexia or anorexia, excessive renal losses, transcellular shift due to chronic metabolic acidosis, and activation of the renin-angiotensin-aldosterone system due to dietary sodium restriction.[45,46] Hypokalemia often manifests as polymyopathy. Clinical signs include decreased activity and muscle weakness or classically as an inability for the patient to lift its head while sitting sternally (**Fig. 2**). Additionally, hypokalemia may result in hyporexia or anorexia and progression of CKD.[2] The target for plasma or serum potassium concentration should be in the middle to upper half of reference range for the laboratory. Once hypokalemia is present, whole body potassium content is low and it is difficult to replete in patients with CKD.[47]

Diets formulated for use in patients with CKD are supplemented with potassium, typically using potassium citrate as it is a source of potassium and an alkalinizing

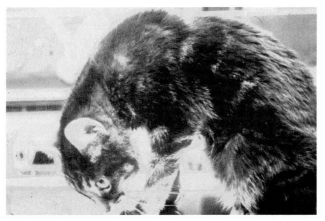

Fig. 2. Hypokalemic polymyopathy in an 18-year-old, castrated male domestic shorthair cat with chronic kidney disease. Serum potassium concentration was 1.8 mEq/L.

agent. This is based, in part, on diets low in potassium and high in acid content being implicated in impairing renal function and promoting development of lymphoplasma-cytic tubulointerstitial lesions in cats.[47–51] Potassium may be supplemented orally using potassium gluconate or potassium citrate. If patients are receiving subcutane-ously administered fluids, potassium may be added to the fluids up to 30 mEq/L as potassium chloride.[7] Irritation at injection site may occur with concentrations above this. Potassium chloride may also be added to fluids administered intravenously depending on blood potassium concentration (**Table 4**). Rate of administration should not exceed 0.5 mEq/kg/h because cardiotoxicity may occur. Potassium may be supplemented orally as well as gluconate or citrate salts; potassium citrate is used more often as it provides alkalization as well. Potassium gluconate (dogs and cats, 2 mEq/kg po q 12 hours)[19] or potassium citrate (dogs and cats, 75 mg/kg po q 12 hours)[19] may be administered; dosage is adjusted to achieve a serum or plasma potassium concentration in the middle to upper half of the reference range. If hypokalemic polymyopathy is present, it usually resolves within 1 to 5 days after initiating parenteral or oral potassium supplementation. Typical commercial modified diets for CKD in dogs and cats contain 0.4% to 0.8% potassium on a dry matter basis for dogs and 0.7% to 1.2% potassium on a dry matter basis for cats.[52]

Table 4
Suggested guidelines for intravenous potassium supplementation

Serum Potassium (mEq/L)	Amount of Potassium to Add to Lactated Ringer's Solution (mEq/L)	Maximum Fluid Rate (mL/kg/h)
<2.0	80	6
2.1–2.5	60	8
2.6–3.0	40	12
3.1–3.5	28	18
3.6–5.0	20	25

Blood sodium concentrations are typically normal in patients with CKD. Sodium retention may occur with CKD because of intravascular volume contraction. This may promote systemic arterial hypertension, in part; therefore, dietary sodium restriction may be beneficial in patients with CKD. Furthermore, there is evidence that excessive sodium intake may be harmful to the kidneys and excessive salt intake may impair effectiveness of antihypertensive therapy.[53] Excessive dietary sodium restriction may be detrimental, however. In one study of experimentally induced CKD in cats, dietary sodium restriction to 50 mg sodium/kg of diet promoted hypokalemia due to activation of the renin-angiotensin-aldosterone system.[46] Additionally, in one study, dietary intake of sodium at 1.1% as fed was associated with increased azotemia in cats with CKD[54]; however, other studies did not find this.[55] Typical commercial modified diets for CKD in dogs and cats contain 0.3% sodium or less on a dry matter basis for dogs and 0.4% sodium or less on a dry matter basis for cats.[52]

P pH of Blood (Acid-Base Status)

Metabolic acidosis occurs commonly with CKD due to retention of acids that are excreted normally by the kidneys. It has been reported that metabolic acidosis occurs in less than 10% of cats with stage 2 or 3 CKD but in nearly 50% of cats with uremia.[56,57] With CKD, there is increased retention of metabolic acids, increased production of ammonia, and decreased bicarbonate reclamation with CKD. Metabolic acidosis is associated with hyporexia/anorexia, hypokalemia, and muscle weakness, Bicarbonate therapy in human beings with CKD has been reported to slow progression and improve nutritional status.[58] Transcellular shifting of potassium occurs with metabolic acidosis because the increased hydrogen ion concentration in blood results in movement of hydrogen ions into cells in exchange for potassium ions that leave the cell and enter the circulation. Potassium is then excreted resulting, in part, a propensity for hypokalemia. Acid-base status may be assessed by measuring blood pH and bicarbonate concentration on an arterial or venous blood gas analysis. Measurement of plasma or serum bicarbonate, also called total carbon dioxide, gives a measure of acid-base status. The goal of treatment is to maintain a normal concentration; in human beings with stage 3 or 4 CKD, a low or high serum bicarbonate concentration is associated with increased mortality.[59] There are several treatments for metabolic acidosis. Many renal failure diets are formulated to contain an alkalinizing agent usually potassium citrate, which is also a source of potassium. Because metabolism of dietary protein results in production of organic acids, dietary protein restriction decreases amount of organic acid that must be excreted by kidneys. Supplemental alkalinizing agents may be administered including potassium citrate or sodium bicarbonate. Potassium citrate (dogs and cats, 75 mg/kg po q 12 hours initially)[19] is preferred because it provides potassium in addition to its alkalinizing properties. Sodium bicarbonate (dogs and cats, 8–12 mg/kg po q 8–12 hours)[19] administration provides alkalization but may worsen systemic arterial hypertension and fluid retention due to the sodium load.

P Proteinuria

Proteinuria occurring in association with CKD in dogs and cats is associated with progression.[5,6,60] Proteinuria is considered a hallmark of glomerular disease; however, proteinuria appears to be nephrotoxic even without overt primary glomerular disease.[61] In humans with CKD, reducing proteinuria slows progression; however, no such evidence exists for dogs and cats with CKD.[62–65] Proteinuria may promote progressive renal injury by several mechanisms including mesangial toxicity, tubular overload and hyperplasia, toxicity from specific filtered proteins (eg, transferrin), and induction of proinflammatory molecules (eg, monocyte chemoattractant protein-1). Excessive proteinuria may injure renal tubules via toxic or receptor-mediated pathways or an overload of lysosomal degradative mechanisms. The abnormally excessive filtered proteins accumulate in proximal tubular lumens, are endocytosed into proximal tubular cells, and contribute to tubulointerstitial injury through upregulation of vasoactive and inflammatory genes and by secretion into peritubular tissue where they incite inflammation.[66] Additionally, components of complements may enter filtrate and initiate interstitial injury, and filtered proteins may form casts obstructing tubular flow.

Proteinuria is often detected by a positive semiquantitative test on routine urine dipsticks. It is further localized to pre-renal, renal, or postrenal causes. The most common causes of proteinuria are postrenal including urinary tract infection or inflammation (exudation of plasma proteins into the urine) and hematuria (loss of plasma proteins with red blood cells). Prerenal causes of proteinuria include hemolysis (hemoglobinuria) and hyperglobulinemia (eg, plasma cell myeloma). Proteinuria is localized to renal causes after prerenal and postrenal causes have been ruled out. Renal proteinuria is often considered glomerular in nature; however, tubular disorders (eg, Fanconi syndrome) and interstitial disorders result in proteinuria as well albeit to a lesser degree. Once prerenal and postrenal causes have been excluded, verification and quantitation of renal proteinuria are made by determining a UPC. Healthy dogs and cats have a UPC less than 0.2; between 0.2 and 0.4 in cats and 0.5 in dogs is borderline proteinuria, and greater than 0.4 in cats and 0.5 in dogs is abnormal. In dogs and cats with CKD, treatment is indicated when the UPC is greater than 2.0 in stage 1 CKD and when the UPC is greater than 0.4 in cats and greater than 0.5 in dogs in stages 2 through 4 CKD.[8] In humans with CKD, reducing proteinuria slows progression; however, no such evidence exists for dogs and cats with CKD.[62-65]

Treatment of renal proteinuria involves decreasing filtration and loss of proteins, principally albumin. Feeding a protein-restricted diet decreases the degree of renal proteinuria.[8,67] Angiotensin-converting enzyme inhibitors (enalapril and benazepril: dogs and cats, 0.25–0.1.0 mg/kg po q 12–24 hours)[19] have also been shown to decrease proteinuria in dogs and cats.[62-64] Benazepril has been advocated over enalapril because benazepril's biliary excretion may compensate for reduced renal clearance in patients with CKD. Serum/plasma creatinine concentration should be evaluated approximately 7 days after initiating therapy with angiotensin-converting enzyme inhibitors. An increase of greater than 0.2 mg/dL indicates a decrease in glomerular filtration rate secondary to therapy and the dosage should be adjusted. Omega-3 fatty acids, specifically eicosapentaenoic acid (EPA) and docosahexaenoic acid (DHA), are also beneficial with renal proteinuria.[31-34] An omega-6–to–omega-3 fatty acid ratio of 3:1 to 5:1 appears to be beneficial and is present in many renal failure diets. Omega-3 fatty acids may also be supplemented to dogs and cats, if necessary (300 mg of EPA + DHA per 10–22 kg po q 24 hours). Immunosuppressive therapy may be considered for dogs with primary glomerular proteinuria as approximately 50% of evaluated renal biopsies from dogs with glomerular proteinuria have an immune-mediated basis.

H Hydration

Patients with CKD are polyuric due to decreased ability to concentrate urine from decreased nephron mass. Polyuria is offset by polydipsia. Because of polyuria, dehydration may occur if water loss exceeds water intake. This occurs more often in cats than in dogs with CKD. In patients that are dehydrated, parenteral fluid is administered.[68] Intravenous administration is preferred over other parenteral routes.

Intravenous fluid therapy is composed of 3 components: amount necessary for rehydration, maintenance fluid requirements, and amount to treat additional losses (eg, vomitus, diarrhea, etc).

- Amount needed for rehydration in milliliters is estimated by multiplying estimated percentage of dehydration by BW in kilograms and multiplying the resultant product by 1000.
- Maintenance fluid requirements are estimated to be 2.2 mL/BW$_{kg}$/h
- Amount necessary to replace fluid lost by other routes can be measured or estimated to be 1.1 mL/BW$_{kg}$/h.

Dehydration may be prevented by increasing oral water intake by having clean and fresh water available at all times, by feeding canned formulated diets, or by adding water to dry formulated diets. Cats may drink more if circulating water fountains are used. In some patients, particularly cats, supplemental fluid may be provided by subcutaneous route as they are unable to maintain hydration by oral intake. Subcutaneously administered fluids are administered using a syringe or bag of fluids with an extension set and a 20- or 22-gauge needle. The easiest site to administer fluids subcutaneously is to insert the hypodermic needle in the loose skin located along the dorsal aspect of the body between the scapulae. Cats that require supplemental subcutaneously administered fluids often require 75 to 150 mL administered every 12 to 72 hours. Lactated Ringer's solution is used most often; however, other types of fluids may be used. Potassium as potassium chloride may be added to fluids administered subcutaneously up to a concentration of 20 mEq/L; above this concentration, administration of the fluid results in discomfort. Some patients do not tolerate subcutaneously administered fluids. Feeding tubes, such as nasogastric or more preferred esophagostomy or gastrostomy, may be placed and used. Esophagostomy and gastrostomy feeding tubes include may also be used for diet delivery and medication administration if the oral route is unavailable.

R Retention of Substances

With CKD, substances that are eliminated normally in urine are retained. These substances include nitrogenous compounds (blood urea nitrogen and creatinine) among others. Elimination of nitrogenous compounds is a major function of the kidneys and retained nitrogenous compounds are associated with clinical signs of CKD. Azotemia is a hallmark of CKD. Thus, restriction of dietary protein is logical. Results of studies are contradictory concerning the influence of dietary protein restriction on progression of CKD.[69–72] Restricting dietary protein may be associated with a decreased degree of azotemia, decreased dietary phosphorous as meat-based protein is also high in phosphorous, decreased metabolic acids generated from dietary protein, and decreased stimulus for gastric hydrochloric acid production and may reduce dosage of antihypertensive agents and decrease requirement for erythropoietin.[73] Modified diets for managing CKD in dogs and cats typically contain 14% to 20% protein on a dry matter basis for dogs and 28% to 35% protein on a dry matter basis for cats.[52]

There are 3 studies of dietary intervention in dogs and cats with spontaneously occurring CKD: 2 in cats and 1 in dogs.[74–77] In these studies, a diet formulated to contain lower quantities of protein, phosphorous, and sodium and higher quantities of potassium, B vitamins, calories, alkalization potential, and omega-3 fatty acids were compared with a diet that was formulated to be similar to maintenance over-the-counter adult dog or cat foods. Results of these studies showed benefit in dogs and cats with CKD: patients lived longer, had fewer episodes of uremia, time to onset of first uremic episode was longer, and owners perceived quality of life was better. Although diets formulated for renal failure are lower in protein than over-the-counter maintenance adult foods, they are still adequate and typically contain higher biologic value protein.

Prebiotics and probiotics have been suggested to redistribute a small amount of nitrogen into the gastrointestinal tract for elimination, thus decreasing the degree of azotemia. Prebiotics are dietary fiber, typically soluble fiber that promotes proliferation of beneficial bacteria in the colon that metabolizes nitrogen and urea intraluminal. The proliferation of bacteria also promotes uptake and utilization of intraluminal nitrogen by the bacteria resulting in less absorption from the colon. Probiotics are live, nonpathogenic bacteria that are presumed to populate the gastrointestinal tract, providing the same benefit. One such probiotic (Azodyl; Vetoquinol, Lure Cedex, France) is commercially available and marketed as "enteric dialysis." A small uncontrolled study showed decreased degree of azotemia; however, a controlled study evaluating administration of the probiotic with and without food failed to show a benefit.[78]

O Other Renal Insults—Avoid

Circumstances, drugs, toxins, and infections may compound CKD by inducing a prerenal azotemia (dehydration) or by affecting remaining nephrons. Dehydration due to any cause not only is associated with worsening azotemia (prerenal) but may also precipitate acute kidney injury resulting in progression of CKD. Patients in CKD are less tolerant of dehydration. Drugs, such as aminoglycosides, urinary acidifiers, amphotericin, nonsteroidal anti-inflammatory drugs, angiotensin-converting enzyme inhibitors, and catabolic drugs (eg, glucocorticoids and immunosuppressive drugs) may be nephrotoxic. These should be used cautiously or not at all in patients with CKD. Patients with CKD have a higher incidence of bacterial urinary tract infections, which has been reported to be 20%. There are several reasons for increased risk of bacterial urinary tract infections with CKD including dilute urine, premature apoptosis of white blood cells, decreased white blood cell recruitment and function, and decreased immunoglobulin concentration in urine. Clinical signs of bacterial urinary tract infection may be absent. If the infection ascends from the urinary bladder to the kidneys, it may promote progression of CKD. Prophylactic antimicrobial therapy should be avoided, if possible, as it may select for multidrug resistant microorganisms. Some antimicrobial agents (eg, aminoglycosides) may be nephrotoxic and many are excreted renally; therefore, pharmacokinetic parameters may be altered. Additionally, some antimicrobial agents may cause hyporexia/anorexia, vomiting, and/or diarrhea that can induce dehydration. Many active bacterial urinary tract infections in patients with CKD are not associated with pyuria or hematuria; therefore, aerobic microbial culture of urine collected by cystocentesis may be necessary to document an active bacterial urinary tract infection.

N Neuroendocrine Function

There are 3 abnormalities of neuroendocrine function that may occur with CKD: renal secondary hyperparathyroidism, hypoproliferative anemia, and systemic arterial hypertension.

Renal secondary hyperparathyroidism

Renal secondary hyperparathyroidism occurs commonly with CKD, and the more advanced the CKD, the more advanced is the renal secondary hyperparathyroidism.[76,79–84] In extreme cases, renal secondary hyperparathyroidism results in fibrous

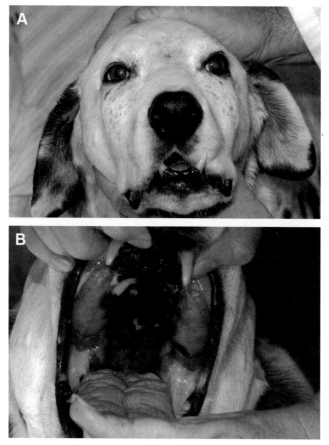

Fig. 3. Renal secondary hyperparathyroidism and fibrous osteodystrophy in an 8-year-old castrated male Dalmatian with CKD. (*A*) The maxilla and mandible are enlarged and the patient cannot close his mouth. (*B*) Excessive fibrous tissue replacing bone in the maxilla and mandible in the patient.

osteodystrophy, particularly of the mandible and maxilla; this occurs more commonly in dogs with congenital or juvenile-onset CKD but may occur in adult patients (**Fig. 3**). It occurs, in part, because of phosphorous retention and decreased calcitriol (1,25-dihydroxy vitamin D3) metabolism. Renal tubular cells contain 1α-hydroxylase, which is the enzyme that converts 25-hydroxyvitamin D to the active 1,25-dihydroxyvitamin D3. Calcitriol stimulates gastrointestinal absorption of calcium and phosphorous and inhibits parathyroid hormone production. Parathyroid hormone stimulates renal reabsorption of calcium and excretion of phosphorous, stimulates calcium and phosphorous release from bone, and stimulates calcitriol production. With CKD, there is decreased enzyme activation of calcitriol. In response to decreased calcitriol, parathyroid hormone production and secretion are increased. Parathyroid hormone may be considered a uremic toxin. With decreased glomerular filtration rate, hyperphosphatemia occurs, which may result in dystrophic mineralization and progression of CKD and further inhibits calcitriol production. Hyperphosphatemia is associated with progression of CKD and shortened survival.

Treatment of renal secondary hyperparathyroidism is aimed at decreasing serum phosphorous concentrations and possibly parathyroid hormone concentrations. The goal is to achieve a serum phosphorous concentration of less than 4.5 mg/dL with stage 2, less than 5.0 mg/dL with stage 3, and less than 6.0 mg/dL with stage 4. Serum phosphorous concentration may be decreased by feeding a low phosphorous diet, administering phosphate binders, and possibly administering calcitriol. Typical commercial modified diets for CKD in dogs and cats contain 0.2% to 0.5% phosphorous on a dry matter basis for dogs and 0.3% to 0.6% phosphorous on a dry matter basis for cats.[52]

There are several phosphate binders that may be used. Conventionally, aluminum hydroxide (dogs and cats, 30–100 mg/kg po q 24 hours divided and administered with meals)[19] has been used. Primary side effects are constipation and anorexia, although aluminum toxicity has been reported with very high dosage. Calcium-containing phosphate binders, such as calcium acetate (PhosLo; Nabi Biopharmaceuticals, Rockville, MD; dogs and cats, 60–90 mg/kg po q 24 hours divided and administered with meals)[19] and chitosan with calcium carbonate (Epakitin; Vetoquinol; dogs and cats: 200 mg/kg po mixed with meals)[19] may be used. The chitosan with calcium carbonate phosphate binder has been shown to decrease serum phosphorous concentrations in cats with spontaneously occurring CKD.[85] In addition to the aforementioned side effects, hypercalcemia may occur particularly if used in association with calcitriol. Non–calcium- and non–aluminum-containing phosphate binders include sevelamer hydrochloride (Renalgel; Genzyme, Cambridge, MA, USA; dogs and cats, 400–1600 mg po q 8–12 hours)[19] and lanthanum carbonate (Fosrenal; Shire, Wayne, PA, USA, and Renalzin; Bayer, Newbury, UK; dogs and cats, 30–90 mg/kg po divided and administered with meals).[19] Both of these appear to have minimal side effects in dogs and cats; however, they have not been evaluated in a controlled fashion.

Hypovitaminosis D occurs in dogs and cats with CKD, but not until an advanced stage (stages 3 and 4).[80] Benefits of calcitriol therapy in patients with CKD has been thought to be mediated by its effects on parathyroid hormone and mineral metabolism[86]; however, other beneficial renal effects have been recognized including suppression of activity of the renin-angiotensin-aldosterone system, systematic activation of vitamin D receptors, and reducing podocytes loss associated with glomerular hypertrophy.[87–90] Calcitriol supplementation (dogs and cats: initial dose of 2.0–2.5 ng/kg po q 24 hours, increase if parathyroid hormone concentrations do not normalize and decrease if hypercalcemia occurs; do not exceed 5 ng/kg po q 24 hours)[7,19] may help decrease serum phosphorous concentration and parathyroid hormone concentration. Because calcitriol enhances intestinal absorption of calcium and phosphorous, it should not be given with meals; administration in the evening on an empty stomach reduces the risk of hypercalcemia.[7] When calcitriol therapy is associated with hypercalcemia, the daily dose may be doubled and given every other day reducing calcitriol-induced intestinal absorption.[91] Calcitriol supplementation may increase appetite, activity, and quality of life.[86] To date, it has been shown to improve survival in dogs with stage 3 or 4 CKD, but not in stages 1 and 2, and it has not been shown to be beneficial in cats with any stage CKD.[1]

Hypoproliferative anemia. A normocytic, normochromic, nonregenerative anemia often occurs in patients with CKD. Causes of the anemia include decreased renal production of erythropoietin, nutritional imbalances because of hyporexia/anorexia, reduced red blood cell life span, and blood loss due to uremic gastroenteritis.[92,93] There is evidence that anemia may be associated with progression of CKD due to decreased blood flow and oxygen delivery, oxidative stress, and induction of fibrosis.[94,95] It has been shown that patients with CKD have increased survival if the hematocrit is above 35%. Treatment includes maintaining good nutritional status, minimizing gastrointestinal blood loss, and stimulating red blood cell production.

Patients with CKD may have blood loss due to uremic gastroenteritis. Hypergastrinemia occurs with CKD and gastrin stimulates hydrochloric acid production by gastric parietal cells resulting in gastric hyperacidity.[18,96] Histamine$_2$-receptor–blocking agents may be beneficial in decreasing gastric acid production, although they are not potent and the effect may be transient. Proton pump inhibitors (dogs and cats, omeprazole: 0.7–2.0 mg/kg po q 12–24 hours; esomeprazole: 0.7 mg/kg po q 12 hours)[19] decrease gastric acid secretion by inhibiting the potassium-hydrogen pump located in the cell membrane; they are the most potent antacids. Sucralfate is also an antacid that has phosphate binding properties and is used to treat active gastric ulcer disease.

Red blood cell production by bone marrow may be stimulated pharmacologically.[97] Anabolic steroids have been used to stimulate red blood cell production and to stimulate appetite. While they may stimulate appetite and increase lean muscle mass, they have minimal effect in promoting red blood cell production and may induce hepatopathy. In addition to anabolic steroids, other hormones may be supplemented including erythropoietin (dogs and cats, initial dose of 100 IU/kg subcutaneously 3 times per week and adjust based on hematocrit)[19] and darbepoetin, a longer-acting form of erythropoietin (induction phase: 1.5 μg/kg subcutaneously q 7 days and when desired target hematocrit is reached the dosage is decreased to q 14 days; frequency or amount of dosage is adjusted depending on response).[7,97–99] Studies with erythropoietin have shown that dogs and cats with CKD feel better even before hematocrit is increased. The main limitation of erythropoietin administration is development of antierythropoietin antibodies, which occurs in 20% to 70% of patients.[98,100] There have been no controlled studies with darbepoetin. Because of antibody production, it has been recommended to begin erythropoietin therapy when the hematocrit is less than 20% or in patients that do not feel well that are anemic but not to that degree. Darbepoetin may be started at a lesser degree of anemia because of the decreased risk of antibody production. Because uremic gastroenteritis is common, iron should be supplemented to offset the iron deficiency associated with blood loss (ferrous sulfate: dogs, 100–300 mg po q 24 hours; cats, 50–100 mg po q 24 hours; iron dextran: dogs, 10–20 mg IM q 3–4 weeks; cats, 50 mg intramuscularly q 3–4 weeks).[19] Additionally, infections should be treated to minimize iron sequestration that may result in decreased effectiveness of erythropoietin and darbepoetin administration. It is the author's opinion that a hematocrit of 35% to 40% is the goal. This is based on results of a study in cats with CKD where the median packed cell volume in the group with progressive disease was 32% (interquartile range of 29%–36%) compared with the group with nonprogressive disease where the median packed cell volume was 36% (interquartile range of 34%–41%).[101] Once the target is reached, the dosage can be slowly decreased to find the lowest amount necessary to control anemia. Complications of administration may include irritation at injection site, systemic arterial hypertension, and polycythemia.[97] In patients that initially respond but in whom the hematocrit begins to decline, suspect antibody production against the recombinant human erythropoietin. Additionally, ensure iron deficiency has not occurred, which would result in decreased red blood cell production.

Systemic arterial hypertension. Systemic arterial hypertension has been reported to occur in up to 65% to 75% of dogs and cats with CKD.[102] It occurs, in part, because of activation of the renin-angiotensin-aldosterone system, increased vasopressin (antidiuretic hormone) levels, and increased sympathetic tone. Indirect determination

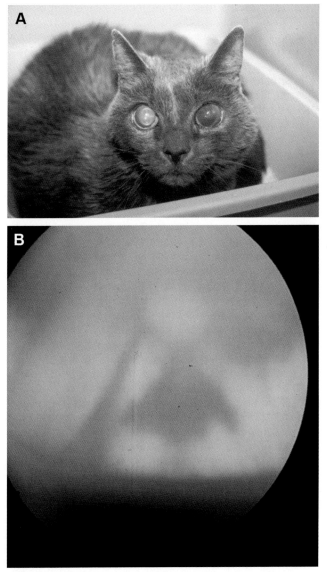

Fig. 4. Hypertensive retinopathy and blindness in a 14-year-old, spayed female domestic shorthair cat with CKD. (*A*) The right pupil is dilated due to retinal detachment and hyphema is present in the left eye. (*B*) Fundic examination of the right eye shows retinal detachment and retinal hemorrhage.

of systemic arterial blood pressure is indicated in all patients diagnosed with CKD and is used to substage CKD. Systemic arterial hypertension may promote progression of CKD and proteinuria; result in left ventricular hypertrophy and possibly left-sided heart failure; neurologic signs such as ischemic encephalopathy, seizures, and death; and ocular disease such as retinal vascular tortuosity and hemorrhage, hyphema, and blindness (**Fig. 4**). The risk is moderate to high with a systolic blood pressure greater than 160 mm Hg. Diagnosis is made by indirect measurement of systemic arterial blood pressure, although direct measurement can be performed by cannulation of the femoral artery. Arterial blood pressure can be determined indirectly using Doppler or oscillometric instruments. Doppler monitors use the Doppler effect to determine systolic blood pressure. Although mean and diastolic blood pressures may be determined using Doppler instruments, they are difficult and inaccurate. Oscillometric instruments measure systolic, mean, and diastolic blood pressures by detecting vibrations of the vascular wall. They are easy to use but require good technique. Indirect blood pressure is usually determined from the palmar, plantar, or coccygeal arteries.

Unless there is evidence of retinal lesions, neurologic signs, unexplained progression of CKD, or systolic blood pressure is greater than 180 mm Hg, the decision to begin antihypertensive therapy is not an emergency. Patients with CKD stages 2 to 4 having arterial systolic blood pressures persistently above 160 mm Hg (AP2; see **Table 1**) or patients with CKD stage 1 with arterial systolic blood pressures persistently exceeding 180 mm Hg (AP3; see **Table 1**) are candidates for treatment.[7] The goal of treatment is to achieve a systolic blood pressure less than 150 mm Hg. Dietary sodium restriction may aid in decreasing systemic arterial blood pressure and may potentiate effects of antihypertensive medications. Calcium channel blockers (amlodipine: dogs, 0.25–0.5 mg/kg po q 12–24 hours; cats, 0.625–1.25 mg po q 12–24 hours)[19] are the most effective antihypertensive drugs used in dogs and cats with CKD. They decrease systemic arterial blood pressure by inducing arterial vasodilation and on average decrease arterial systolic blood pressure by 50 mm Hg.[103] Additionally, they may help to decrease degree of proteinuria, but are not as effective as angiotensin-converting enzyme inhibitors for this. Amlodipine appears safe with few side effects. Angiotensin-converting enzyme inhibitors (enalapril: dogs and cats, 0.25–1.0 mg/kg po q 12–24 hours; benazepril: dogs and cats, 0.25–0.5 mg/kg po q 12–24 hours)[19] decrease enzymatic metabolism of angiotensin I to angiotensin II, resulting in vasodilation and decreased aldosterone production. They are more effective to decrease degree of proteinuria but on average reduce arterial systolic blood pressure by 10 mm Hg.[104] Administration of angiotensin-converting enzyme inhibitors may be associated with an increase in the degree of azotemia and potassium. Laboratory evaluation should be performed 7 to 10 days after initiation or adjustment of angiotensin-converting enzyme therapy. Angiotensin-converting enzyme inhibitors have not been shown to slow down progression of CKD in cats except in patients with UPC greater than 1.0. Calcium channel blockers and angiotensin-converting enzyme inhibitors may be used together. Other treatments for systemic arterial hypertension that may be used include angiotensin receptor blockers (ARBs; irbesartan: dogs, 5 mg/kg PO q 12–24 hours; or losartan: dogs: 1–5 mg/kg PO q 12–24 hours),[19] beta-blockers (atenolol: dogs, 0.25–1.0 mg/kg po q 12–24 hours; cats, 0.5–3.0 mg/kg po q 12–24 hours),[19] alpha-blockers (prazosin: dogs, 1 mg/15 kg po q 12–24 hours; cats: 0.25–0.5 mg po q 12–24 hours),[19] direct arteriolar vasodilators (hydralazine: dogs, 0.5–2.0 mg/kg po q 12 hours; cats, 2.5 mg po q 12–24 hours),[19] and aldosterone receptor antagonists (spironolactone: dogs and cats, 1–2 mg/kg po q 12 hours).[19]

S Serial Monitoring

Because CKD is dynamic and progressive, serial monitoring should be performed on all patients with CKD in order to adjust treatment. Monitoring should include body condition, BW, muscle condition, thoracic auscultation, assessment of hydration status, indirect measurement of systemic arterial blood pressure, complete blood count, biochemical analysis, urinalysis, and possibly aerobic microbial culture of urine collected by cystocentesis. Frequency and extent of monitoring depend on how rapidly CKD is progressing, any nonrenal influences that may affect renal function, and owner satisfaction and finances.

HOW CAN TREATMENT OF CKD BE IMPROVED?

Early detection of CKD in patients may be an important factor on response to treatment. It may be worthwhile to determine serum creatinine concentration and urine specific gravity at 1 to 2 years of age and yearly beginning at 5 to 10 years of age. This may provide detection of CKD at an early stage and intervention at this point may provide better quality of life and longer quantity of life. It is important to keep in mind that the diagnosis of azotemia using the International Renal Insufficiency Society system may be different than the normal reference ranges used by your laboratory. It is recommended to use the values in the International Renal Insufficiency Society staging system where a serum creatinine greater than 1.6 mg/dL in cats and greater than 1.4 mg/dL in dogs is considered azotemic. Analytical techniques used to measure creatinine are consistent across laboratories; therefore, a change in 0.2 mg/dL is considered significant. Also, significant renal disease may be present without azotemia being present (stage 1). Whenever measuring serum creatinine concentration, a urine specific gravity must be determined at the same time in order to interpret the serum creatinine concentration. A complete urinalysis provides much information concerning urinary tract health and should be collected as part of a minimum database. Use of the International Renal Insufficiency Society staging system is important to guide therapy and monitoring and to permit comparison of a patient's disease with others. However, treatment should be individualized to the patient and owners but avoid overtreatment. Minimize or eliminate nonrenal influences that may affect renal function.

Despite appropriate treatment and monitoring, CKD is ultimately a progressive disease. Early identification and treatment may modify the rate of progression and provide for a better quality and longer quantity of life for the patient. Owners can be educated to evaluate disease by observing changes in water intake, urine volume, food intake, BW, body and muscle condition, activity, and behavior.

WHEN SHOULD DIET BE CHANGED IN A PATIENT DIAGNOSED WITH CKD?

Dietary modification is an important component of treating patients with CKD. Dietary modification can be used to offset many deficiencies and excesses that occur with CKD. It is more than protein restriction as diets formulated for use in patients with CKD are calorically dense, phosphorous and sodium restricted, have increased potassium and B vitamins, contain omega 3 fatty acids, contain soluble fiber, and are alkalinizing. Dietary modification has been shown to increase quality and quantity of life in dogs and cats with azotemic CKD (stage 2 or higher), but there are no studies evaluating dietary modification in patients with stage 1, non-proteinuric CKD. Nonetheless, in most patients the diet should be changed at the time of diagnosis of CKD. Furthermore, it is easier to introduce a therapeutic diet when the patient feels good rather than waiting until the disease process has progressed and introduction of a therapeutic diet is not possible.

SUMMARY

Many strides have been made in diagnosing and treating dogs and cats with CKD including dietary modification and pharmacologic therapy. Use of the International

Renal Insufficiency Society staging system provides a basis for diagnosis and management and for assessing response to treatment as well as comparison of results of studies for application to patients.

REFERENCES

1. Polzin DJ. Chronic kidney disease In: Bartges J, Polzin DJ, editors. Nephrology and urology of small animals. Ames (IA): Wiley-Blackwell; 2011. p. 433–71.
2. DiBartola SP, Rutgers HC, Zack PM, et al. Clinicopathologic findings associated with chronic renal disease in cats: 74 cases (1973-1984). J Am Vet Med Assoc 1987; 190:1196–202.
3. Lulich JP, Osborne CA, O'Brien TD, et al. Feline renal failure: questions, answers, questions. Compen Contin Educ Pract Vet 1992;14:127–52.
4. Elliott J, Barber PJ. Feline chronic renal failure: clinical findings in 80 cases diagnosed between 1992 and 1995. J Small Anim Pract 1998;39:78–85.
5. Jacob F, Polzin DJ, Osborne CA, et al. Evaluation of the association between initial proteinuria and morbidity rate or death in dogs with naturally occurring chronic renal failure. J Am Vet Med Assoc 2005;226:393–400.
6. Syme HM, Markwell PJ, Pfeiffer D, et al. Survival of cats with naturally occurring chronic renal failure is related to severity of proteinuria. J Vet Intern Med 2006;20: 528–35.
7. Polzin DJ. Chronic kidney disease in small animals. Vet Clin North Am Small Anim Pract 2011;41:15–30.
8. Lees GE, Brown SA, Elliott J, et al. Assessment and management of proteinuria in dogs and cats: 2004 ACVIM Forum Consensus Statement (small animal). J Vet Intern Med 2005;19:377–85.
9. Stepien RL. Blood pressure determination In: Bartges JW, Polzin DJ, editors. Nephrology and urology of small animals. Ames (IA): Wiley-Blackwell; 2011. p. 86–90.
10. Baldwin K, Bartges J, Buffington T, et al. AAHA nutritional assessment guidelines for dogs and cats. J Am Anim Hosp Assoc 2010;46:285–96.
11. Laflamme D. Devlopment and validation of a body condition score system for dogs. Canine Pract 1997;22:10–5.
12. Laflamme D. Development and validation of a body condition score system for cats: a clinical tool. Feline Pract 1997;25:13–8.
13. Burkholder WJ, Taylor L, Hulse DA. Weight loss to optimal body condition increases ground reactive force in dogs with osteoarthritis. Compen Cotin Educ Pract Vet 2000;23:74.
14. Michel KE, Anderson W, Cupp C, et al. Validation of a subjective muscle mass scoring system for cats. J Anim Physiol Anim Nutr (Berl) 2009;93:806.
15. Bartges JW, Kirk CA, Lauten S. Calculating a patient's nutritional requirements. Vet Med 2004;99:632.
16. Polzin DJ, Osborne CA, Ross S. Evidence-based management of chronic kidney disease In: Bonagura JD, Twedt DC, editors. Kirk's current veterinary therapy XIV. St Louis (MO): Saunders Elsevier; 2008. p. 872–9.
17. Peters RM, Goldstein RE, Erb HN, et al. Histopathologic features of canine uremic gastropathy: a retrospective study. J Vet Intern Med 2005;19:315–20.
18. Goldstein RE, Marks SL, Kass PH, et al. Gastrin concentrations in plasma of cats with chronic renal failure. J Am Vet Med Assoc 1998;213:826–8.
19. Plumb DC. Plumb's veterinary drug handbook. 6th edition. Ames (IA): Blackwell; 2008.

20. Quimby JM, Gustafson DL, Lunn KF. The pharmacokinetics of mirtazapine in cats with chronic kidney disease and in age-matched control cats. J Vet Intern Med 2011;25:985–9.
21. Ljutic D, Perkovic D, Rumboldt Z, et al. Comparison of ondansetron with metoclopramide in the symptomatic relief of uremia-induced nausea and vomiting. Kidney Blood Press Res 2002;25:61–4.
22. Bosworth C, Bartges JW, Snow P. Nasoesophageal and nasogastric feeding tubes. Vet Med 2004;99:590–4.
23. Luhn A, Bartges JW, Snow P. Gastrostomy feeding tubes: percutaneous endoscopic placement. Vet Med 2004;99:612–7.
24. Mesich ML, Bartges JW, Tobias K, et al. Gastrostomy feeding tubes: surgical placement. Vet Med 2004;99:604–10.
25. Thompson K, Bartges JW, Snow P. Gastrostomy feeding tubes: percutaneous, nonsurgical, nonendoscopic placement. Vet Med 2004;99:619–26.
26. Vannatta M, Bartges JW, Snow P. Esophagostomy feeding tubes. Vet Med 2004; 99:596–600.
27. Elliott DA, Riel DL, Rogers QR. Complications and outcomes associated with use of gastrostomy tubes for nutritional management of dogs with renal failure: 56 cases (1994–1999). J Am Vet Med Assoc 2000;217:1337–42.
28. Seaman R, Legendre AM. Owner experiences with home use of a gastrostomy tube in their dog or cat. J Am Vet Med Assoc 1998;212:1576.
29. Brown SA, Finco DR, Crowell WA, et al. Dietary protein intake and the glomerular adaptations to partial nephrectomy in dogs. J Nutr 1991;121:S125–7.
30. Brown SA, Brown CA. Single-nephron adaptations to partial renal ablation in cats. Am J Physiol 1995;269:R1002–8.
31. Brown SA, Brown CA, Crowell WA, et al. Does modifying dietary lipids influence the progression of renal failure? Vet Clin North Am Small Anim Pract 1996;26:1277–85.
32. Brown SA, Brown CA, Crowell WA, et al. Effects of dietary polyunsaturated fatty acid supplementation in early renal insufficiency in dogs. J Lab Clin Med 2000;135:275–86.
33. Brown SA, Finco DR, Brown CA. Is there a role for dietary polyunsaturated fatty acid supplementation in canine renal disease? J Nutr 1998;128:2765S–7S.
34. Brown SA, Brown CA, Crowell WA, et al. Beneficial effects of chronic administration of dietary omega-3 polyunsaturated fatty acids in dogs with renal insufficiency. J Lab Clin Med 1998;131:447-5.
35. Galler A, Tran JL, Krammer-Lukas S, et al. Blood vitamin levels in dogs with chronic kidney disease. Vet J 2012;192:226–31.
36. Agarwal R. Proinflammatory effects of oxidative stress in chronic kidney disease: role of additional angiotensin II blockade. Am J Physiol Renal Physiol 2003;284:F863–9.
37. Brown SA. Oxidative stress and chronic kidney disease. Vet Clin North Am Small Anim Pract 2008;38:157–66, vi.
38. Yu S, Paetau-Robinson I. Dietary supplements of vitamins E and C and beta-carotene reduce oxidative stress in cats with renal insufficiency. Vet Res Commun 2006;30:403–13.
39. Plantinga EA, Everts H, Kastelein AM, et al. Retrospective study of the survival of cats with acquired chronic renal insufficiency offered different commercial diets. Vet Rec 2005;157:185–7.
40. Wei J, Ni L, Yao J. [Experimental treatment of rhubarb on mesangio-proliferative glomerulonephritis in rats]. Zhonghua Nei Ke Za Zhi 1997;36:87–9.
41. Peng A, Gu Y, Lin SY. Herbal treatment for renal diseases. Ann Acad Med Singapore 2005;34:44–51.

42. Hanzlicek AS. The effects of rheum officinale on the progression of feline chronic kidney disease [thesis]. Department of Clinical Sciences, Kansas State University, 2011. p. 54.

43. DiBartola SP. Management of hypokalaemia and hyperkalaemia. J Feline Med Surg 2001;3:181–3.

44. Dow SW, LeCouteur RA, Fettman MJ, et al. Potassium depletion in cats: hypokalemic polymyopathy. J Am Vet Med Assoc 1987;191:1563–8.

45. Dow SW, Fettman MJ, LeCouteur RA, et al. Potassium depletion in cats: renal and dietary influences. J Am Vet Med Assoc 1987;191:1569–75.

46. Buranakarl C, Mathur S, Brown SA. Effects of dietary sodium chloride intake on renal function and blood pressure in cats with normal and reduced renal function. Am J Vet Res 2004;65:620–7.

47. Theisen SK, DiBartola SP, Radin MJ, et al. Muscle potassium content and potassium gluconate supplementation in normokalemic cats with naturally occurring chronic renal failure. J Vet Intern Med 1997;11:212–7.

48. Dow SW, Fettman MJ, LeConteur RA, et al. Potassium depletion in cats: Renal and dietary influences. J Am Vet Med Assoc 1987;191:1569–75.

49. Dow SW, Fettman MJ, Smith KR, et al. Effects of dietary acidification and potassium depletion on acid-base balance, mineral metabolism and renal function in adult cats. J Nutr 1990;120:569–78.

50. Adams LG, Polzin DJ, Osborne CA, et al. Correlation of urine protein/creatinine ratio and twenty-four-hour urinary protein excretion in normal cats and cats with surgically induced chronic renal failure. J Vet Intern Med 1992;6:36–40.

51. DiBartola SP, Buffington CA, Chew DJ, et al. Development of chronic renal disease in cats fed a commercial diet. J Am Vet Med Assoc 1993;202:744–51.

52. Forrester SD, Adams LG, Allen TA. Chronic kidney disease. In: Hand MS, Thatcher CD, Remillard RL, et al, editors. Small animal clinical nutrition. 5th edition. Topeka (KS): Mark Morris Institute; 2010. p. 765–810.

53. Weir MR, Fink JC. Salt intake and progression of chronic kidney disease: an overlooked modifiable exposure? A commentary. Am J Kidney Dis 2005;45:176–88.

54. Kirk CA, Jewell DE, Lowry SR. Effects of sodium chloride on selected parameters in cats. Vet Ther 2006;7:333–46.

55. Xu H, Laflamme DP, Long GL. Effects of dietary sodium chloride on health parameters in mature cats. J Feline Med Surg 2009;11:435–41.

56. Elliott J, Syme HM, Reubens E, et al. Assessment of acid-base status of cats with naturally occurring chronic renal failure. J Small Anim Pract 2003;44:65–70.

57. Elliott J, Syme HM, Markwell PJ. Acid-base balance of cats with chronic renal failure: effect of deterioration in renal function. J Small Anim Pract 2003;44:261–8.

58. de Brito-Ashurst I, Varagunam M, Raftery MJ, et al. Bicarbonate supplementation slows progression of CKD and improves nutritional status. J Am Soc Nephrol 2009;20:2075–84.

59. Navaneethan SD, Schold JD, Arrigain S, et al. Serum bicarbonate and mortality in stage 3 and stage 4 chronic kidney disease. Clin J Am Soc Nephrol 2011;6:2395–402.

60. Finco DR, Brown SA, Brown CA, et al. Progression of chronic renal disease in the dog. J Vet Intern Med 1999;13:516–28.

61. Elliott J, Syme HM. Proteinuria in chronic kidney disease in cats–prognostic marker or therapeutic target? J Vet Intern Med 2006;20:1052–3.

62. King JN, Gunn-Moore DA, Tasker S, et al. Tolerability and efficacy of benazepril in cats with chronic kidney disease. J Vet Intern Med 2006;20:1054–64.

63. Grauer GF, Greco DS, Getzy DM, et al. Effects of enalapril versus placebo as a treatment for canine idiopathic glomerulonephritis. J Vet Intern Med 2000;14: 526–33.

64. Grodecki KM, Gains MJ, Baumal R, et al. Treatment of X-linked hereditary nephritis in Samoyed dogs with angiotensin converting enzyme (ACE) inhibitor. J Comp Pathol 1997;117:209–25.

65. Ohashi Y, Sakai K, Tanaka Y, et al. Reappraisal of proteinuria and estimated GFR to predict progression to ESRD or death for hospitalized chronic kidney disease patients. Ren Fail 2011;33:31–9.

66. Pisoni R, Remuzzi G. Pathophysiology and management of progressive chronic renal failure In: Greenberg A, editor. Primer on kidney diseases. 3rd ed. San Diego (CA): National Kidney Foundation; 2001. p. 385–96.

67. Burkholder WJ, Lees GE, LeBlanc AK, et al. Diet modulates proteinuria in heterozygous female dogs with X-linked hereditary nephropathy. J Vet Intern Med 2004;18: 165–75.

68. Ross LA. Fluid therapy for acute and chronic renal failure. Vet Clin North Am Small Anim Pract 1989;19:343–59.

69. Finco DR, Brown SA, Brown CA, et al. Protein and calorie effects on progression of induced chronic renal failure in cats. Am J Vet Res 1998;59:575–82.

70. Elliott J, Barber PJ, Rawlings JM, et al. Effect of phosphate and protein restriction on progression of chronic renal failure in cats [abstract]. J Vet Intern Med 1998;12:221.

71. Adams LG, Polzin DJ, Osborne CA, et al. Effects of dietary protein and calorie restriction in clinically normal cats and in cats with surgically induced chronic renal failure. Am J Vet Res 1993;54:1653–62.

72. Polzin DJ, Osborne CA, Adams LG. Effect of modified protein diets in dogs and cats with chronic renal failure: current status. J Nutr 1991;121:S140–4.

73. De Santo NG, Perna A, Cirillo M. Low protein diets are mainstay for management of chronic kidney disease. Front Biosci (Schol Ed) 2011;3:1432–42.

74. Elliott J, Rawlings JM, Markwell PJ, et al. Survival of cats with naturally occurring chronic renal failure: effect of dietary management. J Small Anim Pract 2000;41: 235–42.

75. Harte JG, Markwell PJ, Moraillon RM, et al. Dietary management of naturally occurring chronic renal failure in cats. J Nutr 1994;124:2660S–2S.

76. Ross SJ, Osborne CA, Kirk CA, et al. Clinical evaluation of dietary modification for treatment of spontaneous chronic kidney disease in cats. J Am Vet Med Assoc 2006;229:949–57.

77. Jacob F, Polzin DJ, Osborne CA, et al. Clinical evaluation of dietary modification for treatment of spontaneous chronic renal failure in dogs. J Am Vet Med Assoc 2002;220:1163–70.

78. Rishniw M, Wynn SG. Azodyl, a synbiotic, fails to alter azotemia in cats with chronic kidney disease when sprinkled onto food. J Feline Med Surg 2011;13:405–9.

79. Barber PJ, Elliott J. Feline chronic renal failure: calcium homeostasis in 80 cases diagnosed between 1992 and 1995. J Small Anim Pract 1998;39:108–16.

80. Barber PJ, Rawlings JM, Markwell PJ, et al. Effect of dietary phosphate restriction on renal secondary hyperparathyroidism in the cat. J Small Anim Pract 1999;40:62–70.

81. Mattson A, Fettman MJ, Grauer GF. Renal secondary hyperparathyroidism in a cat. J Am Anim Hosp Assoc 1993;29:345–50.

82. Slatopolsky E, Brown A, Dusso A. Calcium, phosphorus and vitamin D disorders in uremia. Contrib Nephrol 2005;149:261–71.

83. Gerber B, Hassig M, Reusch CE. Serum concentrations of 1,25-dihydroxycholecal-ciferol and 25-hydroxycholecalciferol in clinically normal dogs and dogs with acute and chronic renal failure. Am J Vet Res 2003;64:1161–6.
84. Carmichael DT, Williams CA, Aller MS. Renal dysplasia with secondary hyperpara-thyroidism and loose teeth in a young dog. J Vet Dent 1995;12:143–6.
85. Wagner E, Schwendenwein I, Zentek J. Effects of a dietary chitosan and calcium supplement on Ca and P metabolism in cats. Berl Munch Tierarztl Wochenschr 2004;117:310–5.
86. Nagode LA, Chew DJ, Podell M. Benefits of calcitriol therapy and serum phosphorus control in dogs and cats with chronic renal failure. Both are essential to prevent of suppress toxic hyperparathyroidism. Vet Clin North Am Small Anim Pract 1996;26:1293–330.
87. Andress DL. Vitamin D in chronic kidney disease: a systemic role for selective vitamin D receptor activation. Kidney Int 2006;69:33–43.
88. Porsti IH. Expanding targets of vitamin D receptor activation: downregulation of several RAS components in the kidney. Kidney Int 2008;74:1371–3.
89. Freundlich M, Quiroz Y, Zhang Z, et al. Suppression of renin-angiotensin gene expression in the kidney by paricalcitol. Kidney Int 2008;74:1394–402.
90. Shoben AB, Rudser KD, de Boer IH, et al. Association of oral calcitriol with improved survival in nondialyzed CKD. J Am Soc Nephrol 2008;19:1613–9.
91. Hostutler RA, DiBartola SP, Chew DJ, et al. Comparison of the effects of daily and intermittent-dose calcitriol on serum parathyroid hormone and ionized calcium concentrations in normal cats and cats with chronic renal failure. J Vet Intern Med 2006;20:1307–13.
92. Cowgill LD. Pathophysiology and management of anemia in chronic progressive renal failure. Semin Vet Med Surg (Small Anim) 1992;7:175–82.
93. King LG, Giger U, Diserens D, et al. Anemia of chronic renal failure in dogs. J Vet Intern Med 1992;6:264–70.
94. Hoerger TJ, Wittenborn JS, Segel JE, et al. A health policy model of CKD: 1. Model construction, assumptions, and validation of health consequences. Am J Kidney Dis 2010;55:452–62.
95. Gonzalez FF, Fuentes CV, Castro HC, et al. [Economic impact of Losartan use in type 2 diabetic patients with nephropathy]. Rev Med Chil 2009;137:634–40.
96. Ryss ES. [Gastrin and the kidneys]. Klin Med (Mosk) 1984;62:14–7.
97. Chalhoub S, Langston C, Eatroff A. Anemia of renal disease: what it is, what to do and what's new. J Feline Med Surg 2011;13:629–40.
98. Cowgill LD, James KM, Levy JK, et al. Use of recombinant human erythropoietin for management of anemia in dogs and cats with renal failure. J Am Vet Med Assoc 1998;212:521–8.
99. Henry PA. Human recombinant erythropoietin used to treat a cat with anemia caused by chronic renal failure. Can Vet J 1994;35:375.
100. Langston CE, Reine NJ, Kittrell D. The use of erythropoietin. Vet Clin North Am Small Anim Pract 2003;33:1245–60.
101. Chakrabarti S, Syme H, Elliott J. Anemia predicts progression of chronic kidney disease in newly diagnosed azotemic cats. J Vet Intern Med 2010;24:677.
102. Bartges JW, Willis AM, Polzin DJ. Hypertension and renal disease. Vet Clin North Am Small Anim Pract 1996;26:1331–45.
103. Mathur S, Syme H, Brown CA, et al. Effects of the calcium channel antagonist amlodipine in cats with surgically induced hypertensive renal insufficiency. Am J Vet Res 2002;63:833–9.
104. Brown SA, Finco DR, Brown CA, et al. Evaluation of the effects of inhibition of angiotensin converting enzyme with enalapril in dogs with induced chronic renal insufficiency. Am J Vet Res 2003;64:321–7.

Alimentary Neoplasia in Geriatric Dogs and Cats

Michael D. Willard, DVM, MS*

KEYWORDS

- Lymphoma • Carcinoma • Adenocarcinoma • Leiomyoma • Stromal tumor
- Mastocytoma

KEY POINTS

- There are 2 main types of alimentary lymphoma in cats: large cell lymphoblastic and small cell lymphocytic. The former has a poor prognosis, while the latter has a relatively good prognosis.
- It is important to biopsy more than just the duodenum, even when doing biopsies endoscopically. More cases of lymphoma are diagnosed in ileal biopsies than in duodenal biopsies.
- Many tumors previously diagnosed as being leiomyomas and leiomyosarcomas are being reclassified as gastrointestinal stromal tumors based upon immunohistochemical staining.
- Chow chows appear to be predisposed to gastric carcinomas.

Alimentary neoplasia is a common and important problem in geriatric dogs and cats. While there are numerous possible cell types, locations, and associated clinical signs, there are some that are particularly common that should be high on the clinician's "radar screen" when dealing with older pets. This article will focus on the more common neoplastic problems of the esophagus and gastrointestinal tract (GIT) of geriatric dogs and cats.

LYMPHOMA

Lymphoma is the most common neoplasm of the feline GIT and is either the most common or second most common in the canine GIT. Up to 70% of cats with lymphoma have GIT involvment.[1–3] Alimentary lymphoma in cats can be B cell (more commonly but not exclusively in lymphoblastic lymphoma [LBL]) or T cell (more commonly but not exclusively in small cell, lymphocytic lymphoma [SCL]).[4] Different studies have found different preponderances of T- versus B-cell intestinal lymphoma

The author has nothing to disclose.
Department of Small Animal Clinical Sciences, College of Veterinary Medicine, TAMU-4474, Texas A&M University, College Station, TX 77843-4474, USA
* PO Box 12058, College Station, TX 77842.
E-mail address: mwillard@cvm.tamu.edu

in the cat.[2,4–9] Most canine alimentary tract lymphomas are T cell in origin.[10,11] Feline leukemia virus infection and feline immunodeficiency virus infection are important risk factors for feline lymphoma, but most cats with alimentary lymphoma have neither as diagnosed by commonly used assays. However, polymerase chain reaction (PCR) analysis has suggested that feline leukemia virus might be involved in at least some animals that are negative by routine enzyme-linked immunosorbent assay.[1] Cigarette smoke[12] and *Helicobacter* spp infection[13] are also hypothesized to be risk factors for lymphoma in cats. Risk factors in dogs are not clearly identified.

Intestinal Lymphomas

Lymphoma can affect the entire GIT, but it can also be relatively localized to 1 segment. In cats, the small intestine is the most commonly affected site.[14] Small intestinal involvement primarily causes weight loss, often but not invariably associated with diarrhea. Weight loss may precede diarrhea by weeks or months. Hyporexia and/or vomiting may also be seen, especially if there is thickening of the intestinal wall causing obstruction. Large intestinal involvement more reliably causes diarrhea because there is no segment of bowel after it that can mask its involvement. But, severe large bowel involvement can also cause weight loss. If the disease involves extra-GIT sites, clinical signs may vary depending on which other organ or organs are affected. Icterus from hepatic involvement and abdominal enlargement from splenomegaly are especially common. If paraneoplastic hypercalcemia of malignancy is present (primarily in dogs), polyuria-polydipsia may occur.

Cats can have LBL, SCL, epitheliotrophic lymphoma (a subset of SCL), and large granular lymphoma of the GIT. Large granular lymphoma is very aggressive.[15,16] Fortunately, it is rare and will not be discussed further. Dogs primarily have LBL of the GIT. Lymphoblastic lymphoma of the GIT in cats is similar enough to the canine form that they will be discussed together. In both species, LBL tends to be aggressive, growing quickly and producing severe, progressive clinical signs. Alimentary LBL often affects organs outside the GIT; therefore, organomegaly (especially spleen, liver, mesenteric lymph nodes) is common and can sometimes be detected at physical examination.

Most clinical pathology findings tend to be mild or nonspecific (ie, mild anemia, mild neutrophilia, increased hepatic enzymes). However, clinical pathology sometimes helps make a diagnosis. Rarely, circulating lymphoblasts (ie, leukemia) will be found in patients with alimentary lymphoma. Lymphoma is an important cause of protein-losing enteropathy in both the dog and cat; severe hypoalbuminemia (ie, <2.0 g/dL) with or without hypoglobulinemia that is not due to renal losses or hepatic insufficiency mandates consideration of lymphoma.[17] However, lymphoma is not the most common cause of protein-losing enteropathy in dogs (although it might be in cats). Hypercalcemia is uncommon in alimentary lymphoma but is seen more commonly in dogs than cats. Finding hypercalcemia in a patient with GIT signs as mentioned earlier necessitates a careful hunt for neoplasia, especially lymphoma. The ileum is often (not invariably) affected in patients with alimentary lymphoma, and finding hypocobalaminemia may help localize disease to the ileum. However, such ileal disease may be neoplastic or non-neoplastic, and finding a normal serum cobalamin is meaningless when considering whether intestinal disease is present or absent.

Abdominal radiographs can be helpful, but ultrasound is particularly useful in finding changes indicative of infiltrative disease. The majority of cats (~90%) with alimentary lymphoma have been reported to have ultrasonographic changes.[18,19] However, one should never eliminate lymphoma because changes suggestive of infiltrative disease were not found sonographically. While ultrasound is relatively specific for infiltrative diseases, it is potentially insensitive, especially for the less aggressive SCL. Thickened intestinal mucosa in which the normal distinction between different layers is lost is particularly suggestive of lymphoma but is primarily found in the more aggressive LBL. Recently, it is has been found that muscular layer thickening in feline intestines is particularly suggestive of lymphoma.[20] The significance of mesenteric lymphadenomegaly depends on the severity of the enlargement. While major enlargement is suggestive of lymphoma, mild to moderate enlargement can be due to any number of inflammatory abdominal diseases, including inflammatory bowel disease (IBD).[20]

If organomegaly (especially hepatic or splenic) is noted at physical examination or infiltrative disease is suggested by ultrasound, then fine needle aspirate cytology of that organ can sometimes be diagnostic (especially with LBL). Cytologic diagnosis of LBL is easier than cytologic diagnosis of SCL because LBL typically displays obvious signs of malignancy; therefore, it is usually relatively easy to determine that a round cell malignancy is present depending on the adequacy of the sample. Like ultrasonography, fine needle aspiration cytology is very specific with a high positive predictive value but is not always sensitive. You cannot eliminate lymphoma because you did not find it on a fine needle aspirate cytology. Neoplastic lymphoblasts can be very fragile; they can readily rupture during aspiration or preparation of the cytology slide. Only a few cells are necessary to make a diagnosis, but they must be intact. Aspirate cytology of mesenteric lymph nodes poses special difficulties because these lymph nodes are typically reactive since they drain the intestines. Such inflammation may make it difficult to obtain sufficient neoplastic cells to make a diagnosis.

A common source of confusion stems from performing cytology (or histopathology) on a patient that has been receiving corticosteroid therapy for presumptive IBD. If the steroids cause even a partial remission, it can be much harder to make a diagnosis of lymphoma. However, if the steroid therapy has had no beneficial effect or if an initial beneficial effect has been replaced with severe symptomatology, then cytology is more likely to be helpful.

Histopathology (ie, from intestinal biopsy) will be required if a diagnosis cannot be obtained cytologically. Tissue samples may be obtained endoscopically or surgically. There is ongoing controversy as to whether endoscopy or surgery is the preferred technique for intestinal biopsy, the arguments revolving around the quality of tissue samples obtained and access to the different parts of the GIT. While the quality of the tissue sample is probably a major issue when trying to diagnose SCL of cats (see later), it is probably not as major an issue with LBL. Marginal tissue samples often allow histologic diagnosis because the infiltrate is usually extensive in the affected areas and cellular characteristics of malignancy are often obvious. What is important with any intestinal disease (not just lymphoma) is to recognize that the affected portion of the intestine must be biopsied. Some patients with severe infiltrative intestinal disease have no localizing changes on ultrasound or physical examination. If imaging does not localize the lesion, then it behooves the clinician who chooses endoscopic biopsy to access as much of the GIT as possible. Lymphoma may affect all of the GIT or only 1 section (eg, ileum or jejunum) or it may "skip" sections. Furthermore, even when a particular section of the intestines (eg, duodenum) is affected, that does not mean that all the biopsy samples from that portion of the intestine will have the lesion. One can take 6 or 8 duodenal tissue samples endoscopically and only find lymphoma in a subset of the samples, even if all the samples are of adequate quality. How often this occurs is unknown, but the author has seen occasional cases in which this occurred.

Many patients with small intestinal disease undergoing endoscopy only receive gastroduodenoscopy. Ileal biopsy may be particularly important for a variety of intestinal diseases; lymphoma has been diagnosed in the ileum many times when there was no evidence of neoplasia in the duodenum.[21,22] A competent endoscopist should be able to biopsy the ileum in almost all patients. Therefore, endoscopic biopsy of the ileum should be routinely performed unless there is good reason to believe that the duodneum is affected with the same disease process. The gross endoscopic appearance of intestinal mucosal lymphoma varies[9]; therefore, one should biopsy all segments of the bowel, regardless of their appearance.

If laparotomy is performed instead of flexible endoscopy, one should generally biopsy the duodenum, jejunum, ileum, mesenteric lymph node, and liver (plus any other organ or structure that appears abnormal). If the patient is severely hypoalbuminemic, special consideration should be given to preventing suture line dehiscence. If obstruction occurs because of lymphomatous infiltrates, it must be removed if the patient is going to be treated although surgery will not be curative. Furthermore, it is possible that there will be neoplastic infiltration at the suture line (even when it appears normal), making dehiscence an important risk when performing full-thickness biopsy samples.

The prognosis for patients with alimentary LBL is poor. A combination of cyclophosphamide, doxorubicin, vincristine, and prednisolone (CHOP) is a well-accepted protocol for affected cats. Approximately 70% of cats with LBL respond to this chemotherapy with less than 50% achieving complete remission. In cats, the medial survival time is 4 to 6 months with chemotherapy. Abdominal radiation has been used with some success as a rescue therapy in affected cats.[23] Dogs treated with combination chemotherapy (ie, cyclophosphamide, doxorubicin, vincristine, L-asparaginase, prednisolone, lomustine, procarbazine, mustargen) have approximately a 50% response rate, and responders have a median survival time of approximately 110 days.[11] Diarrhea is a negative prognostic factor for dogs with alimentary lymphoma. Colorectal lymphoma may have a somewhat better prognosis.[10]

Patients with substantial, transmural neoplastic infiltration seem to have more complications from chemotherapy (ie, vomiting, diarrhea, perforation with subsequent peritonitis) than patients being treated for multicentric lymphoma. Hypocobalaminemic cats may benefit substantially from cobalamin injections as supportive therapy.

SCL of Cats

SCL of the GIT is relatively unique to the cat, and the following discussion will be for the cat only. This form of lymphoma is generally T-cell. In some studies, it was the most common form of feline intestinal lymphoma,[17,24] while in other studies it was less common than LBL.[4,25] This difference in incidence of SCL versus LBL may represent different epidemiologic factors predisposing cats to lymphoma in different geographic areas. Epitheliotropic intestinal lymphoma tends to be a subset of SCL, although some patients have intermediate-sized lymphocytes.[8] It is unknown if this subset responds differently than the nonepitheliotropic form of SCL.

SCL tends to have a much less aggressive course than patients with LBL. SCL patients are often characterized by chronic weight loss and diarrhea. Organomegaly is rare, and diagnosis is more difficult than with LBL. Major diseases to differentiate from SCL are IBD and hyperthyroidism.

Histopathology of good samples of intestinal tissue (ie, full thickness of mucosa and oriented so that one can see from the tips of the villi to the base of the crypts) is critical because it is impossible to diagnose SCL on cytologic criteria (ie, the small lymphocytes have no malignant characteristics). It has been suggested that endoscopy is sufficient to make a diagnosis of SCL in approximately 70% of the cases,[1] but there are no critical studies that document this statement or that meaningfully compare diagnosis of endoscopic biopsies versus surgical biopsies. The controversy between endoscopic biopsies and surgical biopsies centers around the ability to endoscopically obtain tissue samples with minimal stress (especially in ill, debilitated patients) versus the common problem of obtaining tissue samples that are superficial and do not allow evaluation of the entire thickness of the mucosa, much less the muscularis mucosa. Unfortunately, poor tissue samples are commonly obtained by endoscopists, especially novices or individuals who have not been trained in taking good tissue samples.

It is also clear that lymphoma may only affect 1 section of the intestines. Ileal biopsies seem particularly important in the diagnosis of feline SCL, but it is not clear that ileal biopsies will guarantee diagnosis. One study stated that full-thickness samples were superior to endoscopic samples.[21] However, careful reading of the report reveals that in each case in which a full-thickness, laparoscopic sample provided a diagnosis that was missed by an endoscopic sample, the endoscopic sample was from the duodenum while the full-thickness sample was from the ileum. While ileal biopsies are clearly useful for diagnosing lymphoma, the importance or lack thereof of biopsying the jejunum when looking for SCL is an issue that has not been critically addressed. Jejunal samples may be found to be as or even more important than ileal samples. There is a report of 17 cats with SCL in which jejunum samples were diagnostic in 15 of 15 cats while ileal samples were diagnostic in 13 of 14 cases[26]; however, this is a relatively small study. While the proximal jejunum can be accessed endoscopically in some cats, there are many patients in which endoscopy cannot reach the jejunum.

Laparotomy not only allows jejunal biopsy but also allows biopsy of liver, mesenteric lymph nodes, and other organs (eg, spleen) that might contain neoplastic infiltrates. At this time, there is some thought that laparoscopic biopsy of the intestines may be an advantageous compromise (ie, full-thickness samples of the different sections of intestine but less stress in debilitated patients). While laparoscopy allows full-thickness biopsy of jejunum and ileum as well as liver, it can be very hard to biopsy mesenteric lymph nodes using this technique.

In distinction to LBL (which is generally easy to diagnose), SCL can be a difficult diagnosis even with an excellent tissue sample. Finding infiltrates in the submucosa and muscularis has been suggested to be an important indicator of SCL, but some patients with IBD will have lymphocytic infiltrates in the same places, albeit less marked. Immunohistochemical staining and PCR analysis may be needed. In particular, enteric-associated T-cell infiltration may be especially difficult to distinguish from lymphocytic lymphoma since all the cells will be of the same phenotype.[27] In addition, some SCL have mixed populations of B-cells and T-cells. Therefore, simply obtaining full-thickness samples of intestine does not reliably allow one to distinguish IBD from neoplasia.

Adding to the confusion is the fact that alimentary lymphoma and alimentary inflammation often coexist in the same patient.[26,28] Immunohistochemical staining (eg, immunophenotyping by staining for CD3 and CD79a) will result in diagnosing some patients that initially appeared to have IBD as in fact having lymphoma (primarily SCL) and vice versus.[6] However, immunohistochemical staining is not always sufficient for clear-cut differentiation.[28] PCR testing for gene rearrangement (ie, clonality) is also available and appears to be necessary for definitive diagnosis in some patients.[5] Each assay has advantage and disadvantages. While the sensitivity of these assays is reported for other forms of lymphoma, we do not know what it is for alimentary lymphoma, especially with endoscopic biopsies. The subject is complex and beyond what we will approach here. Suffice it that these resources should be considered whenever the patient or the patient's response to therapy does not clearly fit in the histopathologic diagnosis. The reader is referred to other publications for a discussion on advantages and pitfalls of these techniques.[29–33]

There is ongoing debate about whether IBD can be a risk factor for cats developing SCL. As of this writing, it is not clear whether IBD can transform into SCL. However, it is interesting that distinguishing SCL from IBD is a focal point of the controversy about the best way to biopsy feline intestines. Adding to the confusion is the fact that cats may have SCL in one section of the bowel but IBD in another section.

The prognosis for intestinal SCL is much better than that for LBL, and the drugs used to treat it tend to have fewer side effects than the combination chemotherapy mentioned earlier for LBL. Chlorambucil and prednisolone form the mainstay of treatment and may be administered in various ways. Median survival time of patients that respond to prednisolone plus chlorambucil ranges from 1.5 to 2 years with an excellent quality of life.[26,34,35] Interestingly, this is the same treatment used for severe lymphocytic IBD, and anecdotally the outcome is about the same.

Gastric Lymphoma

The stomach may be infiltrated with lymphoma in association with intestinal lesions, or it may be the only site in the GIT that is affected. The primary clinical sign of gastric lymphoma is typically hyporexia. Vomiting typically comes later, only in the more advanced stages, unless the tumor involves the pylorus and causes vomiting early due to obstruction. Solitary gastric lymphomas are almost always B-cell in origin.[25] *Helicobacter pylori* infection in people is documented to cause low-grade mucosal lymphoma. The question is whether the species of *Helicobacter* found in the feline stomach (eg, *H felis*, *H helmanii*, etc) can cause gastric lymphoma.[13] Anecdotally, some cats with solitary gastric lymphoma have been cured with surgery; this might represent lymphoma caused by *Helicobacter* spp.

CARCINOMA/ADENOCARCINOMA

Carcinomas, including adenocarcinomas, are the most common tumor of the canine stomach and the second most common intestinal tumor in the cat. They occur about as frequently as lymphomas in the canine small intestinal tract but are the most common large intestinal malignancy in the dog. German shepherds and Siamese cats appear predisposed to intestinal carcinomas; Chow-chow dogs appear predisposed to gastric carcinomas.[36]

Esophageal Carcinomas

Esophageal carcinomas are relatively uncommon in dogs and cats, but carcinomas are the most common primary esophageal tumor of cats.[37] There are no recognized predisposing causes. Clinical signs (ie, regurgitation, anorexia, halitosis) are usually absent until the tumor is relatively large or has caused obstruction. Some animals with carcinomas at the lower esophageal sphincter seem to have a more generalized esophageal dysfunction, but this is anecdotal. Plain radiographs may be helpful in diagnosing esophageal carcinomas, but barium contrast esophagrams will usually reliably demonstrate the lesion. Esophagoscopy is definitive because it can locate the lesion and obtain diagnostic tissue samples. The prognosis is very poor. These cancers are usually not diagnosed until they are advanced, at which time they are typically difficult to impossible to resect. They metastasize early. Photodynamic therapy has been tried, but with modest results.[38]

Gastric Carcinomas

Gastric tumors in dogs are usually adenocarcinomas which are often scirrhous in nature. Any part of the stomach may be affected, but the incisura angularis and antrum/pylorus are frequently affected sites. Breeds at increased risk include the Chow-chow,[36] rough collies, Staffordshire bull terriers,[39] and Belgium shepherds.[40] These tumors are locally invasive plus they metastasize to regional lymph nodes early.

Anorexia (and attendant weight loss) is often the first abnormality noted by the client and can predate vomiting by months unless the lesion is very close to the pylorus (in which case vomiting may occur early due to outflow obstruction). When vomiting occurs, hematemesis may or may not be present.[41] Laboratory changes are usually nonspecific (ie, anemia of chronic disease, increased serum alkaline phosphatase). If alimentary blood loss has been sufficiently chronic and severe, iron-deficiency anemia (microcytic, hypochromic) may occur. However, such an anemia is not especially common, and its absence does not lessen the likelihood of a gastric carcinoma.[39]

Plain abdominal radiographs rarely reveal a gastric mass. Barium contrast gastrograms can often document infiltrative disease of the gastric wall, but these contrast studies are cumbersome and take relatively long to perform (especially when a double contrast study is requested). Furthermore, it can take over 24 hours for the barium to leave the stomach sufficiently to allow meaningful gastroscopy. Abdominal ultrasound may reveal an infiltrative lesion in the gastric wall.[42,43] However, it can be hard to adequately examine the entire gastric wall because of luminal contents (especially gas) and gastric motility. Therefore, ultrasound is specific for infiltrative gastric wall lesions but insensitive. Sometimes, it is easier to find gastric lymphadenomegaly secondary to metastasis than the primary gastric lesion. Percutaneous fine needle aspiration of enlarged lymph nodes or thickened gastric wall often allows diagnosis (especially when malignant epithelial cells are found in lymph node). Endoscopic ultrasound allows more reliable evaluation of gastric tumors,[44] but the technique is not widely available.

Endoscopy is typically the most sensitive and specific way to diagnose gastric carcinomas short of exploratory surgery.[45] A careful, methodical examination of the gastric mucosa typically reveals an area that is irregular and eroded or ulcerated, usually on the lesser curvature or near the pylorus.[41,46] More advanced cases of scirrhous carcinomas will typically have a large ulcer with a black center. It can be hard to make a definitive diagnosis endoscopically because the scirrhous nature of many tumors makes it difficult to obtain adequate tissue samples with flexible endoscopic forceps. Although much has been made of the idea that biopsying the margin of the ulcer typically allows diagnosis, that has not been the experience of the author. However, the characteristic appearance of scirrhous gastric adenocarinomas allows the endoscopist to make a presumptive diagnosis when the tumor is advanced. It is also important to recognize that if the lesion is not ulcerated, it is easy for endoscopic forceps to just obtain normal gastric mucosa that is overlying the neoplasia. Cytologic and histologic diagnoses are typically relatively easy. Recently, galectin-3 has been found in canine gastric carcinomas.[47] It may have a pathologic role in tumorogenesis.

Gastric carcinomas have a terrible prognosis. Surgery is the only potentially curative therapy, but it is rare that all the local disease can be surgically resected.[41] A gastric wall resection that does eliminate all local disease typically results in such a small gastric lumen that the patient cannot function. Furthermore, gastric carcinomas have typically metastasized before they have been diagnosed.[48]

Intestinal Carcinomas

Carcinomas may occur anywhere in the canine or feline intestine. Small intestinal carcinomas typically develop as solitary intestinal masses with a propensity to quickly metastasize to regional lymph nodes. Large intestinal carcinomas and adenocarcinomas in dogs are primarily found in the rectum, while large intestinal carcinomas in cats are more commonly found elsewhere in the colon.[49] Benign colonic polyps in dogs (these are rare in cats) are also primarily found in the rectal area. Malignant transformation of benign rectal polyps into carcinomas is reported but rare in dogs (as opposed to people, where it is a common problem).[50] However, it is critical to accurately distinguish the two.

Intestinal carcinomas can cause anorexia, vomiting, obstruction, diarrhea, weight loss, bleeding, and/or intussusception. Rectal adenocarcinomas tend to have different signs. Classically found in older German shepherd dogs, the major clinical signs of rectal adenocarcinoma are tenesmus, dyschezia, hematochezia, and finally constipation.[51] Stools can become "ribbon-like" as the rectal lesion progressively constricts the lumen. Digital rectal examination is the most sensitive test to find rectal lesions; it is more sensitive than proctoscopy or ultrasonography for early lesions. Digital examination is so important that chemical restraint is indicated if the patient strenuously objects to the examination. If a mass lesion or a deep infiltrative lesion is noted during digital examination, then proctoscopy and biopsy are indicated. For rectal lesions, rigid proctoscopy is often superior to flexible endoscopy. Rigid proctoscopy typically provides better visualization of rectal lesions, but more importantly it allows use of rigid biopsy forceps. Proper use of these forceps routinely allows one to obtain excellent tissue samples containing generous amounts of submucosa, which is where malignant cells are most reliably found. Such deep biopsies are especially critical for distinguishing benign polyps from adenocarcinomas.

Carcinomas in the ascending or descending colon are more difficult to diagnose than are rectal neoplasms. Ultrasonography can often find such colonic carcinomas. Colonoscopy tends to be more sensitive than ultrasound for finding colonic tumors and will allow definitive diagnosis (which ultrasound will not). If the lesion is in the descending colon, rigid colonoscopy is typically superior to flexible endoscopy for the same reasons as mentioned earlier for rectal lesions. However, rigid endoscopy will not allow examination of the transverse or ascending colon, nor will it allow examination of the entire descending colon in larger dogs. Abdominal ultrasound is almost always indicated before colonoscopy because finding lymphadenomegaly with metastatic carcinoma cells may obliviate the need for colonoscopy and the attendant colonic cleaning and anesthesia.

Treatment of small intestinal carcinomas preferentially consists of surgical resection. Resection is possible for large intestinal carcinomas, but the colon is more prone to dehiscence than the small intestine. Pubic and/or ischial osteotomy is possible for malignant lesions in the caudal colon,[52] and polyps as well as malignant lesions can be surgically resected or removed endoscopically with polypectomy.[53,54] Rectal lesions are easier to expose and resect.[55,56] Surgical cure of malignant lesions is possible, but regional metastasis is common. Adjunctive chemotherapy is reasonable but palliative. Treatment of rectal adenocarcinoma is particularly difficult because surgical resection (ie, rectal pull through) is often associated with fecal incontinence. If the patient does not experience complications, tumor resection may palliate the patient for months. Resection with concurrent colostomy is possible, but requires a dedicated owner because subsequent patient management can require substantial effort. Radiation therapy has been reported but is not commonly performed.[57] Placement of a stent to alleviate rectal obstruction may be tried, but is a palliative maneuver that has only been attempted a few times.[58] Anecdotally, administration of nonsteroidal anti-inflammatory drugs may help palliate some rectal carcinomas.

MESENCHYMAL TUMORS

Leiomyomas and leiomyosarcomas have classically been the connective tissue tumor diagnosed in the canine GIT. Recently, immunohistochemistry has allowed pathologists to distinguish stromal tumors (ie, those that originate from the interstitial cells of Cajal) (GIST) from leiomyomas (ie, those that originate from smooth muscle).[59] GIST are positive for CD117 and CD34, while leiomyomas and leiomyosarcomas are negative for these antigens but positive for smooth muscle actin and/or desmin.[60–62] The clinical importance of this reclassification is uncertain at this time.

Esophageal Tumors

Leiomyomas and leiomyosarcomas seem to have a predisposition for the canine lower esophageal sphincter (LES),[63] also called the lower esophageal high pressure zone. They are reported in older beagles[64] but may be found in any breed. These neoplasms may be on the gastric side or the esophageal side of the LES. Signs (eg, regurgitation) are usually absent until the tumor is relatively large and causing obstruction. Ultrasound, especially through an abdominal window, may often reveal submucosal infiltration at the LES. Endoscopy is typically the most sensitive technique for finding a mass in this location. However, it is hard to impossible to obtain diagnostic tissue samples with a flexible endoscope because this tumor is typically completely submucosa and covered with normal mucosa. The endoscopist must usually presume the diagnosis based upon the endoscopic appearance and location; definitive diagnosis typically requires surgery. However, it is important to have an experienced surgeon for tumors near the LES. This region is very unforgiving of any technical errors during surgery. Obstruction from cicatrix formation and gastroesophageal reflux from LES dysfunction are 2 potentially devastating postoperative complications. Successful surgery is typically curative.[63,65]

Fibrosarcomas may occur secondary to *Spirocerca lupi* infections.[66] Diagnosis is typically delayed because clinical signs like regurgitation do not occur until late in the clinical course. Microcytic anemia occasionally occurs due to chronic bleeding.[66] Occasionally hypertrophic osteopathy may be the first sign noted. Diagnosis may be made fortuitously when the chest is radiographed for some other reason. Retention of air in the esophagus may be the first abnormality noted on plain radiographs.[67] Definitive diagnosis requires biopsy, and these tumors are easy to sample with a flexible endoscope. Surgical resection is rarely curative but may be palliative (eg, 2–20 months) as these tend to be slower growing than carcinomas.[68]

Gastric and Intestinal Tumors

Clinical signs due to direct involvement of the GIT include anorexia, vomiting, diarrhea, and/or weight loss. Perforation and subsequent septic peritonitis are reported with these tumors, especially with cecal involvement in the dog.[60] However, paraneoplastic syndromes are well reported with these tumors. Hypoglycemia is associated with the larger tumors, and polyuria-polydipsia due to nephrogenic diabetes insipidus is recognized to be associated with this tumor.[69,70] Erythrocytosis may occur as a paraneoplastic syndrome[71] but, paradoxically, anemia is a particularly important problem associated with these tumors. GIT bleeding due to ulceration of the tumor can be responsible for life-threatening hemorrhagic shock. Gastric tumors in particular are known for bleeding; however, intestinal tumors are also prone to ulceration and hemorrhage. Because these tend to be larger, more bulky tumors, they are usually relatively easy to diagnose. Plain abdominal radiographs may be helpful, but ultrasonographic imaging typically detects them best. Fine needle aspiration cytology is not as helpful for diagnosing these tumors because they exfoliate poorly. Endoscopically, these tumors often appear as hard masses covered with normal mucosa. There may or may not be ulceration. When these tumors are ulcerated, there is usually obvious hemorrhage.

Treatment consists of surgical resection. Assuming no post-operative surgical complications, the prognosis is relatively good with patients often living 2 years or more.[69] Regional lymph nodes, mesentery and liver are the most common sites for metastasis. The presence of metastasis does not clearly impact prognosis; but hepatic leiomyosarcoma has a poor prognosis.[72]

FELINE INTESTINAL MAST CELL TUMOR

Mast cell tumor of the GIT is the third most common intestinal tumor of cats.[73] It may occur in any section of the small bowel (large bowel involvement is less common) but is usually not associated with cutaneous lesions. Abdominal palpation can often detect a mass lesion. It is a highly malignant tumor with a high rate of metastasis. Clinical pathology findings tend to be nonspecific, but abdominal effusions with mast cells may occur. Mastocytosis is infrequently seen (as opposed to splenic mastocytosis in which mastocytosis is more common). Eosinophilia may be seen in some patients.[74] Radiographs and ultrasound typically find infiltrative lesions. Cytology or biopsy will allow diagnosis; however, sometimes the histopathology will suggest eosinophilic enteritis.[75] Treatment consists of surgical resection, but it is invariably palliative for a relatively short time.

SUMMARY

Lymphomas, carcinomas, leiomyomas, and stromal tumors are the most common tumors found in the canine and feline GIT. Endoscopic and surgical biopsies are often the mainstays of diagnosis. SCL of the feline intestines poses a special diagnostic dilemma and may require immunohistochemistry as well as PCR to distinguish it from lymphocytic-plasmacytic enteritis.

REFERENCES

1. Richter KP. Feline gastrointestinal lymphoma. Vet Clin N Am 2003;33:1083–98.
2. Gabor LJ, Malik R, Canfield PJ. Clinical and anatomical features of lymphosarcoma in 118 cats. Aust Vet J 1998;76:725–32.
3. Louwerens M, London C, Pedersen N, et al. Feline lymphoma in the post-feline leukemia virus era. J Vet Int Med 2005;19:329–35.
4. Gabor L, Canfield P, Malik R. Immunophenotypic and histological characterisation of 109 cases of feline lymphosarcoma. Aust Vet J 1999;77:436–41.
5. Callanan JJ, Jones BA, Irvine J, et al. Histologic classification and immunophenotype of lymphosarcomas in cats with naturally and experimentally acquired feline immunodeficiency virus infections. Vet Pathol 1996;33:264–72.
6. Waly N, Gruffydd-Jones T, Stokes C, et al. Immunohistochemical diagnosis of alimentary lymphomas and severe intestinal inflammation in cats. J Comp Pathol 2005;133:253–60.

7. Vail DM, Moore AS, Ogilvie GK, et al. Feline lymphoma (145 cases): proliferation indices, cluster of differentiation 3 immunoreactivity, and their association with prognosis in 90 cats. J Vet Int Med 1998;12:349–54.

8. Carreras JK, Goldschmidt M, Lamb M, et al. Feline epitheliotropic intestinal malignant lymphoma: 10 cases (1997–2000). J Vet Int Med 2003;17:326–31.

9. Miura T, Maruyama H, Sakai M, et al. Endoscopic findings on alimentary lymphoma in 7 dogs. J Vet Med Sci 2004;66:577–80.

10. Frank J, Reimer S, Kass P, et al. Clinical outcomes of 30 cases (1997–2004) of canine gastrointestinal lymphoma. J Am Anim Hosp Assoc 2007;43:313–21.

11. Rassnick K, Moore A, Collister K, et al. Efficacy of combination chemotherapy for treatment of gastrointestinal lymphoma in dogs. J Vet Int Med 2009;23:317–22.

12. Bertone ER, Snyder LR, Moore AS. Environmental tobacco smoke and risk of malignant lymphoma in pet cats. Am J Epidemiol 2002;156:268–73.

13. Bridgeford E, Marini R, Feng Y, et al. Gastric Helicobacter species as a cause of feline gastric lymphoma: a viable hypothesis. Vet Immun Immunopath 2008;123:106–13.

14. Rissetto K, Villamil J, Selting K, et al. Recent trends in feline intestinal neoplasia: an epidemiologic study of 1,129 cases in the veterinary medical database from 1964 to 2004. J Am Anim Hosp Assoc 2011;47:28–36.

15. Roccabianca P, Vernau W, Caniatti M, et al. Feline large granular lymphocyte (LGL) lymphoma with secondary leukemia: primary intestinal origin with predominance of a CD3/CD8 alpha alpha phenotype. Vet Pathol 2006;43:15–28.

16. Krick E, Little L, Patel R, et al. Description of clinical and pathological findings, treatment and outcome of feline large granular lymphocyte lymphoma (1996–2004). Veterinary and Comparative Oncology 2008;6:102–10.

17. Fondacaro JV, Richter KP, Carpenter JL. Feline gastrointestinal lymphoma: 67 cases. Eur J Compar Gastroenterol 1999;4:69–74.

18. Penninck DG, Moore AS, Tidwell AS, et al. Ultrasonography of alimentary lymphosarcoma in the cat. Vet Radiol Ultra 1994;35(4):299–304.

19. Hittmair K, Krebitz-Gressl E, Kubber-Heiss A, et al. Feline alimentares lymphosarkom (Magen- und Darm-leukose): rontgenologische, sonographische, histologische und virologishe befunde. Wien Tierarzti Mschr 2000;87:174–83.

20. Zwingenberger A, Marks S, Baker T, et al. Ultrasonographic evaluation of the muscularis propria in cats with diffuse small intestinal lymphoma or inflammatory bowel disease. J Vet Int Med 2010;24:289–92.

21. Evans S, Bonczynski J, Broussard J, et al. Comparison of endoscopic and full-thickness biopsy specimens for diagnosis of inflammatory bowel disease and alimentary tract lymphoma in cats. J Am Vet Med Assoc 2006;229:1447–50.

22. Scott KD, Zoran DL, Mansell J, et al. Consistency of endoscopic biopsies obtained from the duodenum and ileum for feline small cell lymphoma (SC-LSA) and inflammatory bowel disease (IBD) [abstract]. J Vet Int Med 2011;25:695–6.

23. Parshley D, LaRue S, Kitchell B, et al. Abdominal irradiation as a rescue therapy for feline gastrointestinal lymphoma: a retrospective study of 11 cats (2001–2008). J Fel Med Surg 2011;13:63–8.

24. Jackson ML, Wood SL, Misra V, et al. Immunohistochemical identification of B and T lymphocytes in formaline fixed paraffin embedded feline lymphosarcomas relation to feline leukemia virus status tumor site and patient age. Can J Vet Res 1996;60:199–204.

25. Pohlman L, Higginbotham M, Welles E, et al. Immunophenotypic and histologic classification of 50 cases of feline gatrointestinal lymphoma. Vet Pathol 2009;46:259–68.

26. Lingard A, Briscoe K, Beatty J, et al. Low-grade alimentary lymphoma: clinicopatho-logical findings and responses to treatment in 17 cases. J Fel Med Surg 2009;11:692–700.

27. Valli VE, Jacobs RM, Norris A, et al. The histologic classification of 602 cases of feline lymphoproliferative disease using the National Cancer Institute working formulation. J Vet Diag Invest 2000;12:295–306.

28. Briscoe KA, Krockenberger M, Beatty JA, et al. Histopathologic and immunohisto-chemical evaluation of 53 cases of feline lymphoplasmacytic enteritis and low-grade alimentary lymphoma. J Comp Pathol 2011;145:187–98.

29. Bienzle D, Vernau W. The diagnostic assessment of canine lymphoma: implications for treatment. Clin Lab Med 2011;31:21–39.

30. Yagihara H, Uematsu Y, Koike A, et al. Immunophenotyping and gene rearrangement analysis in dogs with lymphoproliferative disorders characterized by small-cell lym-phocytosis. J Vet Diagn Invest 2009;21:197–202.

31. Fukushima K, Ohno K, Koshino-Goto Y, et al. Sensitivity for the detection of a clonally rearranged antigen receptor gene in endoscopically obtained biopsy specimens from canine alimentary lymphoma. J Vet Med Sci 2009;71:1673–6.

32. Kaneko N, Yamamoto Y, Wada Y, et al. Application of polymerase chain reaction to analysis of antigen receptor rearrangements to support endoscopic diagnosis of canine alimentary lymphoma. J Vet Med Sci 2009;71:555–9.

33. Kiupel M, Smedley R, Pfent C, et al. Diagnostic algorithm to differentiate lym-phoma from inflammation in feline small intestinal biopsy samples. Vet Pathol 2011;48:212–22.

34. Stein T, Pellin M, Steinberg H, et al. Treatment of feline gastrointestinal small-cell lymphoma with chlorambucil and glucocorticoids. J Am Anim Hosp Assoc 2010;46:413–7.

35. Kiselow M, Rassnick K, McDonough S, et al. Outcome of cats with low-grade lymphocytic lymphoma: 41 cases (1995–2005). J Am Vet Med Assoc 2008;232:405–10.

36. Bilek A, Hirt R. Breed-associated increased occurrence of gastric carcinoma in Chow-Chows. Wien Tierarzti Mschr 2007;94:71–9.

37. Gualtieri M, Monzeglio MG, Di Giancamillo M. Oesophageal squamous cell carcinoma in two cats. J Small Anim Pract 1999;40:79–83.

38. Jacobs TM, Rosen GM. Photodynamic therapy as a treatment for esophageal squamous cell carcinoma in a dog. J Am Anim Hosp Assoc 2000;36:257–61.

39. Sullivan M, Lee R, Fisher EW, et al. A study of 31 cases of gastric carcinoma in dogs. Vet Rec 1987;120:79–83.

40. Scanziani E, Giusti AM, Gualtieri M, et al. Gastric carcinoma in the Belgian shepherd dog. J Small Anim Pract 1991;32:465–9.

41. Gualtieri M, Monzeglio MG, Scanziani E. Gastric neoplasia. Vet Clin N Am 1999;29:415–40.

42. Dvorak LD, Bay JD, Crouch DT, et al. Successful treatment of intratracheal cutere-brosis in two cats. J Am Anim Hosp Assoc 2000;36:304–8.

43. Kaser-Hotz B, Hauser B, Arnold P. Ultrasonographic findings in canine gastric neoplasia in 13 patients. Vet Radiol Ultra 1996;37(1):51–6.

44. Lecoindre P, Chevallier M. Findings on endo-ultrasonographic (EUS) and endoscopic examination of gastric tumors of dogs. Eur J Compar Gastroenterol 1997;2(1):21–8.

45. Hirt R. Endoskopisch diagnostizierte magenkarzinome beim hund. Kleintierpraxis 2000;45:33–43.

46. Lingeman CH, Garner FM, Taylor DON. Spontaneous gastric adenocarcinomas of dogs: a review. J Nat Cancer Inst 1971;47:137–53.

47. Woo HJ, Joo HG, Song SW, et al. Immunohistochemical detection of galectin-3 in canine gastric carcinomas. J Comp Pathol 2001;124:216–8.
48. Swann HM, Holt DE. Canine gastric adenocarcinoma and leiomyosarcoma: a retrospective study of 21 cases (1986–1999) and literature review. J Am Anim Hosp Assoc 2002;38:157–64.
49. Slawienski MJ, Mauldin GE, Mauldin GN, et al. Malignant colonic neoplasia in cats: 46 cases (1990–1996). J Am Vet Med Assoc 1997;211:878–81.
50. Valerius KD, Ppowers BE, McPherron MA, et al. Adenomatous polyps and carcinoma in situ of the canine colon and rectum: 34 cases (1982–1994). J Am Anim Hosp Assoc 1997;33:156–60.
51. Church EM, Mehlaff CJ, Patnaik AK. Colorectal adenocarcinoma in dogs: 78 cases (1973–1984). J Am Vet Med Assoc 1987;191(6):727–30.
52. Yoon H, Mann F. Bilateral pubic and ischial osteotomy for surgical management of caudal colonic and rectal masses in six dogs and a cat. J Am Vet Med Assoc 2008;232:1016–20.
53. Foy D, Bach J. Endoscopic polypectomy using endocautery in three dogs and one cat. J Am Anim Hosp Assoc 2010;46:168–73.
54. Holt P. Evaluation of transanal endoscopic treatment of benign canine rectal neoplasia. J Small Anim Pract 2007;48:17–25.
55. Danova N, Robles-Emanuelli J, Bjorling D. Surgical excision of primary canine rectal tumors by an anal approach in twenty-three dogs. Vet Surg 2006;35:337–40.
56. Morello E, Martano M, Squassina C, et al. Transanal pull-through rectal amputation for treatment of colorectal carcinoma in 11 dogs. Vet Surg 2008;37:420–6.
57. Turrel JM, Theon AP. Single high-dose irradiation for selected canine rectal carcinomas. Vet Rad 1986;27:141–5.
58. Hume D, Solomon J, Weisse C. Palliative use of a stent for colonic obstruction caused by adenocarcinoma in two cats. J Am Vet Med Assoc 2006;228:392–6.
59. Russell K, Mehler S, Skorupski K, et al. Clinical and immunohistochemical differentiation of gastrointestinal stromal tumors from leimyosarcomas in dogs: 42 cases (1990–2003). J Am Vet Med Assoc 2007;230:1329–33.
60. Maas C, Haar G, Gaag I, et al. Reclassification of small intestinal and cecal smooth muscle tumors in 72 dogs: clinical, histologic, and immunohistochemical evaluation. Vet Surg 2007;36:302–13.
61. Gillespie V, Baer K, Farrelly J, et al. Canine gastrointestinal stromal tumors: immunohistochemical expression of cd34 and examination of prognostic indicators including proliferation markers Ki67 and AgNOR. Vet Pathol 2011;48:283–91.
62. Frost D, Lasota J, Miettinen M. Gastrointestinal stromal tumors and leiomyomas in the dog: a histopathologic, immunohistochemical, and molecular genetic study of 50 cases. Vet Pathol 2003;40:42–54.
63. Rolfe DS, Twedt DC, Seim HB. Chronic regurgitation or vomiting caused by esophageal leiomyoma in three dogs. J Am Anim Hosp Assoc 1994;30:425–30.
64. Culbertson R, Branam PE, Rosenblatt LS. Esophageal/gastric leiomyoma in the laboratory Beagle. J Am Vet Med Assoc 1983;183(11):1168–71.
65. Kerpsack SJ, Birchard SJ. Removal of leiomyomas and other noninvasive masses from the cardiac region of the canine stomach. J Am Anim Hosp Assoc 1994;30:500–4.
66. Ranen E, Lavy E, Aizenberg I, et al. Spirocerosis-associated esophageal sarcomas in dogs: a retrospective study of 17 cases (1997–2003). Vet Parasitol 2004;119:209–21.
67. Ridgway RL, Suter PF. Clinical and radiographic signs in primary and metastatic esophageal neoplasms of the dog. J Am Vet Med Assoc 1979;174(7):700–4.

68. Ranen E, Shamir M, Shahar R, et al. Partial esophagectomy with single layer closure for treatment of esophageal sarcomas in 6 dogs. Vet Surg 2004;33:428–34.
69. Cohen M, Post GS, Wright JC. Gastrointestinal leiomyosarcoma in 14 dogs. J Vet Int Med 2003;17:107–10.
70. Cohen M, Post GS. Nephrogenic diabetes insipidus in a dog with intestinal leiomyosarcoma. J Am Vet Med Assoc 1999;215:1818–9.
71. Sato K, Hikasa Y, Morita T, et al. Secondary erythrocytosis associated with high plasma erythropoietin concentrations in a dog with cecal leiomyosarcoma. J Am Vet Med Assoc 2002;220:486–90.
72. Kapatkin AS, Mullen HS, Matthiesen DT, et al. Leiomyosarcoma in dogs: 44 cases (1983–1988). J Am Vet Med Assoc 1992;201(7):1077–9.
73. Antognoni M, Spaterna A, Lepri E, et al. Characteristic clinical, haematological and histopathological findings in feline mastocytoma. Vet Res Commun 2003;27:727–30.
74. Bortnowski HB, Rosenthal RC. Gastrointestinal mast cell tumors and eosinophilia in two cats. J Am Anim Hosp Assoc 1992;28:271–5.
75. Howl JH, Petersen MG. Intestinal mast cell tumor in a cat presentation as eosinophilic enteritis. J Am Anim Hosp Assoc 1995;31:457–61.

Thyroid Disorders in the Geriatric Veterinary Patient

J. Catharine Scott-Moncrieff, MA, MS, Vet MB, MRCVS

KEYWORDS

- Geriatric • Thyroid disorders • Veterinary • Canine • Feline • Hyperthyroidism
- Hypothyroidism

KEY POINTS

- The effects of age, concurrent illness, and administered medications complicate the diagnosis of thyroid dysfunction in geriatric patients.
- The most common thyroid disorder in dogs is acquired hypothyroidism.
- Tests that are most useful in evaluation in dogs with suspected hypothyroidism are the total thyroxine concentration (TT_4), the free thyroxine concentration, and thyroid-stimulating hormone concentration.
- The most common thyroid disorder in cats is benign hyperthyroidism. Diagnosis is most often complicated by the presence of concurrent illness.
- Treatment should be individualized based on individual case characteristics and presence of concurrent illness.
- Some older cats have a palpable goiter months to years before development of clinical signs of hyperthyroidism.

INTRODUCTION

Thyroid disorders are an important cause of morbidity in geriatric dogs and cats. The diagnosis of thyroid dysfunction is more difficult in older animals because of the impact of age, concurrent illness, and administered medications on serum concentrations of thyroid hormone. This article will review the physiology of the thyroid gland specifically focusing on geriatric patients, discuss the most common causes of thyroid disease in geriatric patients, and review the special concerns of diagnosis and treatment in this subset of patients.

THYROID PHYSIOLOGY

Thyroxine (T_4) and triiodothyronine (T_3) are iodine-containing amino acids synthesized in the thyroid gland. Thyroid hormones are highly bound to serum proteins with T_4

The author has nothing to disclose.
Department Veterinary Clinical Sciences, College of Veterinary Medicine, Purdue University, VCS/LYNN, 625 Harrison Street, West Lafayette, IN 47907-2026, USA
E-mail address: scottmon@purdue.edu

Vet Clin Small Anim 42 (2012) 707–725
http://dx.doi.org/10.1016/j.cvsm.2012.04.012
0195-5616/12/$ – see front matter © 2012 Elsevier Inc. All rights reserved.

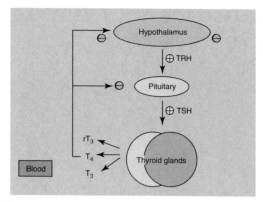

Fig. 1. The hypothalamic-pituitary-thyroid axis. (*From* Ettinger SJ, Feldman EC. Textbook of veterinary internal medicine. 7th edition. Philadelphia: Saunders; 2009. p. 1752; with permission.)

more highly bound than T_3. In the dog, the thyroid-binding proteins are thyroid hormone-binding globulin (TBG), transthyretin, albumin, and apolipoproteins, with most T_4 bound to TBG. Thyroid binding globulin is absent in the cat.[1] Protein-bound hormones are in equilibrium with a small fraction of unbound (free) hormone. Only unbound thyroid hormone enters cells to produce a biologic effect and create a negative feedback effect on the pituitary and hypothalamus. Tri-iodothyronine enters cells more rapidly, has a more rapid onset of action, and is 3 to 5 times more potent than T_4. Thyroid hormones bind to receptors in the nuclei; the hormone receptor complex then binds to DNA and influences the expression of genes coding for regulatory enzymes.

Thyroid hormones have a variety of physiologic effects, which account for the profound clinical effects of thyroid hormone deficiency on the body. Thyroid hormones increase the metabolic rate and oxygen consumption of most tissues. In the heart, thyroid hormones have both a positive inotropic and a positive chronotropic effect, and they increase the number and affinity of beta-adrenergic receptors and enhance the response to catecholamines. Thyroid hormones have catabolic effects on muscle and adipose tissue, stimulate erythropoiesis, and regulate both cholesterol synthesis and degradation.

Thyroid hormone synthesis and secretion are regulated primarily by changes in the circulating concentration of pituitary thyrotropin (thyroid-stimulating hormone [TSH]) (**Fig. 1**). Thyroid hormone metabolism by deiodination is regulated by the relative activity of different deiodinase enzymes and is an important regulatory step in thyroid hormone metabolism. Outer-ring deiodination of T_4 produces T_3, whereas inner-ring deiodination results in formation of biologically inactive reverse T_3. T_4 and T_3 are both concentrated in the liver and secreted in the bile.

EFFECT OF AGE ON THE HYPOTHALAMIC-PITUITARY-THYROID AXIS

In dogs there is a progressive decline in T_4 concentration with age; Serum T_4 concentration is highest in puppies and the T_4 concentration progressively declines during adulthood. In a study of 27 female beagles of different ages, mean serum T_4 concentrations in old dogs were 40% lower than those of young adult dogs.[2] In a larger study of serum collected from 1074 healthy dogs of differing ages, the mean TT_4 concentration was 21% lower in in dogs older than 6 years compared to young adult dogs.[3] In a longitudinal study of 48 Labrador retrievers studied for 12 years, the

Table 1
Mean and median serum TT_4 concentration of samples submitted to a reference laboratory for cats and dogs of different ages

Age, y	Mean T_4, μg/dL	Median T_4, μg/dL	No. of Patients
Dogs			
0–2	1.94	1.9	1043
3–5	1.91	1.8	2773
6–8	1.83	1.6	6975
9–11	1.75	1.5	5064
12–14	1.67	1.4	4016
>14	1.46	1.2	736
All ages	1.78	1.5	20,607
TT_4 reference range	1.0–4.0		
Cats			
0–2	1.93	2.0	414
3–5	2.01	2.1	733
6–8	2.02	2.1	2183
9–11	2.08	2.1	2480
12–14	2.12	2.1	3644
>14	2.13	2.1	4477
All ages	2.08	2.1	13931
TT_4 reference range	0.8–4.7		

Patients with an age listed as 0 were excluded. Samples from cats in which the T_4 concentration was greater than 4.7 μg/dL were excluded from the analysis.
Data was provided by IDEXX Laboratories, Inc., Westbrook, ME.

mean TT_4 decreased by 29% from the age of 6 to 12 years.[4] Similar trends occur for free T_4 (fT_4) and TT_3 concentrations.[3,4] Middle-aged and older dogs also have a blunted T_4 response to TSH compared to young animals.[2] Changes in other parameters of thyroid function have been less studied but increases in anti-T_4 antibody in older dogs have been reported.[4] Although older dogs as a group have lower total T_4 (TT_4) concentrations than younger animals, the mean and median TT_4 concentrations still fall within the lower end of most reference ranges (**Table 1**). None of the studies cited above reported a range for TT_4 in healthy geriatric dogs; it is likely that for many geriatric dogs a TT_4 below the reference range is a normal age-related change. Reasons for the decline in thyroid hormone concentrations with age in dogs are not fully understood; proposed reasons include effect of concurrent illness, change in responsiveness of the thyroid gland to TSH, subclinical thyroid pathology (fibrosis, atrophy, degenerative changes), and decreased biologic activity of TSH with age.

There are no published studies on how thyroid hormone concentration changes with age in cats. In a group of more than 13,000 cats of varying ages that had TT_4 concentrations within or below the reference range, there was no decline in TT_4 with age (see **Table 1**).

EFFECT OF CONCURRENT ILLNESS ON HYPOTHALAMIC-PITUITARY-THYROID AXIS

In nonthyroidal illness, total thyroid hormone concentrations tend to decrease, with the change being more severe with increasing severity of illness. Changes in hormone

Table 2	
Mechanisms by which drugs influence thyroid function in humans	
Mechanism	**Example**
Decrease TSH secretion	Glucocorticoids
Change thyroid hormone secretion	Amiodarone
Decrease gastrointestinal absorption	Sucralfate
Alter serum binding	Phenylbutazone
Change hepatic metabolism	Phenobarbital
Inhibit thyroid peroxidase	Sulfonamides

binding to serum carrier proteins (eg, decreased protein concentration, reduced binding affinity, circulating inhibitors of binding) or peripheral hormone distribution and metabolism (eg, reduced 5′-deiodinase activity), inhibition of TSH secretion, and inhibition of thyroid hormone synthesis are proposed to contribute to this change. Cytokines such as interleukin-1, interleukin-2, interferon gamma, and tumor necrosis factor alpha decrease TT_4 concentrations in dogs.[5] The magnitude of decrease depends on disease severity and is a predictor of mortality.[6,7] Thyroid hormone supplementation does not improve survival in euthyroid humans with decreased thyroid hormone concentrations or increase survival in euthyroic dogs with congestive heart failure.[8] Medical conditions reported to decrease TT_4 concentrations in dogs include hyperadrenocorticism, diabetic ketoacidosis, hypoadrenocorticism, renal failure, hepatic disease, peripheral neuropathy, generalized megaesophagus, heart failure, neoplasia, critical illness or infection, and surgery or anesthesia.[9–15]

EFFECT OF DRUGS ON THE HYPOTHALAMIC-PITUITARY-THYROID AXIS

Many drugs influence the thyroid gland by a variety of mechanisms (**Table 2**). The effect of comonly used drugs on thyroid function in dogs is shown in **Table 3**.[16–22] Glucocorticoids influence peripheral metabolism of thyroid hormones and inhibit TSH secretion. The effect of glucocorticoids depends on the dose and specific preparation. Oral administration of glucocorticoids at immunosuppressive doses causes rapid decreases in TT_4, fT_4, and T_3 but little change in serum TSH. Thyroid hormone concentrations return to normal within 1 week after stopping treatment if dosing is for 3 weeks or less. Longer treatment may prolong duration of suppression. Sulfonamides block iodination of thyroglobulin and in dogs can cause clinical hypothyroidism in a dose- and duration-dependent manner. Effects are reversible within 2 to 4 weeks of discontinuation of therapy. Phenobarbital administration in dogs causes decreased TT_4 and fT_4 concentrations and mild increases in TSH concentration without clinical evidence of hypothyroidism. The effect of drugs other than methimazole on thyroid hormone concentrations in cats has received little attention.

EFFECT OF BREED ON THE HYPOTHALAMIC-PITUITARY-THYROID AXIS

Most laboratories report reference ranges based on measurement of thyroid hormone concentrations in groups of dogs of various breeds and ages; however, there are significant differences between breeds in regard to thyroid hormone concentration. In a study of young healthy greyhounds, 91% of the dogs had a TT_4 concentration below the non–breed-specific reference range and 16% had TT_4 concentrations that were either at or below the limit of detection of the assay.[23] fT_4 was lower than the

Table 3
Drugs that have been demonstrated to influence thyroid function in dogs

Drug	TT_4 ($\downarrow$ or N)	fT_4 ($\downarrow$ or N)	TSH ($\uparrow$ or N)	Clinical Signs of Hypothyroidism?	Notes
Glucocorticoids	$\downarrow$	($\downarrow$ or N)	N	No	Effect dose and duration dependent
Phenobarbital	$\downarrow$	$\downarrow$	Slight $\uparrow$	No	TSH not increased outside reference range
Trimethoprim/ sulfonamides	$\downarrow$	$\downarrow$	$\uparrow$	Yes	Effect dose and duration dependent
Non-steroidal antiinflammatory drugs					Effect varies depending on specific drug used
Aspirin	$\downarrow$	N	N	No	
Deracoxib	N	N	N	No	
Ketoprofen	N	N	N	No	
Meloxicam	N	N	N	No	
Carprofen	N	N	N	No	
Tricyclic antidepressant					Effect of other tricyclic antidepressants unknown in dog
Clomipramine	$\downarrow$	$\downarrow$	N	No	
Propanolol	N	N	N	No	
Potassium bromide	N	N	N	No	

Abbreviation: N, no change.

non–breed-specific reference range in 21% of dogs and at or below the limit of detection in 13% of dogs. In the same study, T_3 concentrations were all within the non–breed-specific reference range. The reason for the difference in thyroid hormone concentrations between greyhounds and other breeds has not yet been elucidated, but studies suggest that it is not due to changes in concentration or function of thyroid binding globulin.[24] There are no published studies investigating the change in concentration of TT_4 or fT_4 with aging in greyhounds; however, in salukis and sloughis, TT_4 and fT_4 concentrations decline with age as has been reported in non–sight hound breeds.[25,26] Other breeds in which breed-specific changes in thyroid hormone parameters have been reported are given in **Table 4**.[23-31]

CANINE THYROID DYSFUNCTION

The most common thyroid disorders of geriatric dogs are acquired hypothyroidism and thyroid neoplasia.

Canine Hypothyroidism

Pathogenesis
Hypothyroidism results from decreased production of T_4 and T_3 from the thyroid gland. Acquired primary hypothyroidism is caused by lymphocytic thyroiditis or idiopathic thyroid atrophy. Canine thyroiditis is believed to be the cause of hypothyroidism in approximately 50% of hypothyroid dogs.[32] Lymphocytic thyroiditis has

Table 4
Canine breeds with unique thyroid hormone reference ranges

Breed	TT_4 ($\downarrow$ or N)	fT_4 ($\downarrow$ or N)	TT_3 ($\downarrow$ or N)	TSH ($\uparrow$ or N)
Greyhound	$\downarrow$	$\downarrow$	Variable	N
Whippet	$\downarrow$	N	—	N
Saluki	$\downarrow$	$\downarrow$	$\downarrow$	$\uparrow$
Sloughi	$\downarrow$	$\downarrow$ or $\uparrow$ (ED)	—	$\uparrow$
Conditioned Alaskan sled dogs	$\downarrow$	$\downarrow$	$\downarrow$	Variable

Abbreviations: ED, equilibrium dialysis; N, no change.

been identified as a risk factor for thyroid neoplasia.[33] Secondary hypothyroidism (deficiency of TSH) is regarded as rare in dogs.

Epidemiology

Hypothyroidism is typically a disease of middle-aged to older dogs. Golden retrievers and Doberman pinschers are among the breeds reported to be at higher risk for hypothyroidism while many breeds have been reported to be at higher risk of thyroiditis (**Table 5**). The peak prevalence of detection of anti-thyroglobulin antibodies is 2 to 4 years of age, which fits with the hypothesis that thyroiditis may progress to complete thyroid failure over time.[32] The severity and progression of thyroiditis seem to be dependent on breed, with some breeds having relatively rapid progression to thyroid failure while other breeds such as the beagle progress to thyroid failure much more slowly, if at all.[32] Studies do not suggest a consistent association of hypothyroidism with sex or neuter status.

Clinical signs

Common clinical signs include lethargy, mental dullness, weight gain, sluggishness, and cold intolerance. Dermatologic changes such as dry scaly skin, changes in haircoat quality or color, alopecia, seborrhea, and superficial pyoderma occur in 60% to 80% of hypothyroid dogs. Alopecia is usually bilaterally symmetric and is first evident in areas of wear, such as the lateral trunk, ventral thorax, and tail. The head and extremities tend to be spared. The hair may be brittle and easily epilated, and loss of undercoat or primary guard hairs may result in a coarse appearance or a puppy-like haircoat. Fading of coat color may also occur, and failure of hair regrowth after clipping is common. Other dermatologic changes in hypothyroid dogs include hyperkeratosis, hyperpigmentation, comedone formation, hypertrichosis, ceruminous otitis, poor wound healing, increased bruising, and myxedema.

Neurologic clinical signs are rare but important manifestations of hypothyroidism. Neurologic signs include peripheral neuropathy, cranial nerve dysfunction (facial, trigeminal, vestibulocochlear), and cerebral dysfunction (seizures, disorientation, circling). Cardiovascular abnormalities in hypothyroid dogs include sinus bradycardia, weak apex beat, low QRS voltages, and reduced left ventricular pump function.

Diagnosis

Diagnostic testing for hypothyroidism should only be pursued if there is clinical evidence of thyroid disease based on evaluation of the history and physical examination. Routine screening of asymptomatic dogs for hypothyroidism will increase the

Table 5
Twenty breeds with the highest and 20 breeds with the lowest prevalence of thyroglobulin antibody in 140,821 serum samples submitted for investigation of thyroid disease

Name	Total Sera	TgAA Positive	Prevalence
English setter	585	184	31%
Old English sheepdog	368	86	23%
Boxer	2642	496	19%
Giant schnauzer	263	49	19%
American pit bull terrier	345	64	19%
Beagle	2452	449	18%
Dalmatian	1372	246	18%
German wirehaired pointer	112	20	18%
Maltese dog	594	105	18%
Rhodesian ridgeback	626	107	17%
Siberian husky	483	80	17%
American Staffordshire terrier	151	24	16%
Cocker spaniel	8576	1305	15%
Chesapeake Bay retriever	509	74	15%
Tibetan terrier	106	15	14%
Shetland sheepdog	5765	813	14%
Golden retriever	17,782	2397	13%
Borzoi	266	35	13%
Husky	646	84	13%
Brittany	556	71	13%
Dachshund	3612	115	3%
Basset hound	699	22	3%
Cairn terrier	590	18	3%
Schnauzer, unspec.	1257	38	3%
Wirehaired fox terrier	170	5	3%
Cavalier King Charles spaniel	274	8	3%
Welsh corgi, undet.	457	13	3%
Yorkshire terrier	1178	33	3%
Norwegian elkhound	263	7	3%
Belgian Tervuren	235	6	3%
Chihuahua	611	15	2%
Greyhound	1409	32	2%
Pekingese	407	9	2%
Boston terrier	500	11	2%
Pomeranian	1301	26	2%
Irish wolfhound	210	4	2%
Whippet	114	2	2%
Soft-coated Wheaten terrier	214	3	1%
Bichon frise	657	8	1%
Miniature Schnauzer	828	10	1%

Overall TgAA prevalence in this study was 10%.
Abbreviations: TgAA, thyroglobulin antibody; undet., undetermined; unspec., unspecified.
   From Graham PA, Refsal KR, Nachreiner RF. Etiopathologic findings of canine hypothyroidism. Vet Clin N Am Small Anim Pract 2007;37(4):617–31; with permission.

Table 6
Sensitivity, sensitivity, and accuracy of 4 assays for fT$_4$ in dogs and cats

Assay	Cats			Dogs		
	Sensitivity, %	Specificity, %	Accuracy, %	Sensitivity, %	Specificity, %	Accuracy, %
Analog fT$_4$	87	100	89	80	97	89
MED IVD	87	100	89	92	90	91
MED AN	92	67	89	71	100	86
Two-step Diasorin	89	100	91	96	90	93

The dog population included 56 dogs with clinical signs of hypothyroidism (31 euthyroid, 25 hypothyroid). The cat population included 45 cats with clinical signs of hyperthyroidism (6 euthyroid, 39 hyperthyroid). Assays included the Immulite 2000 Veterinary fT4 (Siemens Healthcare Diagnostics Products Ltd., Llanberis, Gwynedd, UK), Direct free T4 by dialysis (MED IVD; IVD Technologies, Santa Ana, CA, USA), fT$_4$ by equilibrium dialysis (MED AN; Antech Diagnostics, Irvine, CA, USA), and the Gammacoat fT$_4$ (2-step) Radioimmunoassay (Diasorin, Stillwater, MN, USA).

likelihood of a false-positive result, especially in the geriatric population. Measurement of TT$_4$ concentration is a sensitive initial screening test for hypothyroidism. Tests to confirm the diagnosis include measurement of fT$_4$ and thyrotropin (TSH) concentration and provocative thyroid function tests. Evidence of thyroiditis increases suspicion for thyroid dysfunction. Evaluation of response to thyroid hormone supplementation may be necessary to confirm the diagnosis. Clinicopathologic changes that are commonly present in dogs with hypothyroidism such nonregenerative anemia, fasting hypertriglyceridemia, and hypercholesterolemia increase the index of suspicion for hypothyroidism.

TT$_4$ concentration Measurement of a TT$_4$ concentration well within the reference range indicates normal thyroid function; however, a TT$_4$ concentration below the normal range may be caused by other factors such as nonthyroidal illness, drug administration, age, and breed variation.

fT4 concentration Because only the unbound fraction of serum T$_4$ is biologically active, measurement of fT$_4$ should be more sensitive and specific for the diagnosis of hypothyroidism than TT$_4$. There are a number of different assays currently used in dogs for measurement of fT$_4$ and their diagnostic performance varies (**Table 6**).[34] Although measurement of fT$_4$ concentration is believed to be slightly more specific and sensitive for diagnosis of canine hypothyroidism than measurement of TT$_4$, concurrent illness, drug administration, and breed variability may still suppress fT$_4$ concentration.

Total T$_3$ concentration (TT$_3$) Measurement of TT$_3$ is not recommended for routine diagnosis of canine hypothyroidism because T$_3$ concentration frequently fluctuates out of the reference range in euthyroid dogs.

Thyrotropin concentration (TSH) Measurement of canine TSH concentration is helpful to confirm the diagnosis of hypothyroidism in dogs with a low TT$_4$ concentration, because low TT$_4$ in conjunction with high TSH is highly specific for diagnosis of hypothyroidism (**Table 7**).[35–37] The limitation of measurement of TSH is the lack of

Table 7
Performance of various diagnostic tests for hypothyroidism in dogs

Test	Sensitivity, %	Specificity, %	Accuracy, %
TT_4	89–100	75–82	85
fT_4	80–98	93–94	95
TSH	63–87	82–93	80–84
TSH/T_4[a]	63–67	98–100	82–88
TSH/fT_4[a]	74	98	86

[a] A dog was considered to have hypothyroidism only if the T_4 or fT_4 was low and the TSH was high.
The data are compiled from 3 published studies of a total of 100 hypothyroid dogs and 164 euthyroid dogs. Not all studies evaluated all diagnostic tests listed.
Data from Refs.[34–36]

assay sensitivity; approximately 30% of hypothyroid dogs have a TSH concentration within the reference range.

TSH stimulation test The TSH stimulation test is a test of thyroid reserve. It is considered the gold standard test for assessment of thyroid function in dogs, but its use is limited by the expense of TSH. The protocol requires collection of a serum sample for measurement of T_4, administration of 75 to 150 μg/dog IV of human recombinant TSH with an additional blood sample for TT_4 collected after 6 hours. The higher dose is recommended in dogs with concurrent disease and those receiving medication.[38] Hypothyroidism is confirmed by a pre and post TT_4 concentration below the reference range for basal TT_4 concentration. Euthyroidism is confirmed by a post TT_4 concentration greater than 2.5 μg/dL. Interpretation of intermediate results should take into consideration the clinical signs and severity of concurrent systemic disease.

Diagnostic imaging Ultrasonography may be useful in evaluation of dogs with suspected hypothyroidism. The thyroid gland in many hypothyroid dogs has a smaller volume and cross-sectional area compared to euthyroid dogs and tends to be less echogenic. Nuclear scintigraphy also has high discrimination for evaluation of dogs with suspected hypothyroidism; however, it is rarely performed in clnincal practice.[39]

Therapeutic trial Response to therapy is sometimes the most practical approach to confirming a diagnosis of hypothyroidism. After ruling out nonthyroidal illness, supplementation with synthetic sodium L-thyroxine (L-T_4) should be initiated at a dosage of 0.02 mg/kg q 12 hours. If improvement is noted, therapy should be temporarily withdrawn. Recurrence of clinical signs is consistent with a diagnosis of hypothyroidism. If clinical signs do not recur, thyroid responsive disease in which clinical signs improve due to the nonspecific effects of thyroid hormone should be suspected. If there is no response to treatment after 2 to 3 months of appropriate therapy, and 4- to 6-hour post-pill serum TT_4 concentrations are within the appropriate therapeutic range, therapy should be withdrawn and other diagnoses pursued.

Diagnosis of thyroiditis
Dogs with thyroiditis may have serum antibodies directed against thyroglobulin, T_3, or T_4. Anti-thyroglobulin antibodies are present in 36% to 50% of hypothyroid dogs.[40] Anti-T_3 antibodies are detected in 34% of hypothyroid dogs, while anti-T_4 antibodies are found in 15% of hypothyroid dogs.[41] Because dogs with thyroiditis may still have

adequate thyroid reserve, positive antibody titers are not diagnostic of hypothyroidism; however, a positive titer increases the likelihood of thyroid dysfunction in dogs with equivocal thyroid hormone/TSH concentrations.

Treatment

The treatment of choice for hypothyroidism, regardless of the underlying cause, is L-T_4. Administration of L-T_4 with food may decrease bioavailability.[42] Treatment with synthetic T_3 is not recommended because it has a shorter half-life, requires administration 3 times daily, and is more likely to cause iatrogenic hyperthyroidism. Treatment with T_3 may be indicated if there is inadequate gastrointestinal absorption of L-T_4 because T_3 is better absorbed in the gastrointestinal tract. The use of desiccated thyroid extract, thyroglobulin, or "natural" thyroid preparations is not recommended because the bioavailability and T_4:T_3 ratio of these compounds are variable, making consistent dosing difficult.

Twice-daily administration of T_4 at a dosage of 0.02 mg/kg q 12 hours is recommended initially. If clinical signs resolve and T_4 concentrations are within the therapeutic range after 4 to 8 weeks of therapy, the frequency of T_4 administration can be decreased to once daily. Because of Individual variability in T_4 absorption and serum half-life, the dose should be adjusted based on the measured serum T_4 concentration 4 to 6 hours after dosing. Therapeutic monitoring also minimizes the effect of any differences in potency and bioavailability between different brands of L-thyroxine. For otherwise healthy adult dogs, TT_4 concentration should be at the high end or slightly above the reference range 4 to 6 hours after dosing; however, therapy should be individualized based on clinical response, presence of concurrent illness, age, and concurrent drug administration. Improvement in activity should be evident within the first 1 to 2 weeks of treatment; weight loss should be evident within 8 weeks. Achievement of a normal hair coat may take several months and the coat may initially appear worse as telogen hairs are shed. Neurologic deficits improve rapidly after treatment but complete resolution may take 8 to 12 weeks.

Treatment in presence of concurrent illness Concurrent illness is common in the geriatric population. The appropriate therapeutic range for hypothyroid dogs with concurrent nonthyroidal illness or that are being treated with drugs such as phenobarbital is unknown but is likely lower than the range for healthy dogs. Concurrent measurement of serum TSH concentration may be helpful in interpretation of the post-pill TT_4 concentration. A TSH concentration that persists above the reference range suggests inadequate supplementation or poor owner compliance; conversely, if the TSH is suppresssed and clinical signs have resolved, it is not necessary to increase the L-T_4 dose to drive the post-pill T4 concentration into the therapeutic range, especially in geriatric patients. Unfortunately, current assays for TSH are not sensitive enough to identify dogs that are oversupplemented with L-T_4 .

Caution should be used when initiating treatment with thyroid hormone in certain disease states. Thyroid hormone supplementation increases myocardial oxygen demand and may cause cardiac decompensation in dogs with underlying heart disease. For this reason, the initial dose of L-T_4 should be 25% to 50% of the usual starting dose. The dose may then be increased incrementally based on the results of therapeutic monitoring and reevaluation of cardiac function. In dogs with concurrent hypoadrenocorticism, replacement of mineralocorticoid and glucocorticoid deficiency should be initiated before treatment with L-T_4, because increased basal metabolic rate after supplementation may exacerbate electrolyte disturbances.

Treatment failure Incorrect diagnosis of hypothyroidism is the most common reason for treatment failure. Diseases such as hyperadrenocorticism, atopy, and flea hypersensitivity may have clinical signs similar to those of hypothyroidism and may be associated with decreased thyroid hormone concentrations. Many other disorders result in physiologically appropriate decreases in thyroid hormone concentrations. Other less common reasons for a poor response to treatment include poor absorption of T_4 from the gastrointestinal tract or problems with owner compliance. These situations can be identified by therapeutic monitoring.

Canine Thyroid Neoplasia

Canine thyroid tumors are the most common endocrine tumors in dogs and comprise 1.1% of all canine neoplasms.[43] Breeds at increased risk include the beagle, golden retriever, and Siberian husky, and there is no sex predisposition. The risk of thyroid cancer is highest in dogs between 10 and 15 years of age. Clinically significant canine thyroid tumors are usually large, nonfunctional, unilateral, invasive, and malignant, and most are follicular carcinomas or adenocarcinomas, with only 9% being adenomas.[43] Neoplasms metastatic to the thyroid gland are rare. Hypothyroidism is reported in 18% to 35% of malignant thyroid tumors, while 5% to 20% of canine thyroid carcinomas cause hyperthyroidism. Canine thyroid carcinoma is characterized by local tissue invasion and a high rate of metastasis, particularly to the lungs, retropharyngeal lymph nodes, and the liver.

Clinical signs

Clinical signs are most commonly due to a space occupying cervical mass. Affected dogs may exhibit dyspnea, coughing, dysphagia, retching, anorexia, facial edema, and dysphonia. Other clinical signs include vomiting, listlessness, and weight loss. In dogs with functional thyroid tumors, polyuria and polydipsia, restless behavior, polyphagia, weight loss, diarrhea, and tachycardia may be observed. Signs of hypothyroidism may be present if there is complete bilateral thyroid destruction. Physical examination findings include a firm, usually asymmetric mass in the cervical region and often submandibular lymphadenopathy. Dyspnea, cachexia, and neck pain occur less commonly. Cardiac arrhythmias or murmurs may be detected in hyperthyroid dogs.

Diagnosis

Mild nonregenerative anemia, leukocytosis, mild azotemia, and increased serum liver enzyme activities are typical findings on the minimum database. Hypercalcemia may occur due to concurrent primary hyperparathyroidism or as a paraneoplastic syndrome. Thoracic and abdominal radiographs and abdominal ultrasound may identify heart-based, pulmonary, hepatic, or visceral metastases. Up to 60% of dogs with thyroid carcinoma have radiographic evidence of pulmonary metastasis at the time of diagnosis. Cervical ultrasound and computed tomography may be useful in determining the extent of tumor invasion. Thyroid testing is indicated to determine thyroid status. Increased serum thyroid hormone concentrations due to the presence of autoantibodies to T_3 or T_4, are an important differential for increased serum TT_4 concentration.

Sodium pertechnetate is the isotope of choice for imaging of thyroid tumors.[44] Dogs with nonfunctional thyroid carcinomas tend to have poorly circumscribed heterogeneous isotope uptake. Dogs with functional carcinomas usually have intense, well-circumscribed, homogeneous uptake of isotope. Fine-needle aspiration cytology is useful to differentiate thyroid tumors from abscesses, cysts, mucoceles, and lymph node; however, cytology is not helpful in definitively differentiating benign from malignant thyroid neoplasia. Aspirates may be nondiagnostic due to peripheral blood contamination. Use of larger biopsy instruments, such as a large-bore needle or biopsy needle, is not recommended because most thyroid tumors are highly vascular. A surgical biopsy is necessary for differentiation between a thyroid adenoma and carcinoma. If the mass is clearly not amenable to complete surgical excision, an incisional wedge biopsy should be obtained.

Treatment
Surgical resection is the initial treatment of choice for dogs with thyroid tumors, regardless of the functional status of the tumor.[45] Thyroid tumors that are mobile and well circumscribed are the best surgical candidates. Even if complete removal of the tumor is not possible, surgery provides tissue samples for histopathology and may also alleviate some of the clinical signs associated with the tumor. Surgical risks relate to the high vascularity of thyroid tumors and the risk of damage to the recurrent laryngeal nerves, parathyroid glands, and major blood vessels. In dogs with extensive local tumor infiltration or with distant metastases, surgical resection is strictly palliative. Radiation therapy, radioiodine therapy, or adjunctive chemotherapy should be considered in these patients.

External beam radiation therapy is effective for local control of thyroid tumors but is ineffective in prevention of metastatic disease.[46] Treatment with ^{131}I is a viable alternative to external beam irradiation in tumors that concentrate iodine.[47,48] Canine thyroid carcinoma has a guarded prognosis due to the propensity for both local tissue invasion and metastasis to distant sites. Chemotherapy alone is unlikely to result in total remission of thyroid carcinoma. Doxorubicin, cisplatin, and combination therapy utilizing doxorubicin, cyclophosphamide, and vincristine have been used empirically to treat thyroid carcinoma in the dog.

FELINE THYROID DYSFUNCTION

The most common thyroid disorder of geriatric cats is hyperthyroidism due to thyroid adenoma or hyperplasia. Hyperthyroidism due to thyroid carcinoma occurs in less than 2% of hyperthyroid cats, while nonfunctional thyroid neoplasia is extremely rare. Spontaneous hypothyroidism is extremely rare in cats but hypothyroidism may occur following treatment of hyperthyroidism.

Feline Hyperthyroidism

Feline hyperthyroidism is the most common endocrine disease of geriatric cats with a reported hospital prevalence of 3%.[49] The clinical syndrome is due to autonomous secretion of thyroid hormones by the thyroid gland. Histopathology of affected thyroids usually reveals thyroid adenomatous hyperplasia or benign thyroid adenoma. Pathologic changes may affect one or both lobes of the thyroid gland and in 70% of cats the changes are bilateral. Ectopic hyperplastic thyroid tissue is present in up to 20% of cats.

Pathogenesis
Case-control studies have identified risk factors for hyperthyroidism in cats including age, breed (pure bred cats are at decreased risk), use of cat litter (may be a surrogate for indoor lifestyle), and consumption of an increased proportion of canned cat food in the diet. It is currently believed that the cause is multifactorial with numerous nutritional and environmental risk factors such as ingestion of goitrogenic compounds like phalates and bisphenol, high intake of dietary soy, and decreased or increased

intake of dietary iodine potentially playing a role.[50] The cumulative effects of these exposures over many years may lead to mutations in thyroid follicular cells that ultimately result in autonomous thyroid hormone secretion. Mutations that have been identified in thyroid tissue from hyperthyroid cats include TSH receptor gene and G protein mutations.[50]

Epidemiology
Feline hyperthyroidism is a disease of geriatric cats with a mean age of 13 years. The range of age is 6 to 25 years of age, so occasionally the diagnosis is made in a young or middle-aged cat.[51] Most studies have shown no sex or breed predisposition, although pure bred cats are underrepresented and female cats may be at increased risk.[49]

Clinical signs
Clinical signs include weight loss, diarrhea, chronic vomiting, polyphagia, polyuria, polydipsia, muscle weakness, poor hair coat, and hyperactivity. Anorexia and lethargy are reported in some patients. Additional findings on physical examination include tachycardia, heart murmur, tachypnea, cardiac arrhythmias, dehydration, and a palpable thyroid nodule. Other disorders common in older cats such as renal failure, congestive heart failure, gastrointestinal disease, and diabetes mellitus may mimic some of the clinical signs of hyperthyroidism.

Diagnosis
Since hyperthyroidism is a geriatric disease, it is important to investigate for the presence of concurrent disease and to take into account the special needs of geriatric patients when planning therapy. The minimum database should include a detailed history and physical examination, serum TT_4 concentration, complete blood count, biochemical profile, thoracic radiographs, and arterial blood pressure. Other diagnostic tests indicated in some patients include cardiac ultrasound, abdominal ultrasound, ophthalmologic examination, and electrocardiogram. A technetium scan is recommended in hyperthyroid cats undergoing surgical thyroidectomy.

Polycythemia or a stress leukogram may be present on the complete blood count. A biochemical panel usually reveals mild to moderate increases in alanine aminotransferase, aspartate aminotransferase, and alkaline phosphatase. As much as 80% of the increased alkaline phosphatase is due to the bone isoenzyme of alkaline phosphatase.[52] Other common findings include azotemia, hyperphosphatemia, hypokalemia, and increased fasting ammonia concentration.[53] Approximately 10% of cats are azotemic at time of diagnosis and 50% have increased protein:creatinine ratio.[51] Thoracic radiographs may reveal cardiomegaly, pleural effusion, pulmonary edema, pericardial effusion, or concurrent diseases such primary or metastatic neoplasia. Echocardiography usually shows abnormalities consistent with mild hypertrophic cardiomyopathy; however, more severe heart disease is sometimes present. The most common abnormalities on electrocardiogram are sinus tachycardia and increased amplitude of the R wave (lead II). Hypertension is diagnosed in approximately 15% of cats and is significantly correlated with decreased survival time.[51]

TT_4 **concentration** Diagnosis of hyperthyroidism can usually be confirmed by measurement of a single serum TT_4 concentration. In cats with early hyperthyroidism or with concurrent nonthyroidal illness, the TT_4 concentration may be within the upper half of the reference range. If the TT_4 is high normal or borderline, the measurement should be repeated after concurrent diseases have been treated and resolved, or after a period of 4 to 8 weeks, because hyperthyroidism is a chronic progressive disease and serum TT_4 concentrations increase over time. In cases in which a immediate diagnosis is necessary, a fT_4 concentration, T_3 suppression test, or nuclear scintigraphy should be considered.

fT_4 concentration Measurement of fT_4 concentration is slightly more sensitive than the TT_4 concentration for diagnosis of hyperthyroidism; however, some euthyroid cats with concurrent illness have false-positive increases in fT_4 concentration, with resultant poor specificity (Table 6).[54] Thus, the fT_4 concentration should only be interpreted in the context of the TT_4 concentration. If the TT_4 is at the high end of the reference range and the $freeT_4$ is high, a diagnosis of hyperthyroidism can be confirmed. Most cats with a low T_4 concentration and a high fT_4 concentration are not hyperthyroid. If there is strong clinical suspicion of hyperthyroidism, further diagnostic testing such as the T_3 suppression test or technetium scan should be considered.

T_3 suppression test Baseline T_3 and T_4 concentrations are measured and then synthetic liothyronine (T_3) is administered at a dose of 25 μg/cat orally q 8 hours for 7 treatments. T_3 and T_4 concentrations are then measured again 2 to 6 hours after the last treatment. In euthyroid cats, the second T_4 concentration should be less than 1.5 μg/dL or more than 50% lower than the baseline T_4 concentration.[55] Cats with hyperthyroidism fail to suppress. T_3 concentrations are measured before and after T_3 administration to confirm good client compliance and adequate absorption of the drug.

Technetium scan In cats with suspected hyperthyroidism that have severe concurrent illness, a radioisotope scan using sodium pertechnetate is the most reliable diagnostic test for confirmation of hyperthyroidism.[55] As many as 20% of hyperthyroid cats have ectopic thyroid tissue on scintigraphy.[56]

Treatment
Treatment options for feline hyperthyroidism include oral antithyroid therapy, radioactive iodine therapy, surgical thyroidectomy, and dietary iodine restriction. The choice of treatment depends on the presence of other disease states, the age of the cat, the cat's tolerance for hospitalization, tolerance of antithyroid medications, owner preference, and the results of other diagnostic tests (eg, cardiac evaluation, technetium scan).

Antithyroid drugs (thiourylenes) Methimazole is the most common antithyroid drug used in cats in North America. Carbimazole is a prodrug of methimazole that is the most frequently used antithyroid drug in Europe. Treatment with methimazole is indicated in cats with concurrent medical problems, for test therapy in patients with suspected renal dysfunction, and in cases with financial limitations. Methimazole should be initiated at an initial dose of 2.5 mg po q 8 to 12 hours and then titrated to effect. The final dose required ranges from 2.5 to 20 mg/d, and most cats respond within 2 to 3 weeks of starting therapy. The most common adverse effects seen in 20% of cats are anorexia, vomiting, and lethargy. Transdermal administration of methimazole is associated with a lower risk of gastrointestinal side effects.[57] Mild hematologic abnormalities such as leukopenia, lymphocytosis, and eosinophilia are relatively common. More severe hematologic abnormalities such as severe neutropenia and thrombocytopenia occur in a small percentage of cats. Rarely, excoriation of the head and neck, toxic hepatopathy, and bleeding diatheses may occur. Monitoring recommendations for cats treated with methimazole include a complete blood count, platelet count, biochemical profile, and TT_4 concentration every 2 weeks for the first 3 months of therapy. The timing of sample collection for evaluation of TT_4 concentration in relation to time of administration of medication does not appear to be important in assessing response to methimazole.[58] The advantages of antithyroid drugs include low cost and reversibility of the antithyroid effect. Disadvantages include the risk of adverse effects, failure to respond in some patients, poor owner compliance, and control rather than cure of disease. Methimazole is commonly used to evaluate the effect of treatment upon renal function because treatment of hyperthyroidism may unmask underlying renal disease. If indicators of renal function remain stable during treatment with methimazole, it is more likely that definitive therapy will be well tolerated. If clinical signs of renal failure develop or there is a significant worsening of azotemia after establishing euthyroidism, definitive therapy with ^{131}I or thyroidectomy should be avoided and consideration should be given to long-term medical management.

Radioactive iodine ^{131}I is the radionuclide of choice for the treatment of hyperthyroidism. The isotope has a half-life of 8 days and is a beta and gamma emitter. [131]I is administered intravenously or subcutaneously at either a fixed dose (usually 4–6 mCi) or a calculated dose based on the weight of the cat, the size of the thyroid gland, and the T_4 concentration. It is usually recommended that antithyroid drugs are discontinued 7 to 14 days prior to treatment; however, current evidence does not support this recommendation.[59] After injection, ^{131}I is taken up by thyroid follicular cells and concentrated in the colloid. Emission of β particles destroys functional thyroid tissue without causing damage to normal tissues such as the parathyroid glands. Normal thyroid tissue is spared because it is atrophic and does not concentrate iodine. Thyroid hormone concentrations decline in 5 to 10 days, and clinical improvement is usually observed within 2 weeks, although in some cats the response may be delayed. Treatment with ^{131}I is safe and does not require anesthesia; there is no risk of iatrogenic hypoparathyroidism; and thyroid tissue or metastatic thyroid carcinoma can be effectively treated. In cats with thyroid carcinoma, doses of 20 to 30 mCi are used. Disadvantages of ^{131}I are expense, lack of histopathologic evaluation of thyroid tissue, and requirement for isolation for several days after treatment. Radioactive iodine is the treatment of choice for most hyperthyroid cats; however, it should be avoided in patients with other serious medical problems that require therapy during isolation, in cats with renal failure that worsens after treatment with antithyroid drugs, and in patients that do not tolerate hospitalization.

Thyroidectomy Surgical thyroidectomy is less commonly performed for treatment of hyperthyroid cats because of the increasing availability of radioactive iodine treatment. Disadvantages include the need for general anesthesia, the risk of iatrogenic hypoparathyroidism or hypothyroidism after bilateral thyroidectomy, potential for ectopic thyroid tissue,[56] and morbidity associated with the surgical procedure. The advantages include rapid response to treatment, short hospital stay, convenience in the private practice setting, and the opportunity histopathologic evaluation of thyroid tissue. Indications for thyroidectomy are cats with suspected thyroid carcinoma and cats with unilateral thyroid disease confirmed by nuclear scintigraphy.

Iodine restriction Dietary iodine restriction to less than 0.32 parts per million reduces the circulating thyroid hormone concentrations into the normal range in hyperthyroid cats and has potential as a long-term management strategy.[60] Long-term outcome in cats managed by dietary iodine restriction alone has yet to be determined.

Prognosis

Retrospective studies suggest that age, proteinuria, and hypertension are associated with decreased survival times in treated hyperthyroid cats.[51] Cats treated with methimazole alone had a shorter median survival time than cats treated with radioactive iodine alone or methimazole followed by radioactive iodine.[61]

Iatrogenic hypothyroidism contributes to azotemia after treatment of hyperthyroid cats and is associated with reduced survival times.

Hypothyroidism

Hypothyroidism may occur after bilateral thyroidectomy or radioactive iodine therapy. Clinical signs include anorexia, lethargy, weight gain, poor hair coat, and alopecia. In most cases, hypothyroidism is transient and resolves within weeks of treatment, but persistent hypothyroidism 6 months after treatment contributes to azotemia and is associated with reduced survival time.[63]

Nonfunctional thyroid nodules

In older cats, it is not uncommon to palpate an enlarged thyroid gland in an apparently healthy cat. Possible differential diagnoses include early hyperthyroidism in which a goiter is present but the thyroid gland is not fully autonomous, thyroid cyst, thyroid cystadenoma, or nonfunctional thyroid adenoma or carcinoma.[62,63] Nonfunctional thyroid carcinoma is rare in the cat. If an obvious cervical nodule is palpated in a cat with a normal T_4 concentration, a fine needle aspirate should be considered to determine the tissue of origin. Unfortunately, the accuracy of thyroid cytology for differentiation of benign from malignant thyroid disease is poor.

SUMMARY

The effects of age, concurrent illness, and administered medications complicate the diagnosis of thyroid dysfunction in geriatric patients. Interpretation of thyroid hormone testing should take these factors into account. The most common thyroid disorder in dogs is acquired hypothyroidism. Tests that are most useful in evaluation in dogs with suspected hypothyroidism are TT_4, fT_4, and TSH concentration. Therapeutic monitoring should be utilized for monitoring treatment of canine hypothyroidism. The therapeutic range for TT_4 in geriatric dogs with concurrent illness is likely to be lower than that for younger healthy adult dogs. The most common thyroid disorder in cats is benign hyperthyroidism. Diagnosis is most often complicated by the presence of concurrent illness. Treatment should be individualized based on individual case characteristics and presence of concurrent illness. Some older cats have a palpable goiter months to years before development of clinical signs of hyperthyroidism.

REFERENCES

1. Kaplan EM, Hays MT, Ferguson DC. Thyroid hormone metabolism: a comparative evaluation. Vet Clin N Am Small Anim Pract 1994;24(3):431–63.
2. Gonzalez E, Quadri SK. Effects of aging on the pituitary-thyroid axis in the dog. Exp Gerontol 1988;23:151–60.
3. Reimers TJ, Lawler DF, Sutaria PM, et al. Effects of age, sex, and body size on serum concentrations of thyroid and adrenocortical hormones in dogs. Am J Vet Res 1990;51(3):454–7.

4. Lawler DF, Ballam JM, Meadows R, et al. Influence of lifetime food restriction on physiological variables in Labrador retriever dogs. Exp Gerontol 2007;42:204–14.

5. Panciera DL, Helfand SC, Soergel A. Acute effects of continuous infusions of human recombinant interleukin-2 on serum thyroid hormone concentrations in dogs. Res Vet Sci J 1995;58:96–7.

6. Elliott DA, King LG, Zerbe CA. Thyroid hormone concentrations in critically ill canine intensive care patients. J Vet Emerg Crit Care 1995;5:17–23.

7. Mooney CT, Shiel RE, Dixon RM. Thyroid hormone abnormalities in dogs with non-thyroidal illness. J Small Anim Pract 2008;49:11–6.

8. Tidholm A, Falk T, Gundler S, et al. Effect of thyroid hormone supplementation on survival of euthyroid dogs with congestive heart failure due to systolic myocardial dysfunction: a double-blind placebo controlled trial. Res Vet Sci 2003;75:195–201.

9. Kantrowitz LB, Peterson ME, Melián C, et al. Serum total thyroxine, total triiodothyronine, free thyroxine, and thyrotropin concentrations in dogs with nonthyroidal illness. J Am Vet Med Assoc 2001;219:765–9.

10. Nelson RW, Ihle SL, Feldman EC, et al. Serum free thyroxine concentrations in healthy dogs, dogs with hypothyroidism, and euthyroid dogs with concurrent illness. J Am Vet Med Assoc 1991;198:1401–7.

11. Ferguson DC, Peterson ME. Serum free and total iodothyronine concentrations in dogs with hyperadrenocorticism. Am J Vet Res 1992;53:1636–40.

12. Panciera DL, Refsal KR. Thyroid function in dogs with spontaneous and induced congestive heart failure. Can J Vet Res 1994;58:157–62.

13. Von Klopman T, Boettcher IC, Rotermund A, et al. Euthyroid sick syndrome in dogs with idiopathic epilepsy before treatment with anticonvulsant drugs. J Vet Intern Med 2006;20:516–22.

14. Vail DM, Panciera DL, Ogilvie GK. Thyroid hormone concentrations in dogs with chronic weight loss with special reference to cancer cachexia. J Vet Intern Med 1994;8:122–7.

15. Wood MA, Panciera DL, Berry SH, et al. Influence of isoflurane general anesthesia or anesthesia and surgery on thyroid function tests in dogs. J Vet Intern Med 2009;23:7–15.

16. Gulickers KP, Panciera DL. Influence of various medications on canine thyroid function. Compend Cont Educ Pract Vet 2002;24:511–23.

17. Daminet S, Ferguson DC. Influence of drugs on thyroid function in dogs. J Vet Intern Med 2003;17:463–72.

18. Sauve F, Paradis M, Refsal KR, et al. Effects of oral administration of meloxicam, carprofen, and a nutraceutical on thyroid function in dogs with osteoarthritis. Can Vet J 2003;44:474–9.

19. Daminet S, Croubels S, Duchateau, et al. Influence of acetylsalicylic acid and ketoprofen on canine thyroid function tests. Vet J 2003;166:224–32.

20. Panciera DI, Refsal KR, Sennello KA, et al. Effects of deracoxib and aspirin on serum concentrations of thyroxine, 3,5,3′-triiodothyronine, free thyroxine, and thyroid stimulating hormone in healthy dogs. Am J Vet Res 2006;67(4):599–603.

21. Gulickers KP, Panceria DL. Evaluation of the effects of clomipramine on canine thyroid function tests. J Vet Intern Med 2003;17:44–9.

22. Frank LA, Hnilica KA, May ER, et al. Effects of sulfamethazole-trimethoprim on thyroid function in dogs. Am J Vet Res 2005;66(2):256–9.

23. Shiel RE, Brennan SF, Omodo-Eluk, et al. Thyroid hormone concentrations in young healthy pretraining greyhounds. Vet Rec 2007;161:616–9.

24. Shiel E, Nally E, Mooney T. Qualitative and semi-quantitative assessment of thyroxine binding globulin in the greyhound and other dog breeds. J Vet Intern Med 2011;25:1494 [ECVIM Abstract EN-O-15].

25. Shiel RE, Sist M, Nachreiner RF, et al. Assessment of criteria used by veterinary practitioners to diagnose hypothyroidism in sighthounds and investigation of serum thyroid hormone concentrations in healthy salukis. J Am Vet Med Assoc 2010;236 (3) 302–8.

26. Panacova L, Koch H, Kolb S. Thyroid testing in sloughis. J Vet Intern Med 2008;22: 1144–8.

27. Gaughan KR, Bruyette DS. Thyroid function testing in greyhounds. Am J Vet Res 2001;62:1130–3.

28. Van Geffen C, Bavegems V, Duchateau L, et al. Serum thyroid hormone concentrations and thyroglobulin autoantibodies in trained and non-trained healthy whippets. Vet J 2006;172(1):135–40.

29. Lee JA, Hinchcliff KW, Piercy RJ, et al. Effects of racing and nontraining on plasma thyroid hormone concentrations in sled dogs. J Am Vet Med Assoc 2004;224(2): 226–31.

30. Evason MD, Carr AF, Taylor SM. Alterations in thyroid hormone concentrations in healthy sled dogs before and after athletic conditioning. Am J Vet Res 2004;65(3): 333–7.

31. Panciera DL, Hinchcliff KW, Olson J, et al. Plasma thyroid hormone concentrations in dogs competing in a long-distance sled race. J Vet Intern Med 2003;17:593–6.

32. Graham PA, Refsal KR, Nachreiner RF. Etiopathologic findings of canine hypothyroidism. Vet Clin N Am Small Anim Pract 2007;37(4):617–31.

33. Benjamin SA, Stephens LC, Hamilton BF, et al. Associations between lymphocytic thyroiditis, hypothyroidism, and thyroid neoplasia in beagles. Vet Pathol 1996;33: 486–94.

34. Scott-Moncrieff JC, Nelson RW, Campbell KL, et al. Accuracy of serum free thyroxine concentrations determined by a new veterinary chemiluminescent immunoassay in euthyroid and hypothyroid dogs. J Vet Intern Med 2011;25:1493–4 [ECVIM Abstract EN-O-14].

35. Peterson ME, Melian C, Nichols R. Measurement of serum total thyroxine, triiodothyronine, free thyroxine, and thyrotropin concentrations for diagnosis of hypothyroidism in dogs. J Am Vet Med Assoc 1997;211:1396–402.

36. Dixon RM, Mooney CT. Evaluation of serum free thyroxine and thyrotropin concentrations in the diagnosis of canine hypothyroidism. J Small Anim Pract 1999;40:72–8.

37. Scott-Moncrieff JC, et al. Serum thyrotropin concentrations in healthy dogs, hypothyroid dogs, and euthyroid dogs with concurrent disease. J Am Vet Med Assoc 1998;212:387–91.

38. Boretti FS, Sieber-Ruckstuhl NS, Wenger-Riggenbach B, et al. Comparison of 2 doses of recombinant human thyrotropin for thyroid function testing in healthy and suspected hypothyroid dogs. J Vet Intern Med 2009;23:856–61.

39. Diaz Espineira MM, Mol JA, Peeters ME, et al. Assessment of thyroid function in dogs with low plasma thyroxine concentration. J Vet Intern Med 2007;21:25–32.

40. Nachreiner RF, Refsal KR, Graham PA, et al. prevalence of autoantibodies to thyroglobulin in dogs with non-thyroidal illness. Am J Vet Res 1998;59:951–5.

41. Nachreiner RF, Refsal KR, Graham PA, et al. prevalence of serum thyroid hormone autoantibodies in dogs with clinical signs of hypothyroidism. J Am Vet Med Assoc 2002;220:466–71.

42. Le Traon G, Burgaud S, Horspool L, et al. Pharmacokinetics of total thyroxine in dogs after administration of an oral solution of levothyroxine sodium. J Vet Pharmacol Ther 2008;31:95–101.

43. Wucherer KI, Wilke V. Thyroid cancer in dogs: an update based on 636 cases (1995–2005). J Am Anim Hosp Assoc 2010;46:249–54.

44. Marks SL, Koblik PD, Hornof WJ, et al. ^{99m}Tc-pertechnetate imaging of thyroid tumors in dogs: 29 cases (1980–1992). J Am Vet Med Assoc 1994;204(5):756–60.
45. Klein MK, Powers BE, Withrow SJ, et al. Treatment of thyroid carcinoma in dogs by surgical resection alone: 20 cases (1981–1989). J Am Vet Med Assoc 1995;206(7): 1007–9.
46. Theon AP, Marks SL, Feldman ES, et al. Prognostic factors and patterns of treatment failure in dogs with unresectable differentiated thyroid carcinomas treated with megavoltage irradiation. J Am Vet Med Assoc 2000;216(11):1775–9.
47. Turrel JM, McEntee MC, Burke BP, et al. Sodium iodide ^{131}I treatment of dogs with nonresectable thyroid tumors: 39 cases (1990–2003). J Am Vet Med Assoc 2006; 229(4):542–8.
48. Worth AJ, Zuber RM, Hocking M. Radioiodide (^{131}I) therapy for the treatment of canine thyroid carcinoma. Aust Vet J 2005;83:208–14.
49. Edinboro CH, Scott-Moncrieff JC, Janovitz E, et al. Epidemiological study of relationships between consumption of commercial canned cat food and risk of hyperthyroidism in cats. J Am Vet Med Assoc 2004;224:879–86.
50. Peterson ME, Ward CR. Etiopathologic findings of hyperthyroidism in cats. Vet Clin N Am Small Anim Pract 2007;37(4):633–45.
51. Williams TL, Peak KJ, Brodbelt D, et al. Survival and development of azotemia after treatment of hyperthyroid cats. J Vet Intern Med 2010;24:863–9.
52. Archer FJ, Taylor SM. Alkaline phosphatase bone isoenzyme and osteocalcin in the serum of hyperthyroid cats. Can Vet J 1996;37:735–9.
53. Berent AC, Drobatz KJ, Ziemer L, et al. Liver function in cats with hyperthyroidism before and after ^{131}I therapy. J Vet Intern Med 2007;21:1217–23.
54. Peterson ME, Broome MR, Robertson JE. Accuracy of serum free thyroxine concentrations determined by a new veterinary chemiluminescent immunoassay in euthyroid and hypothyroid dogs [abstract]. Proceedings of the 21st ECVIM-CA Congress. Seville (Spain), September 8–10, 2011. Poster No. EN-P-3. p. 239.
55. Shiel RE, Mooney CT. Testing for hyperthyroidism in cats. Vet Clin N Am Small Anim Pract 2007;37(4):672–91.
56. Harvey AM, Hibbert A, Barrett EL. Scintigraphic findings in 120 hyperthyroid cats. J Fel Med Surg 2009;11:96–106.
57. Sartor LL, Trepanier LA, Kroll MM, et al. Efficacy and safety of transdermal methimazole in the treatment of cats with hyperthyroidism. J Vet Intern Med 2004;18:651–5.
58. Rutland BF, Nachreiner RF, Kruger JM. Optimal testing for thyroid hormone concentration after treatment with methimazole in healthy and hyperthyroid cats. J Vet Intern Med 2009;23:1025–30.
59. Omann R, Lunn KF. Outcome of radioactive iodine therapy in cats receiving recent methimazole therapy [abstract]. J Vet Intern Med 2011;25:684.
60. Melendez LM, Yamka RM, Forrester SD. Titration of dietary iodine for reducing serum thyroxine concentrations in newly diagnosed hyperthyroid cats [abstract]. J Vet Intern Med 2011;25:683.
61. Milner RJ, Channell CD, Levy JK, et al. Survival times for cats with hyperthyroidism treated with iodine 131, methimazole, or both: 167 cases. J Am Vet Med Assoc 2006;228:559–63.
62. Wakeling J, Smith K, Scase T, et al. Subclinical hyperthyroidism in cats: a spontaneous model of subclinical toxic nodular goiter in humans? Thyroid 2007;17:1201–9.
63. Phillips DE, Radinsky MG, Fischer JR, et al. Cystic thyroid and parathyroid lesions in cats. J Am Anim Hosp Assoc 2003;39:349–54.

Painful Decisions for Senior Pets

Steven M. Fox, MS, DVM, MBA, PhD[a,b,c,d,*]

KEYWORDS

- Geriatric • Senior pet • Osteoarthritis • Degenerative joint disease • Cancer
- Pain management

KEY POINTS

- A mechanism-based approach to pain management is the most productive way to make significant advancements.
- Osteoarthritis is a "total joint disease," with many different tissue types contributing to the pain response.
- Cyclooxygenase-2, prostaglandin E_2, interleukin-1β, matrix metalliproteinase-13, inducible nitric oxide synthase, and tumor necrosis factor-α are all major players in the catabolic process of degenerative joint disease.
- Osteoarthritis cannot be cured, but can be managed quite effectively with a multi-modal approach.
- As cancer progresses, changing factors may complicate the pain state. Only through an understanding of the mechanisms associated with dynamic cancer pain, can we manage patients' pain with evidence-based confidence.

In 2010, Fleming and colleagues[1] reported on the mortality patterns of North American dogs. Their findings revealed that older dogs tend to die from neurologic and neoplastic causes. In addition, although neoplastic processes were the leading cause of death among adult dogs in the study, degenerative processes ranked 6th overall. Further, increasing breed size was associated with increasing risk of death because of musculoskeletal (or gastrointestinal) system disease. These data suggest a focus on pain management of degenerative joint disease and cancer in the senior/geriatric pet.

MALADAPTIVE PAIN

Pain is both a good and potentially very bad phenomenon. From an advantageous perspective, pain is an early warning sign that we should avoid potential tissue

The author has nothing to disclose.
[a] Fox Third Bearing Inc, 10821 Forest Avenue, Clive, IA 50325, USA; [b] University of Illinois, Urbana, IL 61801, USA; [c] University of Tennessee, Knoxville, TN 37996, USA; [d] Massey University, Palmerston North, New Zealand
* Fox Third Bearing Inc, 10821 Forest Avenue, Clive, IA 50325, USA.
E-mail address: sfoxk9doc@aol.com

Vet Clin Small Anim 42 (2012) 727–748
http://dx.doi.org/10.1016/j.cvsm.2012.04.010
0195-5616/12/$ – see front matter © 2012 Elsevier Inc. All rights reserved.

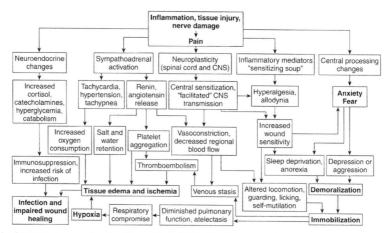

Fig. 1. Consequences of pain. (*From* Muir WM. Physiology and pathophysiology of pain. In: Gaynor JS, Muir WM, editors. Handbook of veterinary pain management. 2nd edition. St Louis (MO): Mosby Elsevier; 2009. p. 31.)

damage. It is the "fight or flight" stimulus. From a negative perspective, pain can lead to stress, distress, and suffering. Maladaptive pain can adversely affect nearly every body system (**Fig. 1**). Our goal should not be to abolish all pain, which is likely not possible in the conscious animal but rather to control maladaptive pain so as to maintain as near normal physiologic functions as is possible and to prevent suffering.

A *mechanism-based approach* to all pathologic conditions, including maladaptive pain, is likely to lead to specific pharmacologic intervention measures for each identified mechanism within a syndrome. Advances in (pain) management are contingent on first determining the symptoms that constitute a syndrome and, then, finding mechanisms for each of these symptoms. The clinical approach for a mechanism-based classification of pain illustrates how a patient with pain could be analyzed from a pain-mechanism perspective (**Fig. 2**). It is the mechanism that needs to be the target for novel drugs, rather than particular disease states. Herein lies the greatest potential for advancement in pain management. However, before addressing mechanism-based pain relief, one needs to review his/her understanding of mechanisms involved in pain.

OSTEOARTHRITIS (DEGENERATIVE JOINT DISEASE)

Osteoarthritis (OA) appears to be mechanically driven, but chemically mediated, with endogenous attempts at aberrant repair. Although clinically apparent, the vicious catabolic/anabolic cycle of OA is not yet comprehensively understood.

Origins of OA Joint Pain

Although the most obvious pathologic changes in an OA joint are usually seen in the articular cartilage, all of the tissues of the joint are involved, including bone, synovium, muscles, nerves, and ligaments. OA is a "total joint" disease.

Degradation and synthesis of cartilage matrix components are related to the release of mediators by chondrocytes and synoviocytes, including the cytokines, interleukin (IL)-1, tumor necrosis factor (TNF), nitric oxide (NO), and growth factors. A minor injury could start the disease process in a less resistant environment, whereas

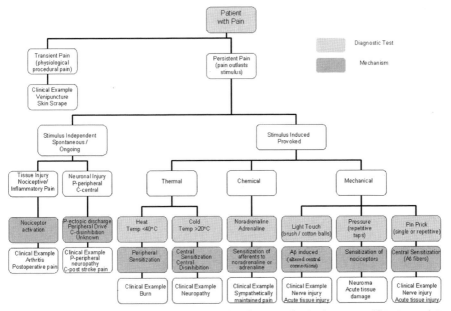

Fig. 2. Clinical approach to a mechanism-based classification of pain. (*From* Woolf CJ, Borsook D, Koltzenburg M. Mechanism-based classifications of pain and analgesic drug discovery. In: Bunter C, Munglani R, Schmidt WK, editors. Pain: current understanding, emerging therapies, and novel approaches to drug discovery. New York: Marcel Dekker; 2003. p. 1–8.)

in other individuals, the joint may be able to compensate for a greater insult. Damage may become irreversible when compensation fails (**Fig. 3**).

For years the focus of OA has been the cartilage; however, the hallmark clinical manifestation of OA is pain (**Fig. 4**), and because cartilage is not innervated and

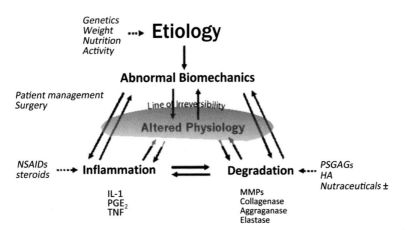

Fig. 3. Etiology of osteoarthritis. Damage may become irreversible when compensation fails. (*From* Fox SM. Pathophysiology of osteoarthritic pain. In: Chronic pain in small animal medicine. London (UK): Manson Publishing; 2010. p. 77.)

A Potentially Viscious Cycle

Joint pain

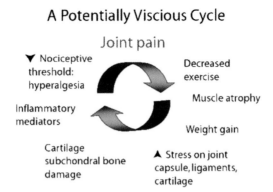

▼ Nociceptive threshold: hyperalgesia

Inflammatory mediators

Cartilage subchondral bone damage

Decreased exercise

Muscle atrophy

Weight gain

▲ Stress on joint capsule, ligaments, cartilage

Fig. 4. Osteoarthritis is a degradative cycle. (*From* Fox SM. Pathophysiology of osteoarthritic pain. In: Chronic pain in small animal medicine. London (UK): Manson Publishing; 2010. p. 76.)

because there is a poor correlation between radiologic signs (narrow joint space and osteophytes) and the occurrence of joint pain, the site of OA pain and the nature of OA pain are of interest (**Table 1**).

In animal studies, most recordings from primary afferent articular nociceptors has been made in either rat or cat, where anatomy of the articular nerves is well understood and the physiologic characteristics of the primary afferent nerve fibers have been investigated.

Inflammatory Mediators Diffuse into the Cartilage via Synovial Fluid

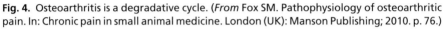

Whereas degradative enzymes and cytokines (cytokines are small cell-signaling protein molecules that are secreted by the glial cell of the nervous system and by numerous cells of the immune system, used extensively in intercellular communication) are normally found within chondrocytes, they are normally inactive or only produced in response to injury. Cytokines further stimulate chondrocytes and synoviocytes to produce and release more degradative enzymes. Cytokines, acting as chemical messengers to maintain the

Table 1
Tissue type and associated pain source

Tissue	Medium of Pain
Hyaline cartilage (?)	Mechanical stress (?)
Subchondral bone	Microfractures, medullary hypertension
Synovium	Inflammation
Osteophytes	Periosteum nerve ending stretch, synovium irritation
Ligaments	Stretch
Enthesis	Inflammation
Joint capsule	Distention, inflammation
Periarticular muscle	Spasm, weakness
Neurons	Decreased threshold, increased response to WDR neurons, silent nociceptor recruitment, central sensitization

Abbreviation: WDR, wide dynamic range.

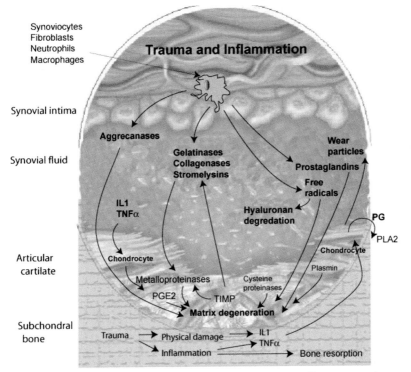

Fig. 5. The catabolic process of osteoarthritis is quite complex, offering several potential quantifiable biomarkers and treatment targets.

chronic phase of inflammation and tissue destruction are upregulated in the OA patient. Collagenases (eg, matrix metalloproteinase [MMP]-13) act on collagen fibers to break down the cartilage framework, while stromelysin (eg, MMP-3) cleaves the aggrecan leading to the loss of matrix proteoglycans (**Fig. 5**).

The lineup of destructive and pathologic factors in OA are extensive (**Table 2**); however, the major players, arguably, are cyclooxygenase (COX)-2, prostaglandin

Table 2	
Inflammatory mediators and their pathologic activity	
Mediator	**Activity**
COX-2	COX-2 gives rise to destructive and painful/inflammatory eicosanoids.
PGE_2	PGE_2 is a major enzyme in the arachidonic acid pathway leading to the pathological features of pain and inflammation.
Il-1β	Il-1β induces hyperalgesia by direct and indirect actions.
MMP-13	MMP-13 cleaves type II collagen of the cartilage matrix.
iNOS	iNOS leads to increased synthesis of NO: associated with cartilage degradation, inhibition of matrix synthesis, and chondrocyte apoptosis.
TNF-α	TNF-α stimulates prostaglandin secretion and increases activity of matrix-degrading proteinases.

(PG)E$_2$, IL-1β, MMP-13, inducible nitric oxide synthase (iNOS), and TNF-α. These inflammatory mediators originate from both the cartilage matrix and the synovium. As the patient loads and unloads the joint with weight-bearing activity, synovial contents move in and out of the cartilage matrix. Herein, the cartilage acts analogous to a sponge emerged in a bucket of water, where the water moves in and out of the sponge as it is squeezed. With weight-loading, inflammatory mediators are forced from the cartilage into the synovial fluid where they contact synovium of the joint intimal lining. Resident synoviocytes respond, like macrophages, producing additional mediators that are released into the synovial fluid. Additional weight-bearing then forces these new (as well as the resident) synovial fluid-bound mediators (back) into the cartilage, as so on. The worse it gets, the worse it gets!

The lineup of destructive and pathologic factors in OA is extensive; however the major players are arguably COX-2, PGE$_2$, IL-1β, MMP-13, iNOS and TNF-α.[2,3] COX-2 is an isozyme of the arachidonic acid (AA) pathway that gives rise to several eicosanoids associated with pain and inflammation—pathologic manifestations of the AA pathway. PGE$_2$ is an end-product of COX-2 metabolism, most frequently recognized for its clinical result in pain and inflammation. IL-1β and TNF-α are the primary cytokines mediating the pathogenesis of OA. Studies have shown that abnormally high levels of IL-1β and TNF-α are present in the synovial fluid, synovium, and cartilage tissue of OA patients.

In vitro studies[4,5] have shown that both IL-1β and TNF-α stimulate secretion of PGs and increase the activity of matrix-degrading proteinases such as collagenase, gelatinase, proteoglycanase, stromelysin, and plasminogen activator. Although IL-1β is physiologically more potent than TNF-α, animal studies[6] suggest the 2 cytokines act synergistically to stimulate cartilage degradation—exceeding the damage observed with either cytokine alone. IL-1β and TNF-α also induce the synthesis of the COX-2 and iNOS enzymes. This leads to elevated levels of PGE$_2$ and NO: upregulating cartilage degradation, inhibition of matrix synthesis, and chondrocyte apoptosis.[7–10] IL-1 also stimulates fibroblasts to produce collagen types I and III. This may contribute to fibrosis of the joint capsule in OA patients.[11]

MMP-13 (collagenase 3) is secreted as an inactive protein, which is activated when cleaved by extracellular proteinases. MMP-13 plays a key role in degradation and remodeling of host extracellular matrix proteins, including degradation of type II collagen. By cleaving the triple helix of type II collagen and core protein of the aggrecan, it induces major irreversible damage to the cartilage matrix structure. In doing so, the biophysical properties of cartilage are modified, reducing its resilience to the abnormal biomechanical forces present in OA. MMP-13 has been shown to be preferentially increased in the deep zone of cartilage (perpendicular zone) and is considered a major catabolic factor in that zone as well as in OA lesional areas.[12–14]

Under the influence of iNOS stimulation by various cytokines, OA cartilage produces an excessive amount of NO. It is proposed[15–20] that NO contributes to the development of arthritic lesions by inhibiting the synthesis of cartilage matrix macromolecules and by inducing chondrocyte death, which could further contribute to the reduction in extracellular matrix in OA. NO is also known to reduce the synthesis of the IL-1 receptor antagonist in chondrocytes, a process possibly responsible for the enhanced IL-1β effect on these cells. Finally, diffusion of NO from the superficial layer of cartilage (tangential zone) to the deeper zone may also contribute to increasing the level of MMP-13 synthesis at the deeper level.[21,22]

Overproduction of cytokines, such as TNF-α, stimulates cartilage matrix degradation by inhibiting the production of proteoglycans and type II collagen while upregulating the production of matrix-degrading enzymes such as MMPs.[23] Such cytokines

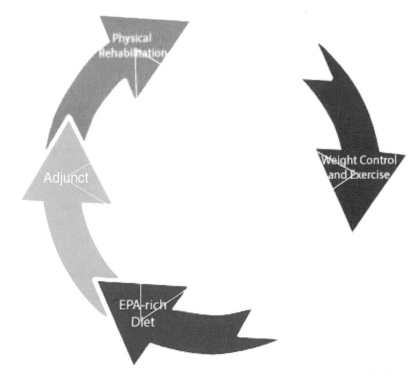

Fig. 6. The multimodal osteoarthritis management "wheel" represents 2 overlapping triangles: pharmaceutical (NSAIDs, chondroprotectant, adjunct drugs) and nonpharmaceutical (weight control and exercise, EPA-rich diet, physical rehabilitation).

also upregulate the expression of COX-2 and iNOS, leading to increased synthesis of PGE_2 and NO.[24,25] Since these inflammatory mediators are the major players in the pathogenesis of OA, they serve as major targets for OA management and treatment. Condroprotective nutraceuticals containing glucosamine, chondroitin sulfate, and avocado soybean unsaponifiables (ASUs) have shown considerable efficacy in abrogating the degradative effect of these mediators when tested in bovine cartilage explants in vitro,[26,27] thereby suggesting their value as prophylaxis in predisposed breeds and in the early stages of OA.

OA cannot be cured but can be managed quite well with a multimodal approach.[28] The multimodal approach suggests 2 overlapping triangles: pharmaceutical (nonsteroidal anti-inflammatory drugs [NSAIDs], chondroprotectant, adjunct drugs) and nonpharmaceutical (weight control and exercise, eicosapentaenoic acid [EPA]-rich diet, physical rehabilitation) (**Fig. 6**).

Intrinsic to the multimodal management concept is that combinations will be synergistic (or at least additive), requiring a reduced amount of each modality and, therefore, there will be less potential for adverse response to any drug in the combination. Selection of drugs within the "cocktail" would be optimal if they collectively blocked all 4 of the physiologic pain processes of transduction, transmission, modulation, and perception. NSAIDs will likely be the foundation for treating canine OA based on their anti-inflammatory, analgesic, and antipyretic properties. They are easy to administer and relatively safe. That said, integration of management

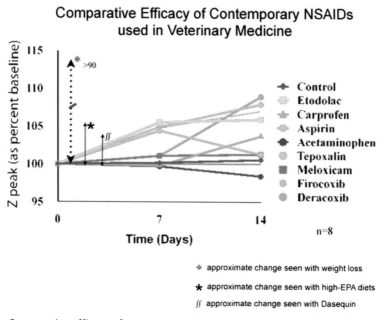

Fig. 7. Comparative efficacy of contemporary NSAIDs, weight loss, high-EPA diets, and ASU nutraceuticals based on force plate gait analysis. (*Data from* Refs.[29–31,77])

modalities can be NSAID-sparing, and some data suggest that the responses to weight loss, high-EPA diet, or ASU nutraceuticals all rival the response seen with NSAIDs as assessed by force plate gait analysis (**Fig. 7**).[29–31] Clinical implementation of the multimodal scheme can be guided by the algorithm provided in **Fig. 8**.

Presuming that cats are "small dogs" in the diagnosis and management of OA is inappropriate. In the cat model of anterior cruciate ligament transsection, the cat quickly (approximately 3 months) reestablishes knee stability, although the progression of OA continues.[32] The actual detailed adaptations responsible for this quick reestablishment of knee stability are not known. It may well be that the disease process in the cat is quite different than in the dog and, accordingly, degenerative joint disease is a much more appropriate term than OA for the cat (**Fig. 9**).

CANCER

The word *cancer* means "crab" and was given to the disease because of its tenacity, a singular ability to cling to its victim like a crab's claws clinging to its prey. The all-important reality of cancer pain is witnessed in John Steinbeck's book *The Grapes of Wrath*, where the character Mrs Wilson, who is dying of cancer, states, "I'm jus' pain covered in skin."

Frank Vertosick, MD, states,[33] "From the Darwinian point of view, cancer is an unimportant disease. Since it preferentially afflicts animals beyond their child-bearing years, cancer poses no threat to animals in the wild, since natural populations experience death in other ways long before they are old enough for cancer to be a concern. We feel the sting of advanced prostate cancer because we are fortunate enough to live into our seventh decade and beyond, a feat rarely achieved even a hundred years ago. During the evolution of the nervous system, we developed pain to

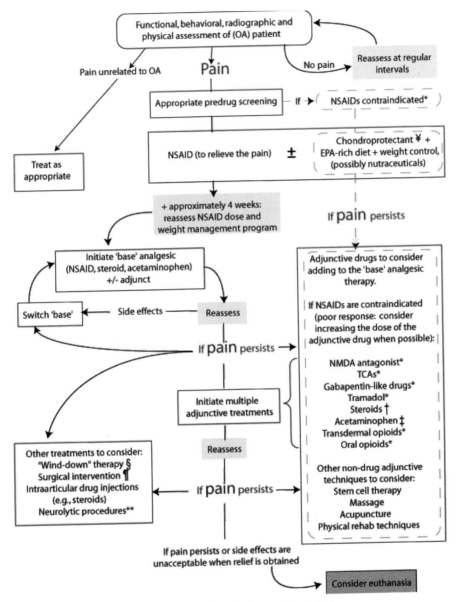

Fig. 8. Algorithm for clinical implementation of the multimodal scheme.

help us heal reversible insults: cracked vertebrae, pinched nerves, temporarily blocked colons, broken legs. To our great sorrow, this same pain also works against us when irreversible diseases like cancer strike; consequently, death becomes a painful affair. We die with all of our pain alarms impotently sounding. It is said that we are all born in another's pain and destined to die in our own."[(pp243–4)] Cancer has become a frightening diagnosis in our culture, and when pets are diagnosed with cancer, the owner's first concern is usually pain.

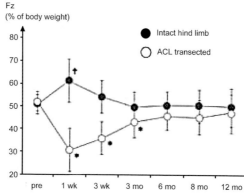

Fig. 9. Approximately 3 months following transsection of the anterior cruciate ligament in the cat's knee, the cat recovers joint stability; however, the disease process of OA progresses. (*From* Maitland ME, Leonard T, Frank CB, et al. Longitudinal measurement of tibial motion relative to the femur during passive displacements in the cat before and after anterior cruciate ligament transection. J Orthop Res 1998;16:448–54.)

Taxonomy

In 1994, the International Association for the Study of Pain (IASP) revised a classification for chronic pain (**Table 3**).[34] This classification includes 5 axes: (1) location of the pain; (2) involved organ or tissue system; (3) temporal pattern of pain; (4) pain intensity and time since onset of pain; and (5) etiology of pain. A distinct group of syndromes, therapies, and other etiologies of pain occur in cancer patients[35] such

Table 3	
Classifications of cancer pain	
Etiologic	Primarily caused by cancer Treatment of malignancy Debility Concurrent pathology
Pathophysiologic	Nociceptive (somatic, visceral) Neuropathic Mixed pathophysiology
Location of cancer pain syndromes	Head and neck Chest Vertebral and radicular pain Abdominal or pelvic Extremity
Temporal	Acute Breakthrough Chronic
Severity-based	Mild Moderate Severe

Data from Eidelman A, Carr DB. Taxonomy of cancer pain. In: de Leon-Casasola OA, editor. Cancer pain: pharmacological, interventional and palliative care approaches. Philadelphia: Saunders Elsevier; 2006. p. 4.

Table 4 Tumors frequently associated with pain	
Tumor	**Remarks**
Bone	Noncompliant tissue tumors are typically painful.
Central nervous system	Tumors arising from neural tissue are not usually painful until late into the course of the disease. Extradural tumors are associated with pain.
Cutaneous (invasive)	Ulcerative, invasive cutaneous tumors tend to be painful.
Gastrointestinal	Distention of the esophagus, stomach, colon, and rectum are painful. Colonic and rectal pain often presents as perineal discomfort.
Intranasal	Bone and turbinate destruction leads to pain.
Intrathoracic and abdominal (eg, mesothelioma, malignant histiocytosis)	Response to intracavity analgesics, such as local analgesics, suggests that these conditions are painful.
Mammary carcinoma (inflammatory)	Dogs consistently show abnormal behavior considered to be pain-induced.
Oral and pharyngeal	Soft tissue tumors of the pharynx and caudal oral cavity are particularly painful, perhaps due to constant irritation from eating. Soft tissue tumors of gingival origin are relatively nonpainful, but become very painful with invasion of bone.
Prostate	This can be quite painful, particularly with bone metastasis.
Surgery	Postoperative pain associated with tumor removal can be greater than anticipated, perhaps due to the presence of neuropathic pain.

Data from Lascelles BDX. Supportive care for the cancer patient. In: Withrow SJ, Vail DM, editors. Withrow & MacEwen's small animal clinical oncology. 4th edition. St Louis (MO): Saunders Elsevier; 2007. p. 292.

that neither the IASP nor any other diagnostic scheme distinguishes cancer pain from nonmalignant causes of chronic pain. Because the classification of cancer pain may have important diagnostic and therapeutic implications, a promising concept is a mechanism-based treatment approach, determining the sequence of analgesic agents based on the underlying causative pathology of cancer pain.

Etiologic Classifications

Some tumor types are more frequently associated with pain (**Table 4**), and four different etiologies of cancer pain are that (1) directly produced by the tumor, (2) due to the various treatment modalities, (3) related to chronic debility, and (4) due to unrelated, concurrent disease processes.[36] Identification of these etiologies is important, as they reflect distinct treatment options and prognoses.

Pain relief from debulking tumors suggests that mechanical distortion of tissues is a component of tumor pain. Compression of a peripheral nerve can cause local demyelination, Wallerian degeneration of the nerve, secondary axon sprouting, and neuroma formation. Physiologic studies have demonstrated that dorsal root ganglion compression can initiate a continuous afferent barrage that becomes self-sustaining. When tumors are identified as a foreign body, they can give rise to paraneoplastic neuropathy.

It is proposed that expression of onconeuronal antigens by cancer cells results in an autoimmunity. When the tumor develops, the body produces antibodies to fight it, by binding to and helping the destruction of tumor cells. Such antibodies may cross-react with epitopes on normal nervous tissue, resulting in an attack on the nervous system. Neoplasms of the spinal cord may be either intramedullary or extramedullary, and primary tumors affecting the paravertebral area may spread and compress the cord, particularly within the intervertebral foramena. An enlarging cancerous lymph node can compress the cord, and cancer that metastasizes to the vertebrae or surrounding tissues may also cause spinal cord compression.

Pain-generating mediators are often released from certain tumors or from surrounding tissues involving invasion or metastasis, thereby producing pain itself.[37] Paradoxically, various cancer therapies may result in pain. Chemotherapeutic agents have been associated with peripheral neuropathies and acute pain in humans,[38] and radiation therapy may injure soft tissue or neuronal structures. Furthermore, immunosuppressive therapy may render some patients at increased risk for secondary infection and complications.

Although psychogenic pain in animals is controversial, nociceptive and neuropathic types of cancer pain are recognized. Stimulated afferent nociceptive pathways in visceral or somatic tissue lead to nociceptive pain. Neuropathic pain is caused by dysfunction of or lesions involving the peripheral or central nervous systems. Differentiating the 2 may influence the selection of a specific therapy. Nociceptive somatic cancer pain arises from soft tissue structures that are nonneurologic and nonvisceral in origin, including skin, muscle, bone, and joints, and often correlates with the extent of tissue damage. Nociceptive visceral cancer pain arises from the deep organs of the abdomen, thorax, or pelvis and is often difficult to localize. Obstruction of hollow viscera, distention of organ walls, stretching of the pancreas or liver capsule, or extension of metastasis into mesentery may induce visceral pain.

Neuropathic Cancer Pain

Neuropathic pain affects the nervous system and may have multiple etiologies, including nerve compression, deafferentation injury, and sympathetically induced origin.[39] Nerve compression has been identified as the most common cause of neuropathic pain in human cancer patients (79%), followed by nerve injury (16%) and sympathetically mediated pain (5%).[40] Neuropathic pain is considered to be relatively less responsive to opioids.[41] Nonopioid adjuncts such as antiepileptic, antidepressant, and antiarrhythmic agents or combinations of these should be considered.[42,43]

It is noteworthy that pain and neurologic deficits result from tumor infiltration or compression of the peripheral nervous system. This may include infiltration of spinal nerve roots, producing radicular symptoms, and invasion of neuronal plexuses. Such invasion or compression may involve a perineural inflammatory reaction that accentuates the nerve pain.[44] Degenerative changes and deafferentation are a consequence of prolonged tumor infiltration or compression.[45] Resultant peripheral sensitization is associated with an increased density of sodium channels in the damaged axons and associated dorsal root ganglion.[46] Ectopic foci of electrical activity arise in injured axons and stimulus thresholds are decreased. Activated peripheral nociceptors release mediators for central sensitization (ie, the amino acid glutamate and neuropeptides, such as substance P and neurokinin A). In turn, these neurotransmitters cause an increase in intracellular calcium and upregulation of N-methyl-D-aspartate receptors. Associated with this increased intracellular calcium comes activation of enzymatic reactions, causing expression of genes that ultimately lower the

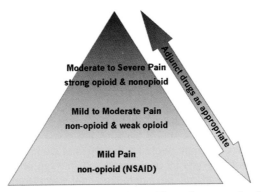

Fig. 10. WHO ladder was adopted in 1986 to give guidance for managing human cancer pain. It has been adopted in veterinary medicine and provides guidance for noncancer pain as well.

excitatory threshold of dorsal horn neurons, exaggerate their response to noxious stimuli, and enlarge the size of their receptor fields (secondary peripheral sensitization).

Anatomy-Based Cancer Pain

Anatomic classification of cancer pain has limited applications since it lacks specificity as to the mechanism of pain; however, it does provide guidance for certain invasive therapies such as external radiation, neurolytic blocks, electrical stimulation, or, perhaps, targeted drug delivery.

Severity-Based Cancer Pain

Severity-based classification of cancer pain reflects the extent of tissue destruction, size of the tumor, or its location. In human patients, metastatic bone lesions and injury to nerves are typically more painful than soft tissue tumors. The severity of cancer pain is dynamic, reflecting the course of the disease and different therapies administered; therefore, it is prudent to review the severity of the pain over time.

The World Health Organization Cancer Pain Ladder

In 1986, the World Health Organization (WHO) developed a simple 3-stage analgesic ladder for treatment of cancer pain that relies on widely available and inexpensive analgesic agents (**Fig. 10**).[47] The WHO analgesic ladder provides clinical guidance from a severity-based pain classification system.

Although the quality of evidence for the WHO ladder approach has been challenged, it has been globally distributed and is considered the standard for cancer pain management in human patients. Contemporary thinking, however, is to use "stronger" analgesics earlier.

Mechanism-Based Treatment

A mechanism-based treatment strategy for managing cancer pain in humans has been studied[48] (ie, neuropathic pain was treated with antidepressants and anticonvulsants, while opioids were integrated into the treatment protocol only after these drugs were considered ineffective). Interestingly, all human patients studied required concurrent therapy with a mean of 3 drug classes, including an opioid, to control their pain. This illustrates the heterogeneity of cancer pain mechanisms and the subsequent value of a "balanced or multimodal analgesia" approach to treatment.

Prevalence of Cancer Pain in Animals

The frequency of cancer pain in animals is difficult to identify as is the prevalence of cancer itself in the pet population. Not all cancers are painful, sensitivity to pain varies between individuals, and the degree of pain may vary during the course of the cancer. Considering that an overall average of about 70% of humans with advanced cancer suffer pain[49] and that many biological systems are common between humans and animals, a conservative estimate might be that 30% of animal cancers are painful.[50] As a rule, pain is more frequently associated with tumors arising in noncompliant tissue (eg, bone). It should not be overlooked that some treatment therapies for cancer may create pain.

Cancer Pain Assessment in Animals

The assessment of cancer pain in animals is particularly challenging, and few reports have been made in this area. Yazbek and Fantoni[51] suggest that a simple questionnaire may be useful in assessing health-related quality of life in dogs with pain secondary to cancer, in that dogs with cancer had significantly lower scores than did healthy dogs. A number of animal pain scales have been proposed, such as visual analogue scales, numerical rating scales, simple descriptive scales, multifactorial pain scales, and composite measure pain scale; however, these are applied to the assessment of acute pain, where some are more valid than others. Physiologic variables such as heart rate, respiratory rate, cortisol levels, temperature, and pupil size are unreliable measures for assessing acute pain,[52,53] and behavioral changes are now considered the most reliable indicator of pain in animals.[54,55] Any change in an animal's normal behavior may be associated with pain. Herein lies the value of integrating the pet owner's observations into the patient's assessment on a continuum of follow-ups. In fact, many clinicians suggest that the owner is a better assessor of their animal's chronic pain than is the veterinarian.

Certain behaviors are worth noting:

- Painful animals are less active.
- Animals in pain do not groom as frequently, especially cats.
- Dogs, in particular, may lick a painful area.
- Both painful dogs and cats may show decreased appetites.
- Painful cats tend to seek seclusion.
- Dogs in pain tend not to yawn, stretch, or "wet dog shake."
- Animals in pain often posture differently.

The most reliable method for identifying pain is the animal's response to analgesic intervention.

Recently, the first animal models of bone cancer pain have been developed. In the mouse femur model, bone cancer pain is induced by injecting murine osteolytic sarcoma cells into the intramedullary space of the femur. These tumor cells proliferate, and ongoing, movement-evoked, and mechanically evoked pain-related behaviors develop that increase in severity over time. These models have allowed elucidation of how cancer pain is generated and how the sensory information is processed when molecular architecture of bone is changed by disease (**Fig. 11**).

Tumor and tumor-associated cells including macrophages, neutrophils, and T-lymphocytes secrete a wide variety of factors including PGs, endothelins, IL-1 and IL-6,

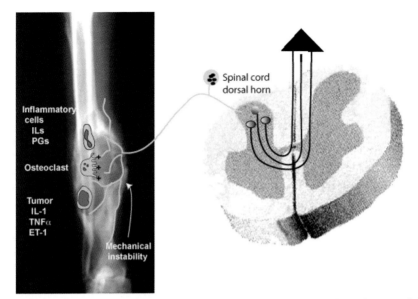

Fig. 11. Bone cancer changes the molecular architecture and bioneurological status of the diseased bone. (ET-1 = endothelin-1).

epidermal growth factor, transforming growth factor, and platelet-derived growth factor, which directly excite primary afferent neurons. Each of these factors may play an important role in the generation of pain associated with various cancers. Pharmaceutical targeting of these factors provides opportunities for pain relief, while anti-PGs and antiendothelins are already commercially available.

Tumor-associated macrophages and several tumor cells express high levels of COX-2, producing large amounts of PGs.[56,57] Although all NSAIDs are anti-PGs, the new COX-2 inhibitors, or coxibs, preferentially inhibit COX-2 and avoid many of the COX-1 inhibition side effects. Additionally, some experiments have suggested that COX-2 is involved in angiogenesis and tumor growth.[58,59] Although further research is required to characterize the effect of coxib-class NSAIDs on different types of cancer, in addition to blocking cancer pain, COX-2 inhibitors may have the added advantage of reducing the growth and metastasis of tumors.

The peptide endothelin-1 is another pharmacologic target for treating cancer pain. A number of small unmyelinated primary afferents express receptors for endothelia,[60] and endothelins may well sensitize or excite nociceptors. Several tumors of humans, including prostate cancer, express high levels of endothelins,[61] and clinical studies have shown a correlation between the severity of the pain in human patients with prostate cancer and endothelin plasma levels.[62]

Tumor-Induced Local Acidosis

Tumor burden often outgrows its vascular supply, becoming ischemic and undergoing apoptosis. Subsequently, an accumulation of acid metabolites prevails, resulting in an acidotic local environment. This is relevant to cancer pain, in that subsets of sensory neurons have been shown to express different acid-sensing ion channels,[63] sensitive to protons or acidosis. Two major classes of acid-sensing ion channels expressed by nociceptors, both sensitive to decreases in pH, are TRPV1 and the

Table 5
Effects of therapy and disease on tissue and nerve injury

	Tissue Injury	Nerve Injury
Iatrogenic		
Chemotherapy		X
Radiation		X
Surgery	X	X
Disease		
Tumor compression		X
Release of active factors	X	
Immune response	X	X

acid-sensing ion channel-3 (ASIC-3). As tumors grow and undergo apoptosis, there is a local release of intracellular ions and inflammation-mediated protons that give rise to a local acidic environment. This neurobiological mechanism is particularly relevant in bone cancer where there is a proliferation and hypertrophy of osteoclasts. Osteoclasts are multinucleated cells of the monocyte lineage that resorb bone by maintaining an extracellular microenvironment of acidic pH (4.0–5.0) at the interface between osteoclast and mineralized bone.[64] Experiments in mice have shown that osteoclasts contribute to the etiology of bone cancer pain[65] and that osteoprotegrin and a bisphosphonate,[66] both of which induce osteoclast apoptosis, are effective in decreasing osteoclast-induced cancer pain. TRPV1 or ASIC antagonists would act similarly but would do so by blocking excitation of acid-sensitive channels on sensory neurons.

Growth Factors from Tumor Cells

Different patients with the same cancer may have vastly different symptoms. Metastases to bone in the same individual may cause pain at one site, but not at a different site. Small cancer deposits in one location may be more painful than large cancers at an unrelated site. Why the variability? One explanation may be that change in the periphery associated with inflammation, nerve injury, or tissue injury are reflected by changes in the phenotype of sensory neurons (**Table 5**).[67] Such changes are, in part, caused by a change in tissue levels of several growth factors released from the local environment at the injury site, including nerve growth factors[68] and glial-derived neurotrophic factor.[69] Likely, the milieu of growth factors to which the sensory neuron is exposed will change as the developing tumor invades the tissue that the neuron innervates.

The mouse sarcoma cell model has also demonstrated that growing tumor cells destroy both the hematopoietic cells of the marrow and the sensory fibers that normally innervate the marrow.[70] This neuronal damage can give rise to neuropathic pain. Gabapentin (often substituted by pregabalin) is a drug originally developed as an anticonvulsant, but it is effective in treating several forms of neuropathic pain and may be useful in treating cancer-induced neuropathic pain.[71]

Summarizing the contributors to bone cancer pain:

◇ Release of cytokines, PGs, and endothelins from hematopoietic, immune, and tumor cells
◇ Osteoclast activity increases → lowered pH → activation of TRVR1 receptor

◇ Bone erosion ⇒ release of growth factors (eg, nerve growth factor)
◇ Tumor growth ⇒ compression of afferent terminals
◇ Neurochemical changes in dorsal root ganglion and spinal cord.

The Moving Target of Cancer Pain

As cancer progresses, changing factors may complicate the pain state. In the mouse model of bone cancer, as the tumor cells begin to proliferate, pain-related behaviors precede any noticeable bone destruction. This is attributed to prohyperalgesic factors such as active nociceptor response in the marrow to PGs and endothelin released from growing tumor cells. At this point, pain might be managed by a coxib-class NSAID or endothelia-antagonist. With continued tumor growth, sensory neurons innervating the marrow are compressed and destroyed, giving rise to neuropathic pain, possibly responsive to gabapentin. Once the tumor becomes invaded by osteoclastic activity, pain might be largely blocked by antiosteoclastogenic drugs such as biphosphonates or osteoprotegerin. As the intramedullary space becomes filled with dying tumor cells, generating an acidic environment, TRPV1 or ASIC antagonists may attenuate the pain. In the later stages of bone destruction, antagonists to the mechanically gated channels and/or adenosine triphosphate receptors in the highly innervated periosteum may alleviate movement-evoked pain. This scenario illustrates how a mechanistic approach to designing more effective therapies for cancer pain should be created based on the understanding of how different stages of the disease impact tumor cell influence on nociceptors; and how phenotype of nociceptors and central nervous system neurons involved in nociceptive transmission change during the course of advancing cancer.

Clearly, the mechanisms associated with cancer pain are complex. However, only through the understanding of these mechanisms can we best manage our patient's pain with evidence-based confidence. The murine bone cancer model has given us insights as to the progressing, dynamic neurobiological changes associated with cancer. These insights further lead us to the conclusion that effective treatment must be multimodal and dynamic.

Visceral Cancer Pain

Many cancers involve internal organs and symptoms are silent until ischemia, compression, or obstruction reaches a given stage, at which time visceral pain is manifest. Pain of visceral cancer origin can be divided into 4 groups: (1) acute mechanical stretch of visceral structures, (2) ischemia of visceral structures, (3) chemical stimuli from an infiltrating tumor or the body's reaction to infiltration, and (4) a compressive form of neuropathic pain that occurs due to direct invasion of nervous structures involving the viscera. Visceral pain can also result from treatment damage of viscera and associated nerves from surgery, chemotherapy, or radiation.

Nutritional Management

Many types of cancer are influenced by nutrition, diet, and nutritional status of the patient. In humans cachexia is seen in 32% to 87% of cases, commonly associated with cancers of the upper gastrointestinal tract.[72] Weight loss can be detrimental to patient quality of life and prognosis, as well as dramatically impact the pharmacokinetics and pharmacodynamics of chemotherapeutics and contribute to increased treatment-related toxicity.[73] Malnutrition is arguably one of the most common causes of death in people with cancer. Association between documented metabolic abnormalities, actual weight loss, and poor prognosis in cats or dogs with cancer has not been convincingly demonstrated. One study[74] from a referral oncology practice showed that only 4% of the dogs were cachectic and 15% of the dogs had detectable and clinically significant muscle wasting. Nevertheless, nutritional assessment of the cancer patient should be part of every treatment plan focusing on history, physical examination, and routine hematologic and biochemical parameters. For the undernourished dog or cat, a liquid nutritional supplement (Recuperation; Viyo Veterinary, Antwerp, Belgium) has been found helpful to encourage water and food consumption.[75]

The following 5 steps have been proposed to define the nutritional requirements for dogs or cats with cancer[76]:

1. Estimate fluid requirements.
2. Estimate energy requirements.
3. Distribute calories (among protein, fat, and carbohydrates).
4. Evaluate remaining nutrients (ie, vitamins, minerals, essential nutrients, etc).
5. Select a method of feeding (voluntary intake being preferred).

END-OF-LIFE CONSIDERATIONS

Reflecting on Dr Vertosick's insight that we are all born in another's pain and destined to die in our own, part of our moral obligation as veterinarians is to relieve pain and suffering in terminally ill cancer patients. Due to the strong human–animal bond built over the pet's lifetime, this obligation often involves assistance for both the pet and its owner. At this point a "pawspice"—end-of-life care program—is a professional obligation. We can, with solidarity, offer pet owners supportive, palliative options for complete care and attention to their pet's special needs when death is eminent. Finally, veterinary medicine is entrusted with the responsibility and option of euthanasia to help animals die in a humane and pain-free manner.

Pet owners don't really care how much you know;
they want to know how much you care.

SUMMARY

OA and cancer are the inevitable consequences of aging, and significantly contribute to the cause of death in cats and dogs. Managing the pain associated with these disease states is the veterinarian's mandate. Many treatment modalities and agents are available for patient management; however, it is only with an understanding of disease neurobiology and a mechanism-based approach to problem diagnosis that the clinician can offer patients an optimal quality of life based on evidence-based best medicine. When treating pain, knowledge is still our best weapon.

REFERENCES

1. Fleming JM, Creepy KE, Promislow DEL. Mortality in North American dogs from 1984 to 2004: an investigation into age-, size-, and breed-related causes of death. J Vet Intern Med 2011;25:187–98.
2. Algner T, Kurz B, Fukui N, et al. Roles of chondrocytes in the pathogenesis of osteoarthritis. Curr Opin Rheumatol 2002;14:578–84.
3. Goldring SR, Goldring MB. The role of cytokines in cartilage matrix degeneration in osteoarthritis. Clin Orthop 2004;427(Suppl):S27–36.
4. Bunning RA, Russell RG. The effect of tumor necrosis factor alpha and gamma-interferon on the resorption of human articular cartilage and on the production of prostaglandin E and of caseinase activity by human articular chondrocytes. Arthritis Rheum 1989;32:780–4.

5. Campbell IK, Piccoli DS, Roberts MJ, et al. Effects of tumor necrosing factor alpha and beta on resorption of human articular cartilage and production of plasminogen activator by human articular chondrocytes. Arthritis Rheum 1990;33:542–52.

6. Henderson B, Pettipher ER. Arthritogenic actions of recombinant IL-1 and tumour necrosis factor alpha in the rabbit: evidence for synergistic interactions between cytokines in vivo. Clin Exp Immunol 1989;75:306–10.

7. Goldring MB, Berenbaum F. Human chondrocyte culture models for studying cyclo-oxygenase expression and prostaglandin regulation of collagen gene expression. Osteoarthritis Cartilage 1999;7(4):386–8.

8. Lotz M. The role of nitric oxide in articular cartilage damage. Rheum Dis Clin North Am 1999;25(2):269–82.

9. Notoya K, Jovanovic DV, Reboul P, et al. The induction of cell death in human osteoarthritis chondrocytes by nitric oxide is related to the production of prostaglandin E2 via the induction of cyclooxygenase-2. J Immunol 2000;165(6):3402–10.

10. Miwa M, Saura R, Hirata S, et al. Induction of apoptosis in bovine articular chondro-cyte by prostaglandin E(2) through cAMP-dependent pathway. Osteoarthritis Carti-lage 2000;8(1):17–24.

11. Lotz M. Cytokines and their receptors. In: Koopman WJ, editor. Arthritis and allied conditions. 13th edition. Baltimore (MD): Williams & Wilkins; 1997. p. 2013.

12. Moldovan F, Pelletier JP, Hambor J, et al. Collagenase-3 (matrix metalloprotease 13) is preferentially localized in the deep layer of human arthritic cartilage in situ: in vitro mimicking effect by transforming growth factor beta. Arthritis Rheum 1997; 40:1653–61.

13. Freemont AJ, Byers RJ, Taiwo YO, et al. In situ zymographic localisation of type II collagen degrading activity in osteoarthritic human articular cartilage. Ann Rheum Dis 1999;58:357–65.

14. Martel-Pelletier J, Welsch DJ, Pelletier JP: Metalloproteases and inhibitors in arthritic diseases. Best Pract Res Clin Rheumatol 2001:805–29.

15. Stefanovic-Racic M, Stadler J, Evans CH. Nitric oxide and arthritis. Arthritis Rheum 1993;36:1036–44.

16. Hickery MS, Palmer RM, Charles IG, et al. The role of nitric oxide in IL-1 and TNFalpha-induced inhibition of proteoglycan synthesis in human articular cartilage. Trans Orthop Res Soc 1994;19:77.

17. Taskiran D, Stefanovic-Racic M, Georgescu HI, et al. Nitric oxide mediates suppres-sion of cartilage proteoglycan synthesis by interleukin-1. Biochem Biophys Res Commun 1994;200:142–8.

18. Järvinen TAH, Moilanen T, Järvinen TLN, et al. Nitric oxide mediates interleukin-1 induced inhibition of glycosaminoglycan synthesis in rat articular cartilage. Mediators Inflamm 1995;4:107–11.

19. Blanco FJ, Guitian R, Vazquez-Martul E, et al. Osteoarthritis chondrocytes die by apoptosis. A possible pathway for osteoarthritis pathology. Arthritis Rheum 1998; 41:284–9.

20. Hashimoto S, Takahashi K, Amiel D, et al. Chondrocyte apoptosis and nitric oxide production during experimentally induced osteoarthritis. Arthritis Rheum 1998;41: 1266–74.

21. Pelletier JP, Mineau F, Ranger P, et al. The increased synthesis of inducible nitric oxide inhibits IL-1Ra synthesis by human articular chondrocytes: possible role in osteoar-thritic cartilage degradation. Osteoarthritis Cartilage 1996;4:77–84.

22. Zaragoza C, Balbin M, Lopez-Otin C, et al. Nitric oxide regulates matrix metallopro-tease-13 expression and activity in endothelium. Kidney Int 2002;61:804–8.

23. Mauviel A, Loyau G, Pujol JP. Effect of unsaponifiable extracts of avocado and soybean (Piascledine) on the collagenolytic action of cultures of human rheumatoid synoviocytes and rabbit articular chondrocytes treated with interleukin-1. Rev Rhum Mal Osteoartic 1991;58:241–5.
24. Henrotin Y, Labasse A, Jaspar JM, et al. Effects of three avocado/soybean unsaponifiable mixtures on metalloproteinases, cytokines and prostaglandin E2 production by human articular chondrocytes. Clin Rheumatol 1998;17:31–9.
25. Boumediene K, Felisaz N, Bogdanowicz P, et al. Avocado/soya unsaponifiables enhance the expression of transforming growth factor beta1 and beta2 in cultured articular chondrocytes. Arthritis Rheum 1999;42:148–56.
26. Chan P-S, Caron JP, Orth MW. Effects of glucosamine and chondroitin sulfate on bovine cartilage explants under long-term culture conditions. AJVR 2007;68:709–15.
27. Au RY, Al-Tallinn TK, Au Ay, et al. Avocado soybean unsaponifiables (ASU) suppress TNF-α, IL-1β, COX-2, iNOS gene expression, and prostaglandin E$_2$ and nitric oxide production in articular chondrocytes and monocyte/macrophages. Osteoarthritis Cartilage 2007;125:1249–55.
28. Fox SM, Millis D. Multimodal management of canine osteoarthritis. London (UK): Manson Publishing; 2010.
29. Millis DL. A multimodal approach to treating osteoarthritis. 2006 Western Veterinary Conference Symposium Proceedings. Las Vegas (NV), February 19–23, 2006.
30. Millis DL. Dasuquin's efficacy may be similar to that of NSAIDs in dogs. Canapp SO, Jr., moderator. Joint health-a roundtable discussion. Vet Med 2010;105(11):1–16. Available at: http://veterinarycalendar.dvm360.com/avhc/Surgery/Dasuquins-efficacy-may-be-similar-to-that-of-NSAID/ArticleStandard/Article/detail/695178.
31. Roush JK. Omega-3 fatty acid effects on force plate analysis & clinical signs. Clinician's Update™, supplement to NAVC clinician's brief®. Hills Pet Nutrition; 2005.
32. Maitland ME, Leonard T, Frank CB, et al. Longitudinal measurement of tibial motion relative to the femur during passive displacements in the cat before and after anterior cruciate ligament transection. J Orthop Res 1998;16(4):448–54.
33. Vertosick FT. Why we hurt: the natural history of pain. New York:Harcourt; 2000.
34. Merskey H, Bogduk N, editors. Classification of chronic pain. 2nd edition. Seattle (WA): IASP Press; 1994.
35. Ventafridda V, Caracen A. Cancer pain classification: a controversial issue. Pain 1991;46:1–2.
36. Caraceni A, Weinstein S. Classification of cancer pain syndromes. Oncology 2001;15:1627–40.
37. Twycross R. Cancer pain classification. Acta Anaesthesiol Scand 1997;41:141–5.
38. Verstappen C, Heimans J, Hoekman K, et al. Neurotoxic complications of chemotherapy in patients with cancer: clinical signs and optimal management. Drugs 2003;63:1549–63.
39. Portenoy R. Cancer pain: pathophysiology and syndromes. Lancet 1992;339:1026–31.
40. Stute P, Soukup, Menzel M. Analysis and treatment of different types of neuropathic cancer pain. J Pain Symptom Manage 2003;26:1123–30.
41. Portenoy R, Foley K, Intumisi C. The nature of opioid responsiveness and its implications for neuropathic pain: new hypotheses derived from studies of opioid infusions. Pain 1990;43:273–86.
42. Chong M, Bajwa Z. Diagnosis and treatment of neuropathic pain. J Pain Symptom Manage 2003;25:S4–11.
43. Caraceni A, Zecca E, Martini C, et al. Gabapentin as an adjuvant to opioid analgesia for neuropathic cancer pain. J Pain Symptom Manage 1999;17:441–5.

44. Martin L, Hagen N. Neuropathic pain in cancer patients: Mechanism syndromes and clinical controversies. J Pain Symptom Manage 1997;14:99–117.
45. Tasker R. The problem of deafferentation pain in the management of the patient with cancer. J Palliat Care 1987;2:8–12.
46. England J, Happel L, Kline D, et al. Sodium channel accumulation in humans with painful neuromas. Neurology 1996;47:272–6.
47. World Health Organization. Cancer pain relief. Geneva (Switzerland): World Health Organization; 1986.
48. Ashby M, Fleming B, Brooksbank M, et al. Description of a mechanistic approach to pain management in advanced cancer. Preliminary report. Pain 1992;51:273–82.
49. Portenoy RK, Lesage P. Management of cancer pain. Lancet 1999;353:1695–700.
50. Lascelles BDX. Relief of chronic cancer pain. In: Dobson JM, Lascelles BDX, editors. BSAVA manual of canine and feline oncology. Quedgeley, Gloucester (UK): BSAVA; 2003. p. 137–51.
51. Yazbek KVB, Fantoni DT. Validity of a health-related quality-of-life scale for dogs with signs of pain secondary to cancer. JAVMA 2005;226:1354–8.
52. Conzemius MG, Hill CM, Sammarco JL, et al. Correlation between subjective and objective measures used to determine severity of postoperative pain in dogs. JAVMA 1997;210:1619–22.
53. Fox SM, Mellor DJ, Lawoko CRO, et al. Changes in plasma cortisol concentrations in bitches in response to different combinations of halothane and butorphanol, with or without ovariohysterectomy. Res Vet Sci 1998;65:125–33.
54. Fox SM, Mellor DJ, Stafford, KJ, et al. The effects of ovariohysterectomy plus different combinations of halothane anaesthesia and butorphanol analgesia on behaviour in the bitch. Res Vet Sci 2000;68:265–74.
55. Hardie EM, Hansen BD, Carroll GS. Behavior after ovariohysterectomy in the dog: what's normal? Appl Anim Behav Sci 1997;51:111–28.
56. Dubois RN, Radhika A, Reddy BS, et al. Increased cyclooxygenase-2 levels in carcinogen-induced rat colonic tumors. Gastroenterology 1996;110:1259–62.
57. Kundu N, Yang QY, Dorsey R, et al. Increased cyclooxygenase-2 (COX-2) expression and activity in a murine model of metastatic breast cancer. Int J Cancer 2001;93:681–6.
58. Masferrer JL, Leahy KM, Koki AT, et al. Antiangiogenic and antitumor activities of cyclooxygenase-2 inhibitors. Cancer Res 2000;60:1306–11.
59. Moore BC, Simmons DL. COX-2 inhibition, apoptosis, and chemoprevention by non-steroidal anti-inflammatory drugs. Curr Med Chem 2000;7:1131–44.
60. Pomonis JD, Rogers SD, Peters CM, et al. Expression and localization of endothelin receptors: implication for the involvement of peripheral glia in nociception. J Neurosci 2001;21:999–1006.
61. Kurbel S, Kurbel B, Kovacic D, et al. Endothelin-secreting tumors and the idea of the pseudoectopic hormone secretion in tumors. Med Hypotheses 1999;52:329–33.
62. Nelson JB, Hedican SP, George DJ, et al. Identification of endothelin-1 in the pathophysiology of metastatic adenocarcinoma of the prostate. Nat Med 1995;1:944–99.
63. Julius D, Basbaum AL. Molecular mechanisms of nociception. Nature 2001;413:203–10.
64. Delaisse J-M, Vales G. Mechanism of mineral solubilization and matrix degradation in osteoclastic bone resorption. In: Rifkin BR, Gay CV, editors. Biology and physiology of the osteoclast. Philadelphia (PA): CRC Press; 1992.
65. Honore P, Menning PM, Rogers SD, et al. Neurochemical plasticity in persistent inflammatory pain. Prog Brain Res 2000;129:357–63.

66. Mannix K, Ahmedazai SH, Anderson H, et al. Using bisphosphonates to control the pain of bone metastases: evidence based guidelines for palliative care. Palliat Med 2000;14:455–61.

67. Honore P, Rogers SD, Schwei MJ, et al. Murine models of inflammatory, neuropathic and cancer pain each generates a unique set of neurochemical changes in the spinal cord and sensory neurons. Neuroscience 2000;98:585–98.

68. Koltzenburg M. The changing sensitivity in the life of the nociceptor. Pain 1999;(Suppl 6):S93–102.

69. Boucher TJ, McMahon SB. Neurotrophic factors and neuropathic pain. Curr Opin Pharmacol 2001;1:66–72.

70. Schwei MJ, Honore P, Rogers SD, et al. Neurochemical and cellular reorganization of the spinal cord in a murine model of bone cancer pain. Neuroscience 1999;19:10886–97.

71. Ripamonti C, Dickerson ED. Strategies for the treatment of cancer pain in the new millennium. Drugs 2001;61:955–77.

72. DeWys WD, Begg C, Lavin PT, et al. Prognostic effect of weight loss prior to chemotherapy in cancer patients. Am J Med 1980;69:491.

73. Langer CI, Hoffman JP, Ottery FD. Clinical significance of weight loss in cancer patients: rationale for the use of anabolic agents in the treatment of cancer-related cachexia. Nutrition 2001;17(Suppl 1):S1–20.

74. Michel KE, Sorenmo K, Shofer FS. Evaluation of body condition and weight loss in dogs presented to a veterinary oncology service. J Vet Intern Med 2004;18:692–5.

75. Rotat C, Lhoest E, Istasse L, et al. Influence of a liquid nutritional supplement on water intake in experimental beagle dogs. Atwerp (Belgium): Viyo Publications; 2010. Available at: www.viyoveterinary.com. Accessed April 10, 2012.

76. Mauldin GE. Nutritional management of the cancer patient. In: Withrow SJ, Vail DM, editors. Small animal clinical oncology. 4th ed. St Louis (MO): Saunders/Elsevier; 2007. p. 307–26.

77. Roush JK, Cross A. University study: effects of feeding omega-3 fatty acids on force plate gait analysis in dogs with osteoarthritis, 3-month feeding study, 2003. Data on file, Hill's Pet Nutrition, Inc. Technical information services 2005.

Cognitive Dysfunction Syndrome
A Disease of Canine and Feline Brain Aging

Gary M. Landsberg, DVM[a,b,]*, Jeff Nichol, DVM[c],
Joseph A. Araujo, BSc[b,d,e]

KEYWORDS

- Cognitive dysfunction syndrome • Brain aging • Behavior • Canine • Feline

KEY POINTS

- Brain aging is a degenerative process that for many dogs and cats ultimately progresses to a loss of one or more cognitive domains or impairment of cognitive function.
- Diagnosis of cognitive dysfunction syndrome (CDS) is based on recognition of behavioral signs and exclusion of other medical conditions and drug side effects, which in some cases can mimic or complicate CDS.
- Clinical categories include disorientation, alterations in social interactions, sleep-wake cycles, elimination habits, and activity, as well as increasing anxiety. Deficits in learning and memory have also been well documented.
- Treatment is aimed at slowing the advancement of neuronal damage and cell death and improving clinical signs. Drugs, diet, and supplements can be used alone or concurrently to improve neurotransmission and reduce oxidative damage and inflammation.

INTRODUCTION

As pets age, behavior changes may be the first indication of declining health and welfare. This is particularly true for some of the most common problems associated with aging, such as pain, sensory decline, and cognitive dysfunction syndrome (CDS). Early identification of these signs provides an opportunity for effective intervention.

GML is an employee of CanCog Technologies Inc. JAA is an employee of InterVivo Solutions Inc and a consultant for CanCog Technologies Inc.
The authors have nothing else to disclose.
[a] North Toronto Animal Clinic, 99 Henderson Avenue, Thornhill, Ontario, Canada L3T 2K9;
[b] CanCog Technologies Inc, 120 Carlton Street, Suite 204, Toronto, Ontario, Canada M5A 4K2;
[c] Veterinary Emergency and Specialty Center of New Mexico, 4000 Montgomery Boulevard NE, Albuquerque, NM 87109, USA; [d] InterVivo Solutions Inc, 120 Carlton Street, Suite 203, Toronto, Ontario, Canada M5A 4K2; [e] Department of Pharmacology and Toxicology, University of Toronto, 1 King's College Circle, Toronto, Ontario, Canada M5S 1A8
* Corresponding author. North Toronto Animal Clinic, 99 Henderson Avenue, Thornhill, Ontario, Canada L3T 2K9.
E-mail address: gmlandvm@aol.com

During veterinary visits, pet owners are likely to report serious behavioral changes, but subtle signs, which may be indicative of declining health or cognition, often go unreported. Family members therefore need assistance in both identifying and reporting any change from normal behavior to their veterinarian. Similarly, clinicians must be proactive in asking about behavioral signs.

The current article focuses on how CDS in dogs and cats parallels neurodegenerative disorders in humans, particularly Alzheimer disease (AD). The goal is to help the practitioner develop a senior care program incorporating behavioral screening to aid in both the recognition of behavior changes consistent with CDS and the implementation of appropriate treatment strategies.

BRAIN AGING AND COGNITIVE DYSFUNCTION

Most mammals show age-related neuropathologic changes. In humans, the most common neurodegenerative disorder is AD, which progressively impairs cognition, behavior, and quality of life. It is increasingly evident that humans, dogs, and cats demonstrate parallels in brain aging associated with cognitive dysfunction. In fact, the aged dog and, to a lesser extent, the aged cat are spontaneous models of AD and therefore can play a valuable role in testing putative AD therapeutics. Conversely, the knowledge gained from studying AD is highly relevant for understanding brain aging and cognitive dysfunction in companion animals.

Lessons Learned from AD Research

Modern medicine has increased the life span across many species, which in turn has increased the incidence of neurodegenerative diseases, such as AD. In humans, AD is generally characterized by initial decline in episodic memory followed by progressive decline across multiple cognitive domains.[1] Ultimately this results in behavioral changes that impair social function and eventually results in death. Classical diagnosis of AD has relied on post-mortem confirmation of 2 hallmark pathologies: the presence of senile plaques, which consist of extracellular deposits of fibrilized amyloid-beta protein (Aβ), and neurofibrillary tangles, which consist of intracellular paired helical fragments of cytoskeletal hyperphosphorylated tau protein.[2] However, it is uncertain if either of these pathologic changes is a causal factor as several other brain changes are documented, including neuronal loss; cortical atrophy including atrophy of the hippocampus; alterations in neurochemical systems such as the cholinergic, glutaminergic, dopaminergic, and GABAergic neurotransmitter systems; and reduced neuronal and synaptic function.[3] Moreover, risk factors associated with the development of AD include genetic, metabolic, and nutritional influences, which may be equally relevant to pet aging.

Recent clinical and research criteria propose there are progressive stages of AD from the preclinical stage (ie, prior to clinical signs) to mild cognitive impairment (MCI; prodromal stage likely to proceed to AD) to a clinical diagnosis of AD based on cognitive-behavioral status.[1] It is suggested that beta-amyloid deposition may occur early in disease progression, followed by neuronal degeneration/synaptic dysfunction (measured by biomarkers of tau pathology or functional imaging). Both of these pathologies likely precede the clinically identifiable stage of MCI or AD in humans.[4] Therefore, clinical AD is now considered a late stage of disease progression, which may explain the limited clinical success of therapeutic interventions (ie, initiated too late in disease progression to improve outcome). Therefore, identification of current and/or novel biomarkers predictive of AD progression will be essential for diagnostic characterization of preclinical and prodromal AD stages and for assessing interventions aimed at prevention or reversing progression of AD. It is theorized that AD risk factors, similar to high blood pressure or increased cholesterol in early diagnosis of cardiovascular disease, will be identified and validated, permitting early intervention and monitoring of disease progression.

Lessons Learned from Senior Dog and Cat Research

Most mammals show evidence of brain aging and consequential cognitive deficits.[5] CDS in companion animals parallels AD progression in several respects. For example, not all aged dogs and cats show behavioral signs consistent with CDS, yet subclinical alterations in cognitive function may be present, which might eventually progress to CDS.[6] Therefore, it is prudent to commence treatment early. Understanding age-related brain pathology and cognitive dysfunction is essential to fully appreciate the potential value of using biomarkers and/or cognitive status in the future diagnosis and treatment of CDS progression.

Effects of Aging on the Brains of Senior Dogs and Cats

In canine aging, frontal lobe volume decreases, ventricular size increases, and there is evidence of meningeal calcification, demyelination, increased lipofuscin, increased apoptic bodies, neuroaxonal degeneration, and reduced neurons.[7,8] In cats, age-related pathologies include neuronal loss, cerebral atrophy, widening of sulci, and increases in ventricular size.[9–11] Perivascular changes, including microhemorrhage or infarcts in periventricular vessels, are reported in senior dogs and cats, which may contribute to signs of CDS.[7,9,12–15] With increasing age, there is an increase in reactive oxygen species leading to oxidative damage in dogs and likely cats.[9,16] Increases in monoamine oxidase B activity in dogs is reported, which may increase catalysis of dopamine with subsequent increases in free radicals.[17] A decline in cholinergic tone occurs in canine aging as evidenced by hypersensitivity to anticholinergics and decreased brain muscarinic receptor density.[18] Diminished cholinergic function is also reported in cats.[10,19] Collectively, these alterations may contribute to working memory deficits or CDS, as well as alterations in motor function and REM sleep.[9,10,20–22]

In aged dogs, cats, and humans, there are similarities in deposition of $A\beta$ in extracellular plaques and perivascular infiltrates; however, dense core plaques seen in AD are not found in dogs or cats, suggesting canine and feline plaques are less mature than those seen in AD.[9,12,14,15,23] Moreover, similar to humans, $A\beta$ plaque load is positively correlated with cognitive impairment in dogs.[13,14,24] By contrast, cats demonstrate more diffuse $A\beta$ plaques than either human or dog.[9,12,15,25,26] Neurofibrillary tangles are not consistently reported in either species; however, hyperphosphorylated tau is reported in brains of aged dogs and cats, which might represent pre-tangle pathology.[7,9,13,25,26]

Overall, both dogs and cats show $A\beta$ brain deposition and pre-tangle pathology with increasing age similar to that seen in AD progression; however, these pathologies do not achieve the severity seen in AD. Nonetheless, brain $A\beta$ deposition may prove to be relatively early predictive biomarker of CDS consistent with preclinical and/or prodromal stages of AD.[4]

Effects of Age on Cognitive Ability of Senior Dogs and Cats

In humans, cognition is composed of multiple cognitive domains that include not only learning and memory but also executive function, language, psychomotor ability, attention, and spatial abilities. In the laboratory, there are protocols to assess many of these domains in dogs and cats. Age-related and domain-specific cognitive decline

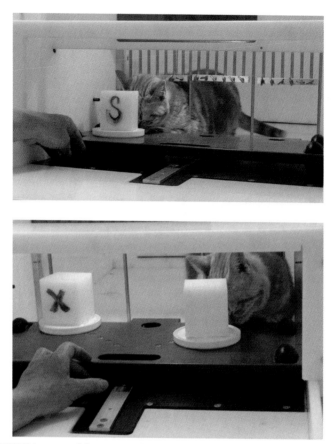

Fig. 1. The DNMP is a test of short-term visuospatial working memory.[27,30] The test consists of 2 phases. In the sample phase, the subject is required to displace an object placed over 1 of 3 possible locations on a food well (*top*); in this case the cat is required to displace block S covering food reward in the well on cat's right. The second stage (*bottom*) occurs after a delay and the subject is presented with 2 objects identical to that used in the sample phase. One object (marked with an X) is located in the same position as the sample object. The correct object is located in one of the remaining 2 positions (the nonmatch), and if the subject displaces the object, it can retrieve the food reward beneath. Initially, subjects are trained using a 5-second delay between the phases, but when the cat learns the rule that the food will always be found under the block in the nonmatch position, gradually longer delays can be introduced to assess memory.

is found in both species, but there is individual variation such that not all subjects are affected.

Using the delayed nonmatching to position (DNMP) memory task (**Fig. 1**), old dogs can be separated into 3 groups—unimpaired, impaired, and severely impaired—which may be analogous to the various stages of AD progression.[27,28] Aged dogs with DNMP impairments also demonstrate altered sleep-wake cycles, increased stereotypy, and decreased social contact with humans, which suggests a link between cognitive impairment and behavioral changes consistent with CDS.[29] Importantly, DNMP impairments can be detected as early as 6 years of age in some

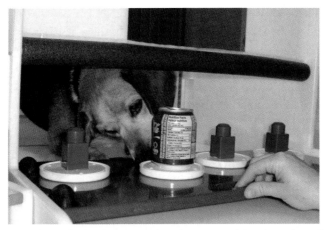

Fig. 2. In the attention task, the dog must select the correct object (covering a food reward), which is presented concurrently with either 1, 2, or 3 incorrect objects (distracters). Studies have demonstrated that performance declines and latency increases with increased distracter number, consistent with a test that assesses selective attention.[33]

dogs, which is consistent with early memory deficits in AD.[30] Also, brain amyloid deposition is reported earliest at 8 to 9 years of age.[23] Collectively, this suggests that memory impairment is an early consequence of canine aging that can precede both clinically relevant behavioral changes and amyloid deposition.

When dogs are repetitively rewarded for approaching 1 of 2 objects that differ substantially (ie, simple object discrimination learning), by contrast, no age effects on learning are evident.[31] However, if the reward contingencies are reversed after learning a simple object discrimination problem such that the dog must learn to respond to the object that previously was not rewarded in the original learning task (reversal learning), aged dogs require significantly more trials to learn to respond to the newly rewarded object than young dogs.[31,32] This impairment is analogous to the diminished executive function observed in human aging, AD, and other species.[32] On the other hand, age-related learning deficits are apparent when complex discrimination learning is assessed (eg, objects more similar or more objects), which may be related to age-related deficits in attention (**Fig. 2**).[33]

Previous studies have identified eyeblink conditioning deficits in aged cats, and a holeboard task revealed age effects on working memory, but not on spatial learning.[34,35] Age-related cognitive impairments are also seen in cats when feline adaptations of canine tests are used (see **Figs. 1** and **2**). Like dogs, cats demonstrate reversal learning and DNMP impairments with increasing age.[36] While there are insufficient data to determine age-of-onset of these impairments, reversal learning impairments were evident in 7.7- to 9-year-old cats compared to 2- to 3.8-year-old cats, suggesting that cognitive deficits precede clinical signs.[37] Similarly, while aged cats demonstrate neuropathologic brain changes similar to those reported in aged humans and dogs, the effect of neuropathologic changes on cognition have not been thoroughly investigated in the cat.[9,26] Overall, both dogs and cats demonstrate age-dependent and domain-specific cognitive decline consistent with those reported in aged humans.

Do Dogs and Cats Get AD?

Dogs and cats show both neuropathologic and cognitive changes that share many attributes of human aging and AD progression. However, late-stage AD progression is associated with impairment in most, if not all, cognitive domains. By contrast, dogs and cats do not show such extensive cognitive impairments (eg, ability to eat is retained), which suggests that the disease progression in pets is more comparable to earlier stages of AD progression. Consistent with this view, aged dogs show declining CSF levels of Aβ42, increased CSF levels of phospho-tau, and atrophy of the hippocampus, all of which are biomarkers being investigated as early diagnostic predictors of AD.[8,38,39] Future research better characterizing the longitudinal interaction among neuropathologic, cognitive, and behavioral changes in aging dogs and cats will be essential in better determining if and how CDS overlaps with AD progression.

COGNITIVE DYSFUNCTION SYNDROME
Clinical Signs of CDS

Classic signs of CDS are summarized by the acronym DISHA, which refers to **d**isorientation; alterations in **i**nteractions with owners, other pets, and the environment; **s**leep-wake cycle disturbances; **h**ousesoiling; and changes in **a**ctivity.[40] Although a decline in activity might be reported, laboratory studies suggest that increased locomotor activity and decreased immobile time are associated with greater cognitive impairment.[29,41] In addition, signs of fear, phobias, and anxiety, which are commonly reported by owners of senior pets, may be analogous to the finding of agitation and anxiety in humans with AD and might also be considered a component of CDS (**Table 1**).[42–46] Finally, memory deficits, which are some of the first recognizable signs of cognitive impairment in humans, have been identified early in the process of brain aging in both dogs and cats.[30,36] Therefore, learning or memory deficits in aged dogs and cats would also be a sign of CDS. However, these are difficult to recognize except perhaps in dogs that have been trained to a high level of performance (eg, service dogs, dogs trained for detection tasks) or by highly perceptive owners. For clinical signs of CDS, see the questionnaire in **Table 1**.

Differentiating Medical and Behavioral Problems from CDS

The determination of either a primary behavioral diagnosis or CDS must first be approached by excluding medical causes (**Table 2**). In the senior pet, this can be particularly challenging because with increasing age, there is an increased likelihood of concomitant medical conditions. Potential behavioral effects of medications must also be considered, especially those known to impact behavior. For example, steroids can increase drinking, appetite, and panting and are also associated with behavioral signs including nervousness, restlessness, irritable aggression, startling, food guarding, avoidance, and increased barking.[47] Additionally, senior pets may be less able to cope with stress, which may make them more susceptible to changes in their environment.

Thus behavioral signs in the senior pet can be due to medical or behavioral causes, cognitive dysfunction, or a combination thereof. For example, disruption of night time sleep in senior pets may be due to CDS, sensory dysfunction, or medical conditions that present with pain, polyuria, or hypertension, as well as alterations in the owner's schedule or home environment. Once problems arise, experience (ie, learning) further influences whether the behavior is likely to be repeated. In establishing a diagnosis of CDS, the clinician must be aware that the characteristic behavioral signs overlap with those of many medical and behavioral disorders.

Table 1 CDS checklist[1]		
Signs: DISHAAL	**Age First Noticed**	**Score 0–3**[a]
D: Disorientation/Confusion—Awareness—Spatial orientation		
Gets stuck or cannot get around objects		
Stares blankly at walls or floor		
Decreased recognition of familiar people/pets		
Goes to wrong side of door; walks into door/walls		
Drops food/cannot find		
Decreased response to auditory or visual stimuli		
Increased reactivity to auditory or visual stimuli (barking)		
I: Interactions—Social Relationships		
Decreased interest in petting/avoids contact		
Decreased greeting behavior		
In need of constant contact, overdependent, "clingy"		
Altered relationships other pets—less social/irritable/aggressive		
Altered relationships with people—less social/irritable/aggressive		
S: Sleep–Wake Cycles; Reversed Day/Night Schedule		
Restless sleep/waking at nights		
Increased daytime sleep		
H: Housesoiling (Learning and Memory)		
Indoor elimination at sites previously trained		
Decrease/loss of signaling		
Goes outdoors, then returns indoors and eliminates		
Elimination in crate or sleeping area		
A: Activity—Increased/Repetitive		
Pacing/wanders aimlessly		
Snaps at air/licks air		
Licking owners/household objects		
Increased appetite (eats quicker or more food)		
A: Activity—Apathy/Depressed		
Decreased interest in food/treats		
Decreased exploration/activity/play		
Decreased self-care (hygiene)		
A: Anxiety		
Vocalization, restlessness/agitation		
Anxiety, fear/phobia to auditory or visual stimuli		
Anxiety, fear/phobia of places (surfaces, locations)		
Anxiety/fear of people		
Separation anxiety		
L: Learning and Memory—Work, Tasks, Commands		
Decreased ability to perform learned tasks, commands		
Decreased responsiveness to familiar commands and tricks		
Inability/slow to learn new tasks		

[a] Score: 0 = none; 1 = mild; 2 = moderate; 3 = severe.
Adapted from Landsberg GM, Hunthausen W, Ackerman L. The effects of aging on the behavior of senior pets. Handbook of behavior problems of the dog and cat. 2nd edition. Philadelphia: WB Saunders; 2003. p. 273; with permission.

Table 2
Medical causes of behavioral signs

Medical Condition/Medical Presentation	Examples of Behavioral Signs
Neurologic: central (intracranial/extracranial) particularly if affecting forebrain, limbic/temporal and hypothalamic; REM sleep disorders	Altered awareness, response to stimuli, loss of learned behaviours, housesoiling, disorientation, confusion, altered activity levels, temporal disorientation, vocalization, change in temperament (fear, anxiety), altered appetite, altered sleep cycles, interrupted sleep
Partial seizures: temporal lobe epilepsy	Repetitive behaviors, self-traumatic disorders, chomping, staring, alterations in temperament (eg, intermittent states of fear or aggression), tremors, shaking, interrupted sleep
Sensory dysfunction	Altered response to stimuli, confusion, disorientation, irritability/aggression, vocalization, house soiling, altered sleep cycles
Endocrine: feline hyperthyroidism	Irritability, aggression, urine marking, decreased or increased activity, night waking
Endocrine: canine hypothyroidism	Lethargy, decreased response to stimuli, irritability/aggression
Endocrine: hyperadrenocorticism/hypoadrenocorticism	Lethargy, house soiling, altered appetite, decreased activity, anxiety
Endocrine: insulinoma, diabetes	Altered emotional state, irritability/aggression, anxiety, lethargy, house soiling, altered appetite
Endocrine: functional ovarian and testicular tumors	Increased androgen-induced behaviors. Males: aggression, roaming, marking, sexual attraction, mounting. Females: nesting or possessive aggression of objects.
Metabolic disorders: hepatic/renal	Signs associated with organ affected: may be anxiety, irritability, aggression, altered sleep, house soiling, mental dullness, decreased activity, restlessness, increase sleep, confusion
Pain	Altered response to stimuli, decreased activity, restless/unsettled, vocalization, house soiling, aggression/irritability, self-trauma, waking at night
Peripheral neuropathy	Self-mutilation, irritability/aggression, circling, hyperesthesia
Gastrointestinal	Licking, polyphagia, pica, coprophagia, fecal house soiling, wind sucking, tongue rolling, unsettled sleep, restlessness
Urogenital	House soiling (urine), polydypsia, waking at night
Dermatologic	Psychogenic alopecia (cats), acral lick dermatitis (dogs), nail biting, hyperesthesia, other self-trauma (chewing/biting/sucking/scratching)

Abbreviation: REM, rapid eye movement.

The practitioner will need to consider physical examination findings (including neurologic, sensory, and pain assessment) along with medical and behavioral signs to select the appropriate diagnostic tests required to reveal the causes and contributing factors of a patient's signs. Identifying all influences on specific behavioral signs is critical for both treatment selection and monitoring of behavioral and medical disorders.

Effects of Stress on Health and Mental Well-Being

Stress is an altered state of homeostasis that can be caused by physical or emotional factors that trigger psychological, behavioral, endocrine, and immune effects. Acute and chronic stress can also impact both health and behavior.[48–50] In addition, senior pets, especially those with medical or behavioral issues, may be more affected by stress and less able to adapt to change. Owners should pay particular attention to their pet's emotional and behavioral state as well as its appetite, sleep, and elimination to evaluate the role of stress. While enrichment can help maintain both physical and mental health, changes in the elderly pet's household or schedule should be made slowly. Natural products or drugs may also be indicated (discussed later).

Prevalence of Behavioral Signs in Senior Pets

Spontaneously reported behavior problems

A number of studies have examined the prevalence of spontaneously reported behavioral signs in senior pets referred to behavioral specialists.[44,45] In 2 canine studies, behavioral complaints related to aggression, or fear and anxiety, were most prevalent. In a similar senior cat study, most displayed signs of marking or soiling; however, cases of aggression, vocalization, and restlessness were also serious enough to solicit referral.[50]

To further examine the distribution of problems reported by owners of senior dogs and cats, the Veterinary Information Network (VIN) database was searched for behavior problems of 50 senior dogs (aged 9–17) and 100 senior cats (aged 12–22 years). Of dogs, 62% had signs consistent with CDS, but most demonstrated anxiety, night waking, and vocalization. In the 100 feline cases reviewed, the most common complaints were related to vocalization, especially at night, and soiling. **Figs. 3** and **4** summarize the distribution of behavioral signs most commonly reported by owners of senior pets across studies.

Solicited reports of behavior problems

Since many of the most common behavioral signs in senior pets go unreported, a more proactive approach is required to establish their prevalence. In 1 study of dogs aged 11 to 16, 28% of 11-to 12-year-old dogs and 68% of 15- to 16-year-old dogs showed at least 1 sign consistent with CDS.[51] In another study of 102 dogs, 41% had alterations in at least 1 category associated with CDS and 32% had alterations in 2 categories.[52] In a more recent study, females and neutered males were significantly more affected than intact males with both prevalence and severity increasing with age, which is consistent with previous reports.[46,53] Moreover, social interactions and house training were the most impaired categories.[46]

In a recent epidemiologic study using an internet survey format of 497 dogs ranging in age from 8 to 19 years, the prevalence of CDS was 5% in 10- to 12-year-old dogs, 23.3% in dogs 12- to 14-year-old dogs, and 41% in dogs older than 14, with an overall prevalence of 14.2%. However, only 1.9% of cases had a veterinary diagnosis of CDS.[54] In 1 study of aged cats presented to veterinary clinics for routine annual care, 28% of 95 cats aged 11 to 15 and 50% of 46 cats older than 15 years were diagnosed with possible CDS.[37]

Prevalences of owner reported signs in senior dogs

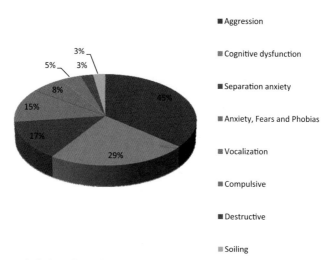

Fig. 3. Fears and phobias (includes generalized anxiety), compulsive includes repetitive and stereotypic behavior; cognitive dysfunction includes disorientation, wandering, waking and anxious at night. Behavior signs were combined from 3 studies: a Spanish study of 270 dogs older than age 7 that were presented for behavior problems, 103 dogs referred to a veterinary behaviorist, and a search of the Veterinary Information Network (VIN) of 50 dogs aged 9 to 17 years.

Importance of Client Education and Screening in the Veterinary Clinic

The data presented above indicate several important findings. First, behavioral signs related to anxiety, vocalization, night waking, soiling in cats, and aggression in dogs are more often spontaneously reported to veterinarians, which is likely related to the impact of these behaviors on the owner. Second, behavioral changes consistent with CDS are reported less frequently but are present in a significant proportion of the population. Third, the prevalence of behavioral signs consistent with CDS increases with age. Finally, because CDS is likely underdiagnosed when solicited reporting is not used, proactive monitoring and assessment of behavioral signs should be components of every veterinary visit involving senior pets. Veterinarians and their staff must inform clients of the health and welfare consequences if these problems are untreated. Handouts and web links on senior care and cognitive dysfunction syndrome can be used to further educate owners. Questionnaires are particularly effective for quick and comprehensive screening. Several are available for screening, including **Table 1**, a scoring system known as age-related cognitive and affective disorders, and a recently published 13-point data-based assessment tool.[40,54]

THERAPEUTIC OPTIONS FOR PETS WITH CDS
Behavioral Support and Environmental Enrichment in the Management of CDS

Canine studies have shown that mental stimulation is an essential component in maintaining quality of life and that continued enrichment in the form of training, play,

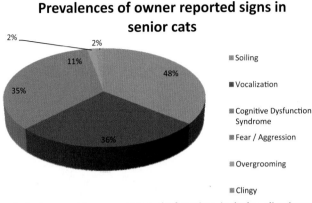

Fig. 4. Soiling includes marking, cognitive dysfunction includes disorientation, restless, wandering and night waking, and fear/aggression (includes fear and hiding). Behavior signs were combined from a VIN data search of 100 cats aged 12 to 22 years and 83 from 3 different behavior referral practices.

exercise, and novel toys can help to maintain cognitive function (ie, use it or lose it).[55] This is analogous to human studies in which increased mental activity and physical exercise have been found to delay the onset of dementia.[56,57]

Environmental enrichment can have positive effects on behavioral health and quality of life in pets and is likely to improve cognitive function.[58] Inconsistency in the management of the senior pet's environment (especially for cats) can cause stress and negatively impact health and behavioral well-being.[40,50] As sensory, motor, and cognitive function decline, new odor, tactile, and/or sound cues may help the pet better cope with its environment. Dogs with increased urine frequency may need more frequent trips outdoors or even the addition of an indoor toilet area. Ramps and physical support devices may be necessary to address mobility issues. For cats, inappropriate elimination may be improved by providing more litter boxes with lower sides and nonslip ramps.

Enrichment should focus on positive social interactions as well as new and varied opportunities for exploration, climbing, perching, hunt-and-chase games, and other stimulating ways to obtain food and treats. Food toys that require pushing, lifting, dropping, batting, pawing, or rolling to release food help older dogs and cats to remain active and alert (**Fig. 5**). By scattering favored food, treats, or catnip in different locations, pets can learn to hunt, search, and retrieve.

Maintenance of a day-night cycle by opening blinds and providing outdoor activities (where practical) to provide daylight during the day and reducing exposure to artificial light at night may be considered. Increased daytime enrichment with several quality interactive sessions, food toys, outdoor exercise (if appropriate), and a final interactive play session prior to bed may help encourage better sleep.

Drug Therapy for CDS

CDS cannot be cured at present, but deterioration may be slowed and clinical signs improved. Assuming concomitant medical and behavior problems are being controlled, various drugs (**Table 3**) may be considered to improve cognitive function or control clinical signs. For each pet, the clinician must weigh potential risks against potential benefits.

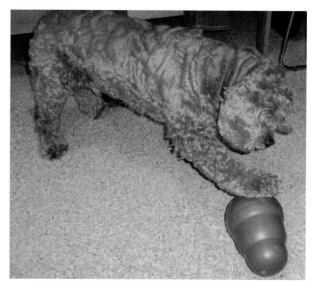

Fig. 5. A food manipulation toy, the Kong Wobbler (Kong Company, Golden, CO, USA). This toy is filled with food pieces and treats that are delivered through the opening as the dog learns to tip the toy.

Selegiline (Anipryl; Pfizer Animal Health, New York, NY, USA) is a selective and irreversible inhibitor of monoamine oxidase B.[59] It may enhance dopamine and other catecholamines in the cortex and hippocampus and has been shown both in the laboratory and clinic to improve signs consistent with CDS in dogs.[59,61] Selegiline

Table 3		
Doses for drugs for behavior therapy of senior pets		
	Dog	**Cat**
Selegiline (CDS)	0.5–1 mg/kg sid in am	0.5–1 mg/kg sid in am
Propentofylline (CDS)	2.5–5 mg/kg bid	¼ of a 50 mg tablet daily
Oxazepam[a]	0.2–1 mg/kg sid–bid	0.2–0.5 mg/kg sid–bid
Clonazepam[a]	0.1–1.0 mg/kg bid–tid	0.02–0.2 mg/kg sid–bid
Lorazepam[a]	0.025–0.2 mg/kg sid–tid	0.025–0.05 mg/kg sid–bid
Diphenhydramine[a]	2–4 mg/kg	1–4 mg/kg
Fluoxetine	1.0–2.0 mg/kg sid	0.5–1.5 mg/kg sid
Paroxetine	0.5–2 mg/kg	0.5–1.5 mg/kg
Sertraline	1–5 mg/kg sid or divided bid	0.5–1.5 mg/kg sid
Buspirone	0.5–2.0 mg/kg sid–tid	0.5–1 mg/kg bid
Trazodone	2–5 mg/kg (up to 8–10) prn–tid	Not determined
Phenobarbital	2.5–5 mg/kg bid	2.5 mg/kg bid
Memantine	0.3–1 mg/kg sid	Not determined
Gabapentin	10–30 mg/kg q 8–12 h	5–10 mg/kg q 12 h

Abbreviation: sid, once daily.

[a] Use single dosing prior to sleep or anxiety-evoking event, up to maximum daily dosing for control of ongoing anxiety.

also may be neuroprotective possibly by reducing free radical production and/or increasing enzymes that scavenge free radicals such as superoxide dismutase and catalase.[59,60] Selegiline is not licensed for use in cats but is used off label with anecdotal reports of improvement in CDS-like signs.[62] Selegiline may require 2 weeks or longer before clinical improvement is seen, should not be used concurrently with other monoamine oxidase inhibitors (eg, amitraz), and should be avoided, or used cautiously, with drugs that may enhance serotonin transmission (such as selective serotonin reuptake inhibitors, tricyclic antidepressants, buspirone, trazodone, tramadol, and dextromethorphan).

Propentofylline (Vivitonin; Merck Animal Health, Milton Keyes, UK) is licensed in some European countries for the treatment of dullness, lethargy, and depressed demeanor in old dogs. Propentofylline may increase blood flow to the heart, skeletal muscles, and brain and may have neuroprotective properties due to inhibiting the uptake of adenosine and blocking phosphodiesterase. Propentofylline has been anecdotally used in cats, but there is no clinical evidence of efficacy.

Drugs thought to enhance the noradrenergic system, such as adrafinil and modafinil, might be useful in older dogs to improve alertness and help maintain normal sleep-wake cycles (by increasing daytime exploration and activity).[63,64] However, dose and efficacy in dogs are not well established. Newer treatment strategies include the N-methyl-D-aspartate receptor antagonist memantine or hormone replacement therapy, but evidence is currently lacking to make appropriate suggestions for treatment.[65]

In canine and feline CDS, as well as in AD, there is evidence of cholinergic decline (see earlier). Because the elderly are particularly susceptible to anticholinergic drugs, it is prudent to consider therapies with less anticholinergic effects. Drugs and natural products that enhance cholinergic transmission might have potential benefits for improving signs of CDS, but more research is required to select appropriate drugs and doses.[66]

Nutritional and Dietary Therapy for CDS

Nutritional and dietary interventions (**Table 4**) can improve antioxidant defense thereby reducing the negative effects of free radicals. A senior diet (Canine b/d, Hills Pet Nutrition, Topeka, KS, USA) for dogs improves signs and slows the progress of cognitive decline.[67–69] The diet improved performance on a number of cognitive tasks when compared to a nonsupplemented diet as early as to 2 to 8 weeks after the onset of therapy. However, the combined effect of the supplemented diet and environmental enrichment provided the greatest benefit and, when started prior to the onset of behavioral signs, may extend cognitive health.[67]

Another strategy is a diet containing medium-chain triglycerides (MCTs), which are converted to ketone bodies by the liver. Since a decline in cerebral glucose metabolism and reduced energy metabolism are associated with cognitive decline, MCT-induced ketone bodies provide an alternate energy source that can be used by the brain. When compared to control, the diet (Purina One Vibrant Maturity 7+ Formula; Nestlé Purina PetCare, St Louis, MO, USA) significantly improved performance on several cognitive tasks.[70] Supplementation with MCTs also improves mitochondrial function, increases polyunsaturated fatty acids in the brain, and decreases amyloid precursor protein in the parietal cortex of aged dogs.[71,72] Supplementation with MCTs is also approved as a medical dietary supplement for AD patients. Cognitive diets for cats have not yet been developed.

A number of clinical trials have shown improvements in signs associated with CDS in dogs using dietary supplements containing phosphatidylserine, a membrane phospholipid.[73,74] One product (Senilife; CEVA Animal Health, Libourne, France) was

Table 4
Ingredients and doses of natural therapeutics for senior pets

	Ingredients	Dose
Senilife	Phosphatidylserine, *Gingko biloba*, vitamin B6 (pyridoxine), vitamin E, resveratrol	Dogs and cats (see label)
Activait	Phosphatidylserine, omega-3 fatty acids, vitamins E and C, L-carnitine, alpha-lipoic acid, coenzyme Q, selenium	Separate dog and cat products
Activait Cat	Note: no alpha-lipoic acid in feline version	See label
Novifit	S-Adenosyl-L-methionine-tosylate disulfate (SAMe)	Dog: 10–20 mg/kg sid Cat: 100 mg sid
Neutricks	Apoaequorin	Dogs: 1 tablet per 18 kg
Prescription diet b/d Canine aging and alertness	Flavonoids and carotenoids from fruits and vegetables, vitamin E, vitamin C, beta-carotene, selenium, L-carnitine, alpha-lipoic acid, omega 3 fatty acids	Dogs
Purina One Vibrant Maturity 7+ Senior	Medium chain triglycerides (from coconut oil)	Dogs
Melatonin	Endogenous-based peptide	Dogs: 3–9 mg Cats: 1.5–6 mg
Anxitane	Suntheanine	Dogs: 2.5–5 mg/kg bid Cats: 25 mg bid
Harmonease	Magnolia and phellodendron	Dogs: up to 22 kg ½ tablet daily; >22 kg 1 tablet daily Cats: N/A
Zylkene	Alpha-casozepine	Dogs: 15–30 mg/kg/d Cats: 15 mg/kg/d
Pheromones	Adaptil collar, diffuser, or spray for dogs Feliway spray or diffuser for cats	As per label
Lavender	Aromatherapy for dogs	As per label

tested in aged dogs using a cross-over design in which DNMP memory performance was improved after 60 days of treatment with Senilife.[75] Although labeled for use in cats, efficacy studies are not published.

Another product containing phosphatidylserine (Activait; Vet Plus Ltd, Lytham St. Annes, UK) demonstrated significant improvement over placebo on signs of disorientation, social interactions, and house soiling in dogs.[74] A feline version of Activait, with no alpha-lipoic acid, is also available but has not been tested in clinical trials.

Another available supplement for cognitive health (Novifit; Virbac Animal Health, Ft Worth, TX, USA) contains S-adenosyl-L-methionine (SAMe) tosylate, which is found in all living cells and is formed from methionine and adenosine triphosphate. SAMe may help to maintain cell membrane fluidity, receptor function, and the turnover of monoamine transmitters, as well as increase the production of the endogenous antioxidant glutathione.[76] In a recent placebo-controlled trial, greater improvement in activity and awareness was reported in the SAMe group after 8 weeks.[77] Since SAMe might increase central serotonin levels, caution should be used when combining with other drugs that might increase serotonin. On the other hand, SAMe has been used in human patients to enhance the effects of serotonin reuptake inhibitors in the treatment of depressive disorders.[78] In laboratory aged dog and cat studies, SAMe improved measures of executive function and possibly attention.[79,80] In cats, these effects were mainly evident in the least cognitively impaired subjects, suggesting that supplementation with SAMe early in disease progression, rather than in more severely impaired subjects, should be most beneficial.[80]

Apoaequorin (Neutricks; Quincy Animal Health, Madison, WI, USA), recently released in the United States, improved learning and attention in laboratory trials compared to both placebo and selegiline.[81] Apaoequorin is a calcium buffering protein that has been postulated to provide neuroprotection in aging and consequently have positive effects on signs of brain aging.

Last, curcumin, an antioxidant, antiamyloid, and antiinflammatory compound found in the turmeric and catechin spices, is postulated to be helpful.[82]

Adjunctive Therapies for Anxiety and Night Waking

Because behavioral signs associated with anxiety and night waking are highly prevalent in senior pets and greatly impact the owner-pet bond, it is prudent for the practitioner to rapidly address them. Drugs and natural remedies that help reduce anxiety and aid in reestablishing normal sleep-wake cycles can also be of benefit in senior pets alone or in conjunction with drugs for CDS (see **Tables 3** and **4**).

Melatonin is best given to dogs 30 minutes before bedtime. Diphenhydramine, phenobarbital, or trazodone can also promote sedation. For the dog or cat that has difficulty settling at night but then sleeps well, situational use of anxiolytics can be helpful. Benzodiazepines have rapid onset, are generally short acting, and have sedative effects at the higher end of the recommended dosage range. In pets where liver function is compromised, clonazepam, lorazepam, or oxazepam is recommended because they have no active metabolites. Since pain may contribute to unsettled sleep or night waking, gabapentin can be added both as an adjunctive therapy for pain management and for its behavioral calming effects.

For senior pets with generalized anxiety, noise phobias, or separation anxiety, buspirone or selective serotonin reuptake inhibitors like fluoxetine (Reconcile; Elanco, Greenfield, IN, USA) and sertraline may be considered because of their low risk of side effects. Paroxetine and tricyclic antidepressants have varying degrees of anticholinergic effects and therefore should not be a first-choice therapeutic. However, these drugs should not be used concurrently with selegiline.

Natural compounds that may reduce anxiety and help pets settle at night include suntheanine (Anxitane; Virbac Animal Health, Ft Worth, TX, USA), honokiol and berberine extracts (Harmonease; VPL, Phoenix, AZ, USA), alpha casozepine (Zylkene; Vetoquinol Canada, Lavaltrie, PQ, Canada), pheromones (Adaptil and Feliway; CEVA Animal Health, Libourne, France), and lavender essential oils.[40]

SUMMARY

CDS is an underdiagnosed behavioral problem that affects a substantial number of aged pets. Because changes in behavior are often early indicators of medical or behavior problems in senior pets, the veterinarian faces the challenge of ruling out the influence of medical problems, sleep disturbances, anxiety, concurrent medications, and pain before a diagnosis of CDS can be made. While there are several options for treatment of CDS, many therapeutics have not been adequately tested. Moreover, early intervention is likely to be most beneficial. As we learn more about biomarkers of brain aging, objective tests for identifying pets likely to progress to CDS may be developed. In the meantime, a proactive approach for early identification and monitoring of behavioral signs is essential for establishing a diagnosis and monitoring treatment success.

REFERENCES

1. McKhann GM, Knopman DS, Chertkow H, et al. The diagnosis of dementia due to Alzheimer's disease: recommendations from the National Institute on Aging-Alzheimer's Association workgroups on diagnostic guidelines for Alzheimer's disease. Alzheim Dem 2011;7:263–9.
2. Jakob-Roetne R, Jacobsen H. Alzheimer's disease: from pathology to therapeutic approaches. Angew Chem Int 2009;48:3030–59.
3. Reinikainen KJ, Soininen H, Riekkinen PJ. Neurotransmitter changes in Alzheimer's disease: implications to diagnostics and therapy. J Neurosci Res 1990;27:576–86.
4. Jack CR, Knopman DS, Jagust WJ, et al. Hypothetical model of dynamic biomarkers of the Alzheimer's pathological cascade. Lancet Neurol 2010;9:119–28.
5. Berchtold NC, Cotman CW. Normal and pathological aging: from animals to humans. In: Bizon JL, Woods A, editors. Animal models of human cognitive aging. New York: Humana Press; 2009. p. 1–28.
6. Salvin HE, Greevy PD, Sachdev PS, et al. Growing old gracefully-behavioral changes associated with "successful aging" in the dog. Canis familiaris. J Vet Behav 2011;6:313–20.
7. Borras D, Ferrer I, Pumarola M. Age related changes in the brain of the dog. Vet Pathol 1999;36:202–11.
8. Tapp PD, Siwak CT, Gao FQ, et al. Frontal lobe volume, function, and beta-amyloid pathology in a canine model of aging. J Neurosci 2004;24:8205–13.
9. Gunn-Moore D, Moffat K, Christie LA, et al. Cognitive dysfunction and the neurobiology of ageing in cats. J Small Anim Pract 2007;48:546–53.
10. Zhang C, Hua T, Zhu Z, et al. Age related changes of structures in cerebellar cortex of cat. J Biosci 2006;31:55–60.
11. Dobson H, Denenberg S. Ageing and imaging based neuropathology in the cat. In: Programs and abstracts of the 17th Congress of ESVCE and 1st Congress of ECAWBM. Avignon: 2011.
12. Cummings BJ, Satou T, Head E, et al. Diffuse plaques contain C-terminal AB42 and not AB40: evidence from cats and dogs. Neurobiol Aging 1996;17:653–9.
13. Cummings BJ, Head E, Afagh AJ, et al. B-Amyloid accumulation correlates with cognitive dysfunction in the aged canine. Neurobiol Learn Mem 1996;66:11–23.
14. Colle M-A, Hauw J-J, Crespau F, et al. Vascular and parenchymal beta-amyloid deposition in the aging dog: correlation with behavior. Neurobiol Aging 2000;21:695–704.
15. Nakamura S, Nakayama H, Kiatipattanasakul W, et al. Senile plaques in very aged cats. Acta Neuropathol 1996;91:437–9.
16. Head E, Liu J, Hagen TM, et al. Oxidative damage increases with age in a canine model of human brain aging. J Neurochem 2002;82:375–81.
17. Ruehl WW, Bruyette WW, DePaoli DS, et al. Canine cognitive dysfunction as a model for human age-related cognitive decline, dementia, and Alzheimer's disease: clinical presentation, cognitive testing, pathology and response to l-deprenyl therapy. Prog Brain Res 1995;106:217–25.
18. Araujo JA, Nobrega JN, Raymond R, et al. Aged dogs demonstrate both increased sensitivity to scopolamine and decreased muscarinic receptor density. Pharmacol Biochem Behav 2011;98(2):203–9.
19. Zhang JH, Sampogna S, Morales FR, et al. Age-related changes in cholinergic neurons in the laterodorsal and the pedunculo-pontine tegmental nuclei of cats: a combined light and electron microscopic study. Brain Res 2005;1052:47–55.

20. Araujo JA, Studzinski, CM, Milgram NW. Further evidence for the cholinergic hypothesis of aging and dementia from the canine model of aging. Prog Psychopharmacol Biol Psychiatry 2005;29:411–22.
21. Araujo JA, Chan ADF, Winka LL, et al. Dose-specific effects of scopolamine on canine cognition: impairment of visuospatial memory, but not visuospatial discrimination. Psychopharmacology 2004;175:92–8.
22. Pugliese M, Cangitano C, Ceccariglia S, et al. Canine cognitive dysfunction and the cerebellum: acetylcholinesterase reduction, neuronal and glial changes. Brain Res 2007;1139:85–94.
23. Head E, McCleary R, Hahn FF, et al. Region-specific age at onset of beta-amyloid in dogs. Neurobiol Aging 2000;21:89–96.
24. Näslund J, Haroutunian V, Mohs R et al. Correlation between elevated levels of amyloid β-peptide in the brain and cognitive decline. JAMA 2000;283:1571–7.
25. Gunn-Moore DA, McVee J, Bradshaw JM, et al. β-Amyloid and hyper-phosphorylated tau deposition in cat brains. J Fel Med Surg 2006;8:234–42.
26. Head E, Moffat K, Das P, et al. Beta-amyloid deposition and tau phosphorylation in clinically characterized aged cats. Neurobiol Aging 2005;26:749–63.
27. Adams B, Chan A, Callahan H, et al. Use of a delayed non-matching to position task to model age-dependent cognitive decline in the dog. Behav Brain Res 2000;108:47–56.
28. Adams B, Chan A, Callahan H, et al. The canine as a model of human brain aging: recent developments. Prog Neuropsychopharmacol Biol Psychiatry 2000;24:675–92.
29. Siwak CT, Tapp PD, Milgram NW. Effect of age and level of cognitive function on spontaneous and exploratory behaviours in the beagle dog. Learn Mem 2001;8:65–70.
30. Studzinski CM, Christie L-A, Araujo JA et al. Visuospatial function in the beagle dog: An early marker of cognitive decline in a model of human cognitive aging and dementia. Neurobiol Learn Mem 2006;86(2):197–204.
31. Milgram NW, Head E, Weiner E, et al. Cognitive functions and aging in the dog: acquisition of nonspatial visual tasks. Behav Neurosci 1994;108:57–68.
32. Tapp PD, Siwak CT, Estrada J, et al. Size and reversal learning in the beagle dog as a measure of executive function and inhibitory control in aging. Learn Mem 2003;10:64–73.
33. Snigdha S, Christie L, De Rivera C, et al. Age and distraction are determinants of performance on a novel visual search task in aged Beagle dogs. Age (Dordr) 2012;34(1):67–73.
34. Harrison J, Buchwald J. Eyeblink conditioning deficits in the old cat. Neurobiol Aging 1983;4:45–51.
35. McCune S, Stevenson J, Fretwell L, et al. Aging does not significantly affect performance in a spatial learning task in the domestic cat (Felis silvestris catus). Appl Anim Behav Sci 2008;3:345–56.
36. Milgram NW, Landsberg GM, De Rivera C, et al. Age and cognitive dysfunction in the domestic cat. In: Proceedings of the ACVB/AVSAB Symposium. St Louis; 2011. p. 28–9.
37. Landsberg G, Denenberg S, Araujo J. Cognitive dysfunction in cats. A syndrome we used to dismiss as old age. J Fel Med Surg 2010;12:837–48.
38. Head E, Pop V, Sarsoza F, et al. Amyloid-beta peptide and oligomers in the brain and cerebrospinal fluid of aged canine. J Alzheimer Dis 2010;20:637–46.
39. Araujo JA, Higgins GA, de Rivera C, et al. Evaluation of translation Alzheimer's disease biomarkers in the aged dog: the effects of age and BACE inhibition on CSF amyloid. In: Abstracts of the Alzheimer's Association International Conference. Paris; 2011.

40. Landsberg GM, Hunthausen W, Ackerman L. The effects of aging on the behavior of senior pets. In: Handbook of behavior problems of the dog and cat. 3rd edition. Philadelphia: WB Saunders; in press.

41. Rosado B, Gonzalez MA, Pesini P, et al. Effects of age and severity of cognitive dysfunction on spontaneous behaviour in companion dogs. In: Abstract in ESVCE-ECAWBM Congress. Avignon; 2011.

42. Senanarong V, Cummings JL, Fairbanks L, et al. Agitation in Alzheimer's disease is a manifestation of frontal lobe dysfunction. Dement Geratr Cogn Disord 2004;17:14–20.

43. McCurry SM, Gibbons LE, Logsdon RG, et al. Anxiety and nighttime behavioral disturbances. Awakenings in patients with Alzheimer's disease. J Gerontol Nurs 2004;30:12–20.

44. Mariotti VM, Landucci M, Lippi I, et al. Epidemiological study of behavioural disorders in elderly dogs. In: Heath S, editor. Proceedings 7th International Meeting of Veterinary Behaviour Medicine, ESVCE. Belgium: 2009. p. 241–3.

45. Horwitz D. Dealing with common behavior problems in senior dogs. Vet Med 2001; 96:869–87.

46. Azkona G, Garcia-Beleguer S, Chacon G, et al. Prevalence and risk factors of behavioral changes associated with age-related cognitive impairment in geriatric dogs. J Sm Anim Pract 2009;50:87–91.

47. Notari L, Mills D. Possible behavioral effects of exogenous corticosteroids on dog behavior: a preliminary investigation. J Vet Behav 2011;6:321–7.

48. Berteselli GV, Servidaq F, DallAra P, et al. Evaluation of the immunological, stress and behavioral parameters in dogs (Canis familiaris) with anxiety-related disorders. In: Mills D, Levine E, Landsberg G, et al, editors. Current issues and research in veterinary behavioral medicine. West Lafayette (IN): Purdue Press; 2005. p. 18–22.

49. Overall KL. Dogs as "natural" models of human psychiatric disorders: assessing validity and understanding mechanism. Prog Neuropsychopharmacol Biol Psychiatry 2000;24:727–6.

50. Landsberg GM, DePorter T, Araujo JA. Management of anxiety, sleeplessness and cognitive dysfunction in the senior pet. Vet Clin North Am Small Anim Pract 2011;41:565–90.

51. Nielson JC, Hart BL, Cliff KD, et al. Prevalence of behavioral changes associated with age-related cognitive impairment in dogs. J Am Vet Med Assoc 2001;218:1787–91.

52. Osella MC, Re G, Odore R, et al. Canine cognitive dysfunction syndrome: prevalence, clinical signs and treatment with a neuroprotective nutraceutical. Appl Anim Behav Sci 2007;105:297–310.

53. Hart BL. Effect of gonadectomy on subsequent development of age-related cognitive impairment in dogs. J Am Vet Med Assoc 2001;219:51–6.

54. Salvin HE, McGreevy PD, Sachev PS, et al. Under diagnosis of canine cognitive dysfunction; a cross-sectional survey of older companion dogs. Vet J 2011;188: 331–6.

55. McMillan FD. Maximizing quality of life in ill animals. J Am Anim Hosp Assoc 223;39: 227–35.

56. Valenzuela M, Sachdev P. Harnessing brain and cognitive reserve for the prevention of dementia. Ind J Psychiatry 2009;51:16–21.

57. Yonas E G, Roberts RO, Knopman DS, et al. Aging and mild cognitive impairment. A population-based study. Arch Neurol 2010;67:80–6.

58. Head E. Combining an antioxidant-fortified diet with behavioral enrichment leads to cognitive improvement and reduced brain pathology in aging canines: strategies for healthy aging. Ann N Y Acad Sci 2007;1114:398–406.

59. Milgram NW, Ivy GO, Head E, et al. The effect of l-deprenyl on behavior, cognitive function, and biogenic amines in the dog. Neurochem Res 1993;18:1211–9.

60. Carillo MC, Milgram NW, Ivy GO, et al. (–)Deprenyl increases activities of superoxide dismutase (SOD) in striatum of dog brain. Life Sci 1994;54:1483–9.
61. Campbell S, Trettien A, Kozan B. A non-comparative open label study evaluating the effect of selegiline hydrochloride in a clinical setting. Vet Ther 2001;2(1):24–39.
62. Landsberg G. Therapeutic options for cognitive decline in senior pets. J Am Anim Hosp Assoc 2006;42:407–13.
63. Siwak CT, Gruet P, Woehrle F, et al. Behavioral activating effects of adrafinil in aged canines. Pharmacol Biochem Behav 2000;66:293–300.
64. Siwak CT, Gruet P, Woehrle F, et al. Comparison of the effects of adrafinil, propentofylline and nicergoline on behavior in aged dogs. Am J Vet Res 2000;61:1410–4.
65. Martinez-Coria H, Green KN, Billings LM, et al. Memantine improves cognition and reduces Alzheimer's-like neuropathology in transgenic mice. Am J Pathol 2010; 176(2): 870–80.
66. Araujo JA, Greig NH, Ingram DK, et al. Cholinesterase inhibitors improve both memory and complex learning in aged Beagle dogs. J Alzheimer Dis 2011;26:143–55.
67. Milgram NW, Head EA, Zicker SC, et al. Long term treatment with antioxidants and a program of behavioral enrichment reduces age-dependent impairment in discrimination and reversal learning in beagle dogs. Exp Gerentol 2004;39:753–65.
68. Milgram NW, Zicker SC, Head E, et al. Dietary enrichment counteracts age-associated cognitive dysfunction in canines. Neurobiol Aging 2002;23:737–45.
69. Araujo JA, Studzinski, CM, Head E, et al. Assessment of nutritional interventions for modification of age-associated cognitive decline using a canine model of human aging. AGE 2005;27:27–37.
70. Pan Y, Larson B, Araujo JA, et al. Dietary supplementation with medium-chain TAG has long-lasting cognition-enhancing effects in aged dogs. Br J Nutr 2010;103:1746–54.
71. Taha AY, Henderson ST, Burnham WM. Dietary enrichment with medium chain-triglycerides (AC-1203) elevates polyunsaturated fatty acids in the parietal cortex of aged dogs; implications for treating age-related cognitive decline. Neurochem Res 2009;34:1619–25.
72. Studzinski CM, MacKay WA, Beckett TL, et al. Induction of ketosis may improve mitochondrial function and decrease steady-state amyloid-beta precursor protein (APP) levels in the aged dog. Brain Res 2008;1226:209–17.
73. Osella MC, Re G, Odore R, et al. Canine cognitive dysfunction syndrome: prevalence, clinical signs and treatment with a neuroprotective nutraceutical. Appl Anim Behav Sci 2007;105:297–310.
74. Heath SE, Barabas S, Craze PG. Nutritional supplementation in cases of canine cognitive dysfunction-a clinical trial. Appl Anim Behav Sci 2007;105:274–83.
75. Araujo JA, Landsberg GM, Milgram NW, et al. Improvement of short-term memory performance in aged beagles by a nutraceutical supplement containing phosphatidylserine, Ginkgo biloba, vitamin E and pyridoxine. Can Vet J 2008;49:379–85.
76. Bottiglieri T. S-Adenosyl-L-methionine (SAMe): from the bench to the bedside—molecular basis of a pleiotrophic molecule. Am J Clin Nutr 2002;76:1151–7S.
77. Rème CA, Dramard V, Kern L, et al. Effect of S-adenosylmethionine tablets on the reduction of age-related mental decline in dogs: a double-blind placebo-controlled trial. Vet Ther 2008;9:69–82.
78. Papakostas GI, Mischoulon D, Shyu I, et al. S-Adenosyl methionine (SAMe) augmentation of serotonin reuptake inhibitors for antidepressant nonresponders with major depressive disorder: a double-blind, randomized clinical trial. Am J Psychiatry 2010; 167:942–8.

79. Mongillo P, Araujo JA, de Rivera C, et al. The effects of novifit on cognitive function in aged beagle dogs. J Vet Behav 2010;5:39. [In: Abstract of the 7th International IVBM International Veterinary Behavior Meeting. Edinburgh (Scotland), 2009].

80. Araujo JA, Faubert ML, Brooks ML, et al. Novifit (NoviSAMe) tablets improves executive function in aged dogs and cats: implications for treatment of cognitive dysfunction syndrome. Intern J Appl Res Vet Med 2012;10:90–8.

81. Milgram NW, Landsberg GM, Visnesky M. Effect of apoaequroin on cognitive function in aged canines. In: Abstracts of the 17th Congress of ESVCE and 1st Annual Congress of ECAWBM. Avignon; 2011.

82. Ringman JM, Frautschy SA, Cole GM, et al. A potential role of the curry spice curcumin in Alzheimer's disease. Curr Alzheimer Res 2005;2:131–6.

Nutritional Care for Aging Cats and Dogs

D.P. Laflamme, DVM, PhD

KEYWORDS

- Diet • Geriatrics • Nutritional evaluation • Obesity • Osteoarthritis
- Cognitive dysfunction

KEY POINTS

- Before prescribing a dietary change in any patient, a nutritional evaluation should be completed to include assessment of the patient, the current diet, and feeding management.
- Body condition score to assess body fat and muscle score to assess muscle atrophy are key indicators of nutritional and health status in senior pets.
- Cognitive dysfunction is a common condition in aged pets and may respond to dietary management with antioxidants and alternative energy sources, as well as environmental and behavioral enrichment for mental stimulation.
- Multimodal management of osteoarthritis includes a combination of weight management, physical therapy, diet including long chain n-3 polyunsaturated fatty acids from fish oil, other nutraceuticals, and pharmaceutical agents.
- Obesity is associated with increased oxidative stress, inflammation, and insulin resistance, which contribute to a number of health problems.
- Weight loss can be achieved in most pets by creating a negative energy balance and is best achieved using diets with low calorie density, increased protein content, and an overall increased nutrient:calorie ratio.

According to pet owners, most pets, even senior pets, are healthy or generally healthy and do not require therapeutic diets.[1,2] But, all pets must eat. And, despite an increase in the influence of the internet, veterinarians remain the top resource for pet owners for information regarding pet health and nutrition.[2] Therefore, veterinarians need to be prepared to provide nutritional advice for healthy pets as well as for pets that are ill. This is especially true for senior pets, due to their unique needs. This article is designed to provide guidance for nutritional assessment of aging pets, with information about feeding healthy older pets as well as addressing some common age-related, nutrient-sensitive conditions in senior dogs and cats.

Approximately 40% of pet dogs and cats are 7 years of age or older.[1,2] Aging brings with it physiologic changes. Some changes are obvious, like whitening of hair,

Nestlé Purina PetCare Research, Checkerboard Square - 2S, St Louis, MO 63164, USA
E-mail address: dorothy.laflamme@rd.nestle.com

Vet Clin Small Anim 42 (2012) 769–791
http://dx.doi.org/10.1016/j.cvsm.2012.04.002
0195-5616/12/$ – see front matter © 2012 Elsevier Inc. All rights reserved.
vetsmall.theclinics.com

general decline in body and coat condition, and failing senses including sight and hearing. However, other changes are less obvious, and these include alterations in the physiology of the digestive tract, immune system, kidneys, and other organs. There is considerable individual variation in age-related changes. With regard to metabolism and normal age-related changes, cats aged 7 to 11 may be considered "mature" or middle aged, while those 12 years and above may be considered "senior" or "geriatric." For dogs, the effect of age differs, in part, based on breed size. As a general rule, dogs and cats 7 years of age or older may be considered to be at risk for age-related health problems, since this is the age when many age-related diseases begin to be more frequently observed.[3] "Geriatric" screening should be considered as a preventive medicine service, conducted to identify diseases in their early stages, or to head off preventable diseases. An important part of this evaluation is a thorough nutritional assessment.

GERIATRIC NUTRITIONAL EVALUATION

Before instituting a dietary change in any patient, especially an older dog or cat, a nutritional evaluation should be completed. This should include an evaluation of the patient, the current diet, and feeding management.[4,5] The goal of dietary history-taking is to identify the presence and significance of factors that put patients at risk for malnutrition. Understanding how the nutritional needs of older animals may change and a thorough evaluation of the individual patient will allow an appropriate dietary recommendation. Such recommendations should take into account both the needs of the patient and client preferences.

Changes in feeding management should be considered a part of total patient management. As with any aspect of medical management, the patient should be reevaluated at appropriate intervals to ensure achievement of desired results.

Patient Evaluation

A complete medical history should be assessed and a thorough physical examination conducted. A comprehensive geriatric evaluation may identify evidence of clinical or subclinical problems that may benefit from dietary modification. For example, anemia, low serum albumin, low potassium, increased serum creatinine, or increased serum glucose may indicate problems that could benefit from dietary modification as part of medical management.

Body weight and body condition score (BCS)[5-8] are important to assess. Increases or decreases in body weight or condition should trigger further evaluation. A longitudinal study in cats indicated that weight loss is evident in aging cats approximately 2 to 3 years before death from various causes, often well before clinical signs are apparent.[9] Limited data and anecdotal observations suggest that preventing weight loss in nonobese cats can delay terminal conditions. If weight loss is evident in dogs or cats, further evaluation should determine if this is associated with increased or decreased calorie intake. A detailed dietary history and evaluation are warranted.

If the patient shows an increased, or excessive, body condition, it is important to consider current diet and feeding management. Older dogs and middle-aged cats tend to have reduced energy needs. If calorie intake is not adjusted accordingly, weight gain will result. However, unexplained weight gain should be evaluated for predisposing causes, such as hypothyroidism. Animals that are overweight likely will benefit from a weight reduction program.

In addition to BCS, it is important to assess changes in muscle mass, using a muscle condition scoring system.[4,5,10] Animals, especially those that are sick, may be losing lean muscle mass despite an abundance of body fat. Pronounced loss of lean body mass (LBM) is associated with increased morbidity and mortality.[11–13]

Dietary Evaluation

A complete dietary evaluation should include the normal diet, as well as other foods to which the pet has access. Commercially prepared foods should be identified by brand. Any changes to the diet should be identified, as well as the reason for the change. Since many pet owners provide treats and table food, and about 10% of owners provide nutritional supplements, for their pets, these also should be identified by types and amounts.[2,14]

Once the nutritional characteristics of the total diet are known, it should be compared against the individual patient's needs. In general, inactive animals or those that are somewhat overweight should be receiving lower calorie foods, yet may need foods with an increased nutrient:calorie ratio formulated to compensate for increased needs of other nutrients. Feeding such animals a high-calorie food may require an inappropriate reduction in volume of food, resulting in lack of satiation as well as restriction of essential nutrients. On the other hand, feeding a low-calorie food to a pet with high energy needs may require excessive food intake, resulting in loss of body weight or excessive stool volume.

Feeding Management Evaluation

It is important to consider how foods are provided and how they are accepted by the pet. Clients should be asked how much and how often each food is fed. It is also important to identify if pets are fed measured amounts of food, or free choice. Within multiple pet households, determine if pets share a food bowl or have access to other pets' foods.

The diet history should determine if there have been any changes in how the patient is fed, or how it eats. This information is not only important in determining the adequacy of the current dietary situation, it can be important in planning a dietary recommendation that will achieve good client and patient acceptance and compliance.

EFFECTS OF AGING ON NUTRITIONAL REQUIREMENTS
Energy Needs

Maintenance energy requirements (MER) are the energy needs required for the normal animal to survive with normal activity. Individual MER can vary based on genetic potential, health status, and whether the animal is sexually intact or neutered. In addition to these factors, MER appears to decrease with age in most species.[15] In dogs, a decrease of about 25% in MER has been documented as dogs age, with the greatest decrease occurring in dogs greater than 7 years of age.[15,16]

Age-related changes in MER in cats are more controversial. Some report no change in MER with age in senior cats.[15,17] Yet, MER data from cats over a longer period and over a greater age range show a different picture.[18,19] It appears that MER in middle-aged cats (approximately 7–11 years of age) decreases, similar to that observed in other species.[18] However, by about 11 years of age onward, MER per unit of body weight actually increases, with the greatest increases occurring after 13 years of age.[19]

The primary driver of energy requirements in normal pets is LBM, which includes skeletal muscle, skin, and organs and accounts for about 96% of basal energy expenditure.[20] Across species, including dogs and cats, LBM tends to decrease with age.[9,21] This, plus a decrease in activity, can contribute to the reduction in MER seen in aging dogs and middle-aged cats.

If MER decrease, and energy intake does not decrease accordingly, that pet will become overweight. It is this last point that drives the market position of many foods for older dogs and cats. Most commercial foods for geriatric pets contain a reduced concentration of dietary fat and calories.[22] Some have dietary fiber added to further reduce the caloric density. These products may be appropriate for the large number of pets that are overweight or likely to get that way.

Not all older animals are overweight or less active. In fact, while "middle-aged" animals tend to be overweight, a greater proportion of dogs and cats over 12 years of age are underweight compared to other age groups.[9,23,24] This effect is especially pronounced in cats. In addition to an increase in MER in this age group, which may partly explain weight loss, older cats may experience a reduction in digestive capabilities. Approximately one third of cats over the age of 12 may have reduced ability to digest fat, and 1 in 5 cats over age 14 have reduced ability to digest protein.[9] A reduced ability to digest either protein or fat could contribute to weight loss in aging cats.

These patients, and others that are underweight, may benefit from a more energy dense, highly digestible product to help compensate for these age-related changes. A nutritional assessment should be completed on each patient to determine its individual needs, rather than assuming that all older pets need reduced calorie intake. In addition, since weight loss can be an early indicator of chronic disease, especially in cats,[9] unexplained weight loss should be carefully evaluated.

Protein Needs

Protein is another important nutrient for aging pets. For many years veterinarians recommended protein restriction for older dogs in the mistaken belief that this would help protect kidney function.[25] However, research has unequivocally demonstrated that protein restriction is unnecessary in healthy, older dogs.[26–28] On the contrary, protein requirements sufficient to support protein turnover actually increase in older dogs.[29]

Protein turnover is the cycle of catabolism of endogenous protein and synthesis of new proteins needed by the body at any given time, including hormones, enzymes, immune proteins, and others. When dietary protein intake is insufficient, the body responds by decreasing both catabolism and synthesis and by mobilizing protein from LBM to support essential protein synthesis. Normal animals can adapt to this low protein intake and maintain nitrogen balance, yet be in a protein-depleted state associated with gradual loss of LBM. In this situation, animals may appear healthy but have a decreased ability to respond to environmental insults including infections and toxic substances.[28,29] In addition to the direct effect of inadequate protein intake, aging has a detrimental effect on protein turnover and LBM. In one review, 85% of the studies found an age-related decline in endogenous protein synthesis.[30] Inadequate protein intake increases the rate of loss of LBM in aging dogs, while abundant protein slows the loss.[21] There is growing recognition of the importance of this change in body composition. Loss of LBM has been recognized as a predictor of morbidity and mortality in aging subjects.[11–13]

Actual protein needs may vary based on individual factors, such as breed, lifestyle, health, and individual metabolism. In addition, calorie intake affects dietary protein need. Older dogs tend to need fewer calories, thus less food, than younger dogs. Therefore, diets for older dogs should contain a higher percentage of dietary protein, or increased protein:calorie ratio, in order to meet their needs. Diets containing at least 25% of calories from good quality protein should meet the protein needs of most healthy senior dogs. Similar data showing an age effect in cats are lacking; however, cats of all ages have high protein requirements. And, similar to other species, cats need considerably more protein to maintain LBM than is needed to maintain nitrogen balance.

Other Nutrients

All dogs and cats have specific needs for vitamins and minerals, which are normally provided by complete and balanced diets. There is little evidence that the requirements for these nutrients differ in healthy older animals. However, patients with subclinical disease associated with a mild malabsorption syndrome or polyuria may have increased losses of water-soluble nutrients, such as B vitamins, or fat-soluble nutrients, such as vitamins A and E. As noted previously, approximately one third of geriatric cats have a reduced ability to digest dietary fats. In these cats, there is a significant correlation between fat digestibility and the digestibility of other essential nutrients including several B-vitamins, vitamin E, potassium, and other minerals.[9] Geriatric cats with gastrointestinal disease are more likely to be deficient in cobalamin (vitamin B12) compared to younger cats.[31,32] Thus, older cats should be carefully evaluated for possible nutrient deficiencies and may benefit from supplemental amounts of these nutrients.

Oxidative damage plays an important role in many diseases and a deficiency of antioxidant nutrients can have detrimental effects on antioxidant function, immune function, and markers of health.[33–35] Studies in dogs or cats have reported beneficial effects from increased amounts of dietary antioxidants on markers of oxidative status and are beginning to show benefits in certain disease states.[36–39] However, it is difficult to show clear cause-and-effect relations between the diseases and antioxidant status because oxidative damage is subtle, and the associated diseases develop slowly over many years.[40,41] Given the weight of available information, it is reasonable to ensure that aging dogs and cats receive dietary antioxidant nutrients at levels well above the minimum requirements.

DIET-SENSITIVE CONDITIONS IN GERIATRIC DOGS AND CATS

Few diseases in modern pets are "diet-induced." One possible exception to this is obesity, which, while many interactive factors are involved, is ultimately caused by consuming more calories than needed by the dog or cat. However, many other diseases are "diet-sensitive," meaning that diet can play a role in managing the effects of the disease. Examples of diet-sensitive diseases common in aging dogs or cats include chronic renal disease, diabetes mellitus, heart failure, and many others. Information on the management of many of these diseases can be found in other articles in this issue. The remainder of this article will focus on the role of diet in some common problems in aging pets: aging-related cognitive disorders, osteoarthritis (OA), and obesity.

COGNITIVE DYSFUNCTION OF AGING

Older animals often undergo personality changes. Elderly pets can be less mentally alert, have altered sleep patterns and sleep more, and may exhibit varying degrees of cognitive decline. The main behavioral changes associated with cognitive dysfunction in dogs can be grouped into 4 categories: disorientation in the immediate environment; altered interactions with people or other animals; disturbed sleep-wake cycle patterns; and loss of house training.[42–44] Studies suggest that signs of cognitive dysfunction occur in 20% to 30% of dogs over 7 to 9 years of age, increasing to 68% in dogs over 14 years of age.[42–44] Similar categories of behavioral changes have been reported to occur in cats with cognitive dysfunction.[45,46] Behavior problems increase in frequency in aging cats as well, occurring in 50% to 88% of cats 15 to 19 years of age.[46] The severity of cognitive decline in dogs and cats may range from minimal changes to severe dementia and is suggested to be progressive.[47]

There are considerable similarities between human and canine cognitive decline such that what is learned in one may be applicable to the other.[43,48–50] Among the changes are physical atrophy of areas of the brain, as well as increases in oxidative damage and decreases or alterations in mitochondrial energy metabolism in the brain.[45,50,51] Fatty acid composition of the brain phospholipids also are altered in cognitive dysfunction and Alzheimer's disease.[49]

Prevention of cognitive decline in pets focuses on environmental enrichment and mental stimulation, while management might entail pharmaceutical and nutritional care. The use of dietary or supplemental antioxidants has been used to decrease the deleterious effects of free radicals.[39,43] Evidence suggests that free radicals play an important role in aging. The brain is particularly susceptible to the effects of free radicals as it has a high rate of oxidative metabolism, a high content of lipids, and a limited ability for regeneration. Numerous studies have demonstrated improved memory or cognitive performance in aged rodents, and dogs fed antioxidant-enriched diets or supplements coupled with behavioral enrichment.[43,52,53] Long-term feeding of antioxidants appears to help maintain cognitive function and reduce the age-related pathology linked with cognitive dysfunction; however, the effects were maximized when combined with behavioral enrichment.[52–54]

Docosahexaenoic acid (DHA: C22:6 n-3), a long-chain, polyunsaturated omega-3 fatty acid (n3PUFA), plays an important role in normal neural functions. Several studies have shown a decrease in DHA in the aging brain, whereas supplementation with DHA or eicosapentaenoic acid (EPA:C20:5 n-3) from fish oil may act as a defense against Alzheimer's disease and dementia in elderly humans and rodents.[49,55] Supplementation with fish oil results in improved neural development and learning ability in young dogs,[56] but data currently are lacking regarding any benefit from DHA in canine cognitive disorders.

In addition to potential benefits from antioxidants and long-chain omega-3 fatty acids, alternative energy sources may prove beneficial to offset cognitive decline. While glucose is believed to be the primary energy source of neurons in the brain and central nervous system, glucose metabolism becomes less efficient with aging so alternate sources of energy are needed to support the high energy requirements of the brain.[50,57] Lactate, ketones, and short to medium chain fatty acids are alternate energy sources that can be used by neural tissue.[50,51,57–61] Fatty acids from medium-chain triglycerides (MCTs) readily cross the blood-brain barrier and can provide up to 20% of the energy used in normal brain tissue.[58] MCTs also stimulate ketone production, which also cross the blood-brain barrier and provide a source of energy for neural tissue.[50,57] In addition, research in dogs showed that MCT supplementation results in an increase in n3PUFA in brain phospholipids, a benefit that may help offset the age-related decline in these fatty acids.[49] Whether because of changes in fatty acids or its use as an energy source, MCTs have been shown to reduce signs of cognitive dysfunction in human diabetic patients as well as some patients with mild Alzheimer's disease.[60,61] In aging dogs fed a diet containing 5.5% MCTs, cognitive performance was significantly enhanced compared to the age-matched control dogs.[50] In this study, postprandial serum ketone concentrations were increased in dogs fed the MCTs but remained well within the normal physiologic range. In other research, dogs receiving 2 g/kg/d of MCTs for just 2 months showed dramatic improvement in mitochondrial function, reduced oxidative damage, and reduced amyloid proteins that are recognized to contribute to cognitive decline.[57]

In summary, it appears that cognitive disorders are common in aging pets. A combination of mental stimulation through environment enrichment and mental exercises, plus appropriate diet, can help to minimize these age-related effects. Diets that provide an alternate brain energy source, such as MCTs, and antioxidants have been proved helpful in dogs. At this time, no published studies show a dietary benefit for cats with cognitive disorders, although diets enriched with antioxidants and omega-3 fatty acids have been recommended for aging cats.[45,46]

OSTEOARTHRITIS

OA, or degenerative joint disease, is the most prevalent joint disorder in dogs, affecting as many as 20% of adult dogs.[62] The reported prevalence of radiographic evidence of OA in cats has ranged from 16.5% to 91%, with a greater prevalence in older cats.[63] OA is associated with inflammation and increased degradation or loss of proteoglycans from the extracellular matrix, resulting in a morphologic breakdown in articular cartilage.[64] Increases in prostaglandin E_2 (PGE_2), metalloproteinases (MMPs), interleukin (IL)-1β, IL-6, and IL-10, and leukotriene (LT)B_4 occur, as well as markers of oxidative stress, contributing to increased tissue damage in arthritic joints.[64–66]

Obesity is recognized as a risk factor for OA in humans and dogs, and preventing obesity can help reduce both the incidence and severity of OA.[67–69] For example, in a 14-year study on food restriction in dogs, those dogs fed to maintain lean body condition throughout their lifetimes exhibited a delayed need for treatment and reduced severity of OA in the hips and other joints compared to their heavier siblings.[68] One of the most compelling findings from that study was the observation that even a mild degree of excess body weight can adversely affect joint health. This link between obesity and OA is important, since about 34% of adult dogs seen by veterinarians are overweight or obese.[24] The role of obesity in feline OA is less well documented. Many cats with OA are underweight, and the results from epidemiologic studies on obesity are mixed.[63] While one study showed a 3-fold increase in lameness in obese cats, another showed no effect of body condition on lameness or musculoskeletal disease diagnoses.[23,63,70]

The contribution of obesity to joint destruction is more than just physical strain due to weight bearing. Obesity is an inflammatory condition: adipose tissue or associated macrophages produce increased amounts of inflammatory mediators in obesity.[71] Obesity is also associated with an increase in oxidative stress,[72] a feature common with OA. Multiple studies in both humans and dogs have shown that weight loss helps decrease lameness and pain and increase joint mobility in patients with OA.[67,69,73,74] Obesity is discussed in more detail later.

Other than weight management, a primary target of OA treatment is the inhibition of cyclooxygenase (COX) enzymes—especially the COX-2 enzyme—through the use of nonsteroidal anti-inflammatory drugs (NSAIDs).[75,76] COX-2 inhibitors can decrease PGE_2 concentrations and block inflammatory pathways involved in OA, as well as reduce pain and lameness.[75–77] In dogs, there is a strong correlation between PGE_2 concentrations and clinical signs of pain and lameness from OA.[78] Blocking both the COX and lipooxygenase (LOX) enzymes significantly reduces MMPs, IL-1β, LTB$_4$, and PGE_2, resulting in decreased tissue damage in arthritic joints.[79,80]

Another means of reducing PGE_2 and other inflammatory eicosanoids is through the use of dietary n3PUFA containing EPA and DHA. The primary omega-6 fatty acid in cell membranes is arachidonic acid (ArA), which serves as the precursor for the production of the potent inflammatory eicosanoids in OA: PGE_2, thromboxane (TX)A_2, and LTB$_4$. If the diet is enriched with n3PUFA, part of the ArA in cell membranes will be replaced by EPA. EPA may then be used instead of ArA for the production of eicosanoids, resulting in less PGE_2 and production of less inflammatory compounds (eg, PGE_3, TXA_3, and LTB_5 instead of PGE_2, TXA_2, and LTB_4).[81–83] Dietary n3PUFA also suppress the proinflammatory mediators IL-1, IL-2, and tumor necrosis factor in cartilage tissue.[83,84] Thus, substituting n3PUFA for part of the omega-6 fatty acids should reduce inflammation and benefit inflammatory conditions including OA.

A review of studies in arthritic people indicated that most showed positive results from n3PUFA supplementation.[85,86] A number of studies in dogs have also shown benefits from n3PUFA on various measures of OA including subjective (client-perceivable) and objective (blood values and weight bearing measured via force plate) assessments. In one of the earliest studies, 22 dogs with OA of the hip were given a fatty acid supplement marketed for dogs with inflammatory skin conditions.[87] Thirteen of these dogs had noticeable improvement in their arthritic signs within 2 weeks. An open clinical trial using a commercial n3PUFA-enriched diet documented improvement in lameness beginning within weeks, with continued improvement such that 88% of the dogs showed client-perceived improvements by the end of the 2-month study (unpublished observations). Several double-blinded, controlled clinical trials using different diets with n3PUFA documented changes such as reduced plasma PGE_2 and synovial fluid MMPs, reduced markers of lameness, and enhanced weight bearing.[88–91] Diets containing approximately 250 mg n3PUFA from fish oil per 100 Kcal (ME) of the diet appear to provide significant benefits for canine OA.

Only one study evaluating n3PUFA in cats with OA has been published. That study used a diet containing 188 mg n3PUFA/100 Kcal ME, plus green-lipped mussel extract (GLM) glucosamine and chondroitin sulfate fed to cats with evidence of reduced activity and OA.[92] For many of the parameters measured, the control cats improved comparable to the treated cats (placebo effect), but activity increased significantly more in the treated cats than the control cats.

It is important to note that not all n-3 fatty acids have an equivalent anti-inflammatory effect. Although EPA is most effective, both EPA and DHA have anti-inflammatory effects.[93] Shorter chain n-3 fatty acids, such as alpha linoleic acid (ALA) from flax and other vegetable oils, are far less effective for providing EPA and an anti-inflammatory effect due to an inefficient rate of conversion and increased oxidation.[94,95] Therefore, although ALA provides a suitable source of n-3 fatty acids for normal maintenance needs, to achieve the desired anti-inflammatory effect for dogs with OA, n3PUFA from fish oil is preferred over sources of ALA.

Several additional compounds or nutraceuticals appear to be at least somewhat helpful in the management of OA. Among those that have been evaluated in dogs or cats are glucosamine and chondroitin sulfate, elk velvet antler (EVA) powder, GLM, and unsaponifiable lipids from avocado or soybeans (ASU).

A decrease in glucosamine synthesis by chondrocytes has been implicated in OA, whereas supplemental glucosamine has a stimulatory effect on chondrocytes.[96] Many, but not all, studies in human patients show significant improvement in clinical signs of OA in patients consuming 1500 mg glucosamine/d (~21 mg/kg ideal body weight).[97,98] Clinical studies in dogs involving glucosamine alone are lacking but it has been evaluated in conjunction with chondroitin sulfate. Chondroitin sulfate, an endogenously produced polysaccharide found in the joint cartilage matrix, works synergistically with glucosamine to reduce inflammation and slow cartilage deterioration or decrease pain in OA.[98–101] Canine studies using a combination of glucosamine and chondroitin sulfate reported a clinical benefit, similar to that seen in other species.[102–104] In cats, a diet that contained chondroitin sulfate and glucosamine, along with n3PUFA and GLM appeared to show benefit for cats with OA.[92] As individual components were not evaluated, it is not possible to determine which of the components may have been responsible for the benefit.

A limited number of studies in dogs have documented good effects from EVA powder at 14 to 21 g/kg body weight/d[105] or GLM at 20 to 49 mg/kg body weight/d[106,107] compared to placebos. However, another study showed the placebo performed better than the GLM.[108] The difference in results was attributed to inadequate dosing in the nonresponsive dogs, as this trial used only 11 mg GLM/kg body weight.[108]

ASU is an extract from soybean oil and avocado oil. In vitro studies with ASU have documented an anti-inflammatory and antioxidant effect as well as anabolic effect on synovial tissues, resulting in reduced destruction and actual stimulation of articular chondrocytes.[109-111] Specific effects included upregulation of glycosaminoglycan and collagen synthesis.[110] In human clinical trials, ASU was proved more effective than placebo, and equivalent to treatment with chondroitin sulfate, at reducing pain in OA patients.[109,112] Limited studies in dogs have been published. One study evaluated ASU in dogs with induced anterior cruciate ligament rupture.[111] These dogs received a placebo or ASU daily at a dose of 10 mg/kg body weight, which is approximately 2-fold the recommended dosage for human patients with OA. ASU resulted in reduced severity of lesions and markers of OA. Another study, in dogs without OA, compared different dosages of ASU on transforming growth factor (TGF)-β.[113] TGF-β is expressed by chondrocytes and osteoblasts and promotes the production of extracellular matrix in articular cartilage. Using every third day dosing at approximately 4.3 mg/kg body weight (300 mg/dog every 3 days) was equivalent to daily dosing at 4. 3 mg/kg body weight for increasing TGF-β_1 and TGF-β_2. Whether this dose would be appropriate in dogs with OA is unclear.

Arthritis is associated with an increase in oxidative stress and chondrocyte-produced reactive oxygen species and reduced antioxidant capacity.[65,114,115] The severity of arthritic lesions is increased in the face of decreased antioxidant capacity.[115] In vitro studies, rodent studies, and human epidemiologic studies suggest that antioxidant supplements would be of value in managing OA, but human clinical trials have been mixed in results.[116-119] While increased markers of oxidative stress have been confirmed in dogs with OA,[65,120] no peer-reviewed studies have evaluated "classic" antioxidants such as vitamin C or E in dogs or cats with OA. On the other hand, other compounds tested for use in the management of OA have also shown antioxidant effects. For example, the flavoid flaxocoxid (FlexileRx; Primus Pharmaceuticals, Inc., Scottsdale, AZ, USA) is an inhibitor of COX and LOX enzymes but also has strong antioxidant effects.[80] Likewise, glucosaminoglycans, chondroitin sulfate, ASU, and EVA show antioxidant effects or reductions in prooxidants that may contribute to their therapeutic effects.[111,121,122] While additional research is needed, the available evidence to date together suggests a benefit of dietary antioxidants for patients with OA.

In addition to nutrient modifications that may help in the dietary management of OA directly, dogs and cats need appropriately balanced nutrition to support normal maintenance of joints and other tissues. In human OA patients, deficiencies in antioxidant nutrients, B-vitamins, zinc, calcium, magnesium, and selenium are frequently reported.[123,124] While it is not known how many of these deficiencies contribute to OA, these nutrients play a role in the normal maintenance of cartilage and other tissues. Therefore, it is important that pets with OA receive diets that provide complete and balanced nutrition. In addition, protein plays in important role in maintaining LBM and muscle strength. As older dogs and cats tend to lose LBM with age, and insufficient protein intake accelerates this loss,[21] it is important that older pets with OA receive sufficient dietary protein.

In summary, OA is common in aging pets. Multimodal management using a combination of weight management, appropriate physical therapy, diet including n3PUFA from fish oil, other nutraceuticals, and pharmaceutical agents provides numerous options to maximize success for managing this condition.

OBESITY

Overweight and obesity (hyperadiposity) represent the most common forms of malnutrition in dogs and cats in developed countries. The prevalence of hyperadiposity has been reported to range between 34% and 59% of dogs and between 27% and 39% of cats.[23,24,125–129] Hyperadiposity is a contributing or confounding factor in a large number of health problems, including OA, diabetes mellitus, respiratory and cardiovascular problems, neoplasias, and others.[69,130–134] Hyperadiposity is associated with dysregulation of adipose-derived hormones, cytokines, and metabolic regulators, collectively called adipokines, which contribute to a state of insulin resistance, mild inflammation, and oxidative stress and which can contribute to many of the diseases linked with obesity.[135–139]

Prevention of hyperadiposity relies on understanding contributing or associated risk factors and managing them appropriately. Important risk factors in pets include neutering and inactivity.[23,24,126–129] Neutering can reduce MER by 25% to 35%, as well as increase spontaneous food intake and decrease activity.[140–143] Other risk factors for dogs include feeding excess table scraps or treats.[24,129,144] Surprisingly, ad libitum feeding was not a risk factor in either dogs or cats, whereas feeding more frequent meals was a risk factor for excess weight in cats.[126,128] Feeding high-fat diets contributes to increased body fat, especially when fed ad libitum,[23,141,142] and so should be avoided in pets at risk for weight gain.

Active management of obesity depends on first recognizing the problem. The most practical method for clinical assessment of hyperadiposity is a combination of body weight and BCS, using a validated BCS system.[6–8,145] When using the 9-point system, each unit increase in BCS above ideal (BCS = 5) is approximately equivalent to 10% to 15% excess body weight. Therefore, a dog or cat with BCS of 7 is about 20% to 30% over ideal weight. By recording both body weight and BCS, ideal body weight can be reasonably estimated. Animals that are becoming obese can be identified sooner and managed more easily. An illustrated BCS system can provide a useful tool for pet owner education regarding obesity prevention and management. Unfortunately, many veterinarians still do not use a BCS system routinely. In one study, veterinarians weighed dogs in only 70% of cases, assigned a subjective body composition assessment in 29% of cases, and assigned a recognized BCS to less than 1% of cases.[146]

Effective management of obesity depends on creating a negative energy balance. An appropriate diet, behavioral changes regarding feeding management, and increased activity for the pet all contribute to creating the negative energy balance and effective weight loss.

Dietary Factors

The amount of calories needed to induce weight loss will vary greatly among individual animals due to differences in MER as well as their level of activity.[147,148] In addition, MER decreases in response to calorie restriction and weight loss.[149–152] This appears to be due, in part, to metabolic adaptation, as indicated by reduced triiodothyronine concentrations, and reductions in LBM which drive basal metabolism.[149,152] It is, therefore, important that adjustments in calorie allowance are made on a regular basis, such as every month, to maintain ongoing weight loss.

Use of an appropriate diet for weight loss is important, and there are several criteria to consider. While it is ultimately calorie restriction that induces weight loss, it is important to avoid excessive restriction of essential nutrients so a low-calorie product with increased nutrient: calorie ratios should be considered. Further, an important goal for weight loss is to promote fat loss while minimizing loss of LBM, which can be influenced by dietary composition, especially protein.

Consumption of low-calorie diets with increased protein significantly increase fat loss and reduce the loss of LBM during weight loss.[153–157] For example, among cats undergoing weight loss, increasing dietary protein from 35% to 45% of energy resulted in more than 10% greater fat loss, and absolute loss of LBM was cut in half by increasing dietary protein.[155] As LBM is the primary driver of resting energy usage, this effect can be important for long-term weight management.

In addition to preservation of LBM, protein has a significant thermogenic effect so that metabolic energy expenditure is increased in subjects fed high-protein diets.[156,158] The thermic effect of protein results in a small but significant increase in total daily energy expenditure.[156,158] Metabolic adaptation to calorie restriction includes a reduction in resting energy expenditure, which can slow weight loss and may contribute to weight rebound.[149,151] The thermic effect provided by a high-protein diet can help offset this reduction and allow greater consumption of food calories, compared to those fed lower-protein diets, while maintaining a similar rate of weight loss.[156–158] The benefit carries over even after weight loss as consumption of a high-protein diet during weight loss helps with the weight maintenance phase.[156,157] Following weight loss, cats that had been fed a high-protein (11.9 g/100 Kcal, or ~43% of energy) diet during weight loss were able to consume about 12% more calories in the post-loss weight maintenance period without weight gain.[157]

Dietary fiber is an important consideration for weight loss diets. Due to the low digestibility of dietary fiber, it provides little dietary energy so helps to reduce the caloric density of foods. In addition, dietary fiber provides a satiety effect that may be of value in weight management.[159–161] Dietary fiber plus high protein appear to be complementary and provide enhanced satiety over either factor alone.[162] Water can also be used to reduce calorie density in foods and can help reduce calorie intake, at least in the short term.[163] Cats tend to eat a fairly constant volume of food and are slow to adjust to changes in caloric density, whether from high fiber or water dilution. When first fed high-moisture diets, their calorie intake decreases, contributing to weight loss.[163]

Many compounds have been evaluated for use in weight loss diets. A few have demonstrated benefits that may be of some help in weight management. Recently, studies have evaluated soy isoflavones for use in weight management.[164–166] Loss of body fat was enhanced in dogs fed a low-calorie diet containing soy isoflavones: these dogs were more likely to achieve their target body fat, compared to those fed a similar diet without isoflavones.[164] Soy isoflavones can reduce the weight gain or increase in body fat normally associated with castration or spaying.[164,165] In addition, LBM increased in the cats treated with isoflavones.[165] These effects suggest a beneficial metabolic repartitioning associated with the soy isoflavones, which may help reduce weight rebound in animals following weight loss.

Other compounds that have shown some promise for weight management include diacylglycerols (DAG) and L-carnitine.[167,168] DAG are lipids that contain 2 fatty acids per glycerol molecule, unlike triglycerides, which contain 3 fatty acids per glycerol. The fatty acids from DAG are metabolized differently and tend to be oxidized readily.[169] Overweight dogs fed a diet containing 7% DAG lost 2.3% of their starting body weight over 6 weeks, while the control dogs consuming the same amount of calories maintained body weight.[168] Carnitine is produced endogenously from the amino acids lysine and methionine and is important in fat metabolism. Center and colleagues[167] reported a significant increase in rate of weight loss in cats fed a diet supplemented with carnitine compared to a control group (24% vs 20%, respectively, over an 18-week period). Other studies, in other species, have shown little benefit.[170–172] No peer-reviewed studies evaluating the use of carnitine for weight management in dogs have been published. It is suggested that carnitine supplementation is likely to be of greatest benefit when the intake of dietary protein or other precursors are insufficient to promote adequate endogenous production.

Behavioral Factors and Feeding Management

In addition to diet, changes in feeding management are critically important to successful weight management. In both human and pet obesity management, behavioral changes regarding food intake and activity are important for both weight loss and long-term weight management.[173–176] Owners of obese pets are likely to unintentionally feed their pet excessive calories. Effective control strategies are those that will increase the owners' mindfulness regarding feeding behaviors.[177]

Dog owners report that veterinary guidance is important in managing their pet's obesity.[178,179] Effective weight management programs have included specific feeding guidelines, appropriate guidance on feeding of treats, and frequent monitoring with adjustments in food allowance.[173,174] Given the intensity of work involved with supporting weight management, the concept of veterinary "obesity clinics" has been explored. Obesity clinics can be run by trained technicians to perform such important functions as client education, ongoing client support, rechecking of body weight and BCS, updating feeding guidelines, and dispensing food. Clinics can be managed as individual appointments, or as group sessions that provide owners with the additional benefit of a peer support group. Among practices that offer such clinics, 79% noted that it was a valuable service.[179]

Provision of a handout that details the portion of cups or cans of a specific diet (with client input on diet selection) to be fed daily was found to be helpful for clients.[178] There is a limitation to this, however, as there is considerable imprecision even when using measuring cups to weigh food.[180] In small pets, this imprecision could be sufficient to compromise the weight management plan, so it is recommended to use an accurate weight scale rather than measuring cups whenever possible.

Monitoring food intake and activity via use of a daily log is a principal pillar of behavioral modification for human obesity management.[176] Many clients find that keeping a daily diary regarding their pet's food intake and activity is helpful.[178] Where multiple people in a household might feed the pets, use of a daily log can be especially useful to avoid accidental overfeedings.

Most dog owners and many cat owners provide treats to their pets on a regular basis.[2] The creation of a "treat allowance" equal to 10% of the daily calories allows owners to continue this pleasurable activity while also achieving appropriate energy balance. Owners may benefit from a menu of low-calorie foods or commercial treats that would be appropriate to use within the allowed calories.

Increasing exercise can aid in weight management by expending calories and preserving LBM. Wakshlag and colleagues[148] reported that more-active dogs, considering activity in the form of both structured and unstructured activities, were able to consume about 20% more calories yet achieve a similar rate of weight loss compared to less-active dogs. Interactive exercise provides an alternative activity for pet and owner to enjoy together, rather than food-related activities. Activity in cats may be enhanced by interactive play, such as with a toy on a string or a laser light. Food toys provide another option. These are plastic balls or other shapes with holes that dispense kibble or treats as the cat or dog plays with the toy. To avoid an undesired increase in calorie intake, a portion of the allocated meal or predetermined treats can be dispensed via a food ball rather than additional foods.

Gradual weight loss is more likely to allow long-term maintenance of the reduced body weight.[149] Weight rebound can be minimized by providing controlled food intake and adjusting the calories fed to just meet the needs of the pet for weight maintenance.[173] Owners already accustomed to measuring food and monitoring their pet's weight should be encouraged to apply these behavior modifications to long-term weight management. When transitioning from weight loss to weight maintenance, an initial increase of 20% of calorie intake is recommended, with ongoing adjustments as needed.

In addition to measuring food, use of smaller bowls can help reduce the amount of food owners provide for their pets. Food intake was reduced by about 10% when cat owners used a 6-ounce bowl compared to a 12-ounce bowl.[181] Similarly, dog owners placed at least 13% less food into a small bowl using a small scoop, compared to the use of a larger bowl or larger scoop.[182] The use of smaller bowls may help pets with long-term weight maintenance.

Pharmaceutical Management of Obesity

Two new drugs, both microsomal transfer protein inhibitors, were introduced in 2007 to aid in canine weight management.[183–185] Their primary mode of action is to inhibit food intake. The drugs interfere with enzymes involved in fat absorption from the intestines, resulting in both a slight decrease in fat absorption and a physiologic release of satiety factors that inhibit food intake. Both drugs are associated with mild side effects that include vomiting, diarrhea, and increased liver enzymes.[183–185]

Reduced food intake during drug-induced weight loss results in restriction of essential nutrients as well as calories, unless a therapeutic weight loss diet with an increased nutrient/energy ratio is fed. Due to the common side effects from these drugs, however, a new food should not be introduced at the same time as the drug. Once use of the drug is stopped, the dogs' appetites will return, which is associated with weight rebound. In most cases, ongoing control of food intake will be essential to continue weight loss or maintain ideal weight.

In summary, hyperadiposity is associated with numerous health problems, so weight management is an important part of patient care. Weight loss can be achieved in most pets by creating a negative energy balance and is best achieved using diets with low calorie density, increased protein content, and an overall increased nutrient/calorie ratio. Ongoing support and adjustments to food intake are usually necessary and helpful to achieve weight loss and long-term weight management.

SUMMARY

The majority of aging pets are generally healthy but may have special dietary needs. Prior to recommending a diet for a senior pet, a thorough nutritional evaluation should be completed. Over 40% of dogs and cats between the ages of 5 and 10 years are overweight or obese. Such pets may benefit from diets with lower fat and calories and more protein. Although many middle-aged and older pets are overweight, a large percentage of geriatric cats and dogs have a low body condition. Many geriatric cats have a decreased ability to digest fat and/or protein. Thus, geriatric cats (>12 years if age) may need a highly digestible, nutrient-dense diet.

Common age-related nutrient-sensitive conditions in dogs or cats include cognitive disorders, OA, and obesity, among others. Age-related cognitive disorders can benefit from a combination of mental stimulation through environment enrichment and mental exercises, plus appropriate diet. Diets that provide an alternate brain energy source, such as MCTs, and antioxidants have been proved helpful in dogs. OA, an inflammatory condition that occurs in many aging dogs and cats, may benefit from both weight management and nutrients that reduce the inflammatory responses, such as long-chain omega-3 fatty acids. Obesity is thought to contribute to a number of health conditions, so weight management is important. Weight loss can be achieved in most pets by creating a negative energy balance and is best achieved using diets with low calorie density, increased protein content, and an overall increased nutrient/calorie ratio.

Aging pets should be monitored regularly to confirm that the desired nutritional benefits are being achieved, and to assess any need for new dietary changes.

REFERENCES

1. Lund EM, Armstrong PJ, Kirk CA, et al. Health status and population characteristics of dogs and cats examined at private veterinary practices in the United States. J Am Vet Med Assoc 1999;214:1336–41.
2. Laflamme DP, Abood SK, Fascetti AJ, et al. Pet feeding practices among dog and cat owners in the United States and Australia. J Am Vet Med Assoc 2008;232:687–94.
3. Kraft W. Geriatrics in canine and feline internal medicine. Eur J Med Res 1998;3:31–41.
4. Baldwin K, Bartges J, Buffington T, et al. AAHA Nutritional assessment guidelines for dogs and cats. J Am Anim Hosp Assoc 2010;46:285–96.
5. Freeman L, Becvarova I, Cave N, et al. WSAVA nutritional assessment guidelines. J Fel Med Surg 2011;13:516–25.
6. Laflamme DP. Development and validation of a body condition score system for dogs: a clinical tool. Can Pract 1997;22:10–5.
7. Laflamme DP. Development and validation of a body condition score system for cats: a clinical tool. Fel Pract 1997;25:13–8.
8. German AJ, Holden SL, Moxham GL, et al. A simple, reliable tool for owners to assess the body condition of their dog or cat. J Nutr 2006;136:2031S–3S.
9. Perez-Camargo G. Cat nutrition: what's new in the old? Comp Cont Educ Small Anim Pract 2004;26(Suppl 2A):5–10.
10. Michel KE, Anderson W, Cupp C, et al. Correlation of a feline muscle mass score with body composition determined by DEXA. Br J Nutr 2011;106:S57–9.
11. Fujita S, Volpi E. Nutrition and sarcopenia of aging. Nutr Res Rev 2004;17:69–76.
12. Cupp CJ, Kerr WW. Effect of diet and body composition on life span in aging cats. Proceedings of the Nestle Purina Companion Animal Nutrition Summit: focus on gerontology. Clearwater Beach (FL), March 26–27, 2010. St Louis (MO): Nestlé Purina PetCare; 2010.
13. Han SS, Kim KW, Kim KI, et al. Lean mass index: a better predictor of mortality than body mass index in elderly Asians. J Am Geriatr Soc 2010;58:312–7.
14. Freeman LM, Abood SK, Fascetti AJ, et al. Disease prevalence and use of therapeutic diets and dietary supplements among dog and cat owners. J Am Vet Med Assoc 2006;229:531–4.
15. Harper EJ. Changing perspectives on aging and energy requirements: aging and energy intakes in humans, dogs and cats. J Nutr 1998;128:2623S–6S.
16. Laflamme DP, Martineau B, Jones W, et al. Effect of age on maintenance energy requirements and apparent digestibility of canine diets. Comp Cont Educ Small Anim Pract 2000;22(Suppl 9A):113.

17. Bermingham EN, Thomas DG, Morris PJ, et al. Energy requirements of adult cats. Brit J Nutr 2010:103:1083–93.
18. Laflamme DP, Ballam JM. Effect of age on maintenance energy requirements of adult cats. Comp Cont Educ Small Anim Pract 2002;24(Suppl 9A):82.
19. Cupp C, Perez-Camargo G, Patil A, et al. Long-term food consumption and body weight changes in a controlled population of geriatric cats. Comp Cont Educ Small Anim Pract 2004;26(Suppl 2A):60.
20. Elia M. The inter-organ flux of substrates in fed and fasted man, an indicated by arteriovenous balance studies. Nutr Res Rev 1991;4:3–31.
21. Kealy RD. Factors influencing lean body mass in aging dogs. Comp Cont Educ Small Anim Pract 1999;21(11K):34–7.
22. Hutchinson D, Freeman LM, Schreiner KE, et al. Survey of opinions about nutritional requirements of senior dogs and analysis of nutrient profiles of commercially available diets for senior dogs. Intern J Appl Res Vet Med 2011;9:68–79.
23. Lund EM, Armstrong PJ, Kirk CA, et al. Prevalence and risk factors for obesity in adult cats from private US veterinary practices. Int J Appl Res Vet Med 2005;3:88–96.
24. Lund EM, Armstrong PJ, Kirk CA, et al. Prevalence and risk factors for obesity in adult dogs from private US veterinary practices. Int J Appl Res Vet Med 2006;4:177–86.
25. Finco DR. Effects of dietary protein and phosphorus on the kidney of dogs. Proc Waltham/OSU Symposium. Vernon (CA): Kal Kan Foods, Inc.; 1992. p. 39–41.
26. Finco DR, Brown SA, Crowell WA, et al. Effects of aging and dietary protein intake on uninephrectomized geriatric dogs. Am J Vet Res 1994;55:1282–90.
27. Bovee KC. Mythology of protein restriction for dogs with reduced renal function. Comp Cont Educ Small Anim Pract 1999;21(Suppl 11):15–20.
28. Laflamme DP. Issues in pet food safety: dietary protein. Top Comp Anim Med 2008;23:154–7.
29. Wannemacher RW, McCoy JR. Determination of optimal dietary protein requirements of young and old dogs. J Nutr 1966;88:66–74.
30. Richardson A, Birchenall-Sparks MC. Age-related changes in protein synthesis. Rev Biol Res Aging 1983;1:255–73.
31. Williams DA, Steiner JM, Ruaux CG. Older cats with gastrointestinal disease are more likely to be cobalamin deficient. Comp Cont Educ Small Anim Pract 2004; 26(Suppl 2A):62.
32. Simpson KW, Fyfe J, Cornetta A, et al. Subnormal concentrations of serum cobalamin (vitamin B12) in cats with gastrointestinal disease. J Vet Intern Med 2001;15: 26–32.
33. Packer L, Landvik S. Vitamin E: introduction to biochemistry and health benefits. Ann N Y Acad Sci 1989;570:1–6.
34. Freeman LM, Rush JE, Milbury PE, et al. Antioxidant status and biomarkers of oxidative stress in dogs with congestive heart failure. J Vet Intern Med 2005;19:537–41.
35. Yu S, Paetau-Robinson I. Dietary supplements of vitamins E and C and beta-carotene reduce oxidative stress in cats with renal insufficiency. Vet Res Commun 2006;30:403–13.
36. Wedekind KJ, Zicker S, Lowry S, et al. Antioxidant status of adult beagles is affected by dietary antioxidant intake. J Nutr 2002;132:1658S–60S.
37. Brown SA. Oxidative stress and chronic kidney disease. Vet Clin N Am Small Anim Pract 2008;38:157–66.
38. Cupp CJ, Kerr WW, Jean-Philippe C, et al. The role of nutritional interventions in the longevity and maintenance of long-term health in aging cats. Intern J Appl Res Vet Med 2008;6:69–81.

39. Head E. Oxidative damage and cognitive dysfunction: antioxidant treatments to promote healthy brain aging. Neurchem Res 2009;34:670–8.
40. Jacob RA, Burri BJ. Oxidative damage and defense. Am J Clin Nutr 1996;63:985S–90S.
41. Afanas'ev I. ROS and RNS signaling in heart disorders: could antioxidant treatment be successful? Oxid Med Cell Longev 2011;2011:293769.
42. Neilson JC, Hart BL, Cliff KD, et al. Prevalence of behavioral changes associated with age-related cognitive impairment in dogs. J Am Vet Med Assoc 2001;218:1787–91.
43. Heath SE, Barabas S, Craze PG. Nutritional supplementation in cases of canine cognitive dysfunction: a clinical trial. Appl Anim Behav Sci 2007;105:284–96.
44. Zakona G, Garcia-Belenguer S, Chacon G, et al. Prevalence and risk factors for behavioural changes associated with age-related cognitive impairment in geriatric dogs. J Sm Anim Pract 2009;50:87–91.
45. Landsberg G, Denenberg S, Araujo J. Cognitive dysfunction in cats: a syndrome we used to dismiss as 'old age'. J Fel Med Surg 2010;12:837–48.
46. Gunn-Moore D. Cognitive dysfunction in cats: clinical assessment and management. Top Comp Anim Med 2011;26:17–24.
47. Bain MJ, Hart BL, Cliff KD, et al. Predicting behavioral changes associated with age-related cognitive impairment in dogs. J Am Vet Med Assoc 2001;218:1792–5.
48. Cummings BJ, Head E, Ruehl W, et al. The canine as an animal model of human aging and dementia. Neurobiol Aging 1996;17:259–68.
49. Taha AY, Henderson ST, Burnham WM. Dietary enrichment with medium chain triglycerides (AC-1203) elevates polyunsaturated fatty acids in the parietal cortex of aged dogs: implications for treating age-related cognitive decline. Neurochem Res 2009;34(9):1619–25.
50. Pan Y, Larson B, Araujo JA, et al. Dietary supplementation with medium-chain TAG has long-lasting cognition-enhancing effects in aged dogs. Br J Nutr 2010;103:1746–54.
51. Parihar MS, Brewer GJ. Mitogenic failure in Alzheimer disease. Am J Physiol Cell Physiol 2007;292:C8–23.
52. Head E. Oxidative damage and cognitive dysfunction: antioxidant treatments to promote healthy brain aging. Neurochem Res 2009;34:670–8.
53. Pop V, Head E, Hill MA, et al. Synergistic effects of long-term antioxidant diet and behavioral enrichment on β-amyloid load and non-amyloidogenic processing in aged canines. J Neurosci 2010;30:9831–9.
54. Fahnestock M, Marchese M, Head E, et al. BDNF increases with behavioral enrichment and an antioxidant diet in aged dog. Neurobiol Aging 2012;33(3):546–54.
55. Jiang L, Shi Y, Wang L, et al. The influence of orally administered docosahexaenoic acid on cognitive ability in aged mice. J Nutr Biochem 2009;20:735–41.
56. Heinemann KM, Bauer JE. Docohexaenoic acid and neurological development in animals. J Am Vet Med Assoc 2006;228:700–5.
57. Studzinski CM, MacKay WA, Beckett TL, et al. Induction of ketosis may improve mitochondrial function and decrease steady-state amyloid-β precursor protein (APP) levels in the aged dog. Brain Res 2008;1226:209–17.
58. Ebert D, Haller RG, Walton ME. Energy contribution of octanoate to intact rat brain metabolism measured by ^{13}C nuclear magnetic resonance spectroscopy. J Neurosci 2003;23:5928–35.
59. Quistorff B, Secher NH, Van Lieshout JJ. Lactate fuels the human brain during exercise. Fed Assoc Soc Exp Biol J 2008;22:3443–9.

60. Page KA, Williamson A, Yu N, et al. Medium-chain fatty acids improve cognitive function in intensively treated type I diabetic patients and support in vitro synaptic transmission during acute hypoglycemia. Diabetes 2009;58:1237–44.

61. Reger MA, Henderson ST, Hale C, et al. Effects of beta-hydroxybutyrate on cognition in memory-impaired adults. Neurobiol Aging 2004;25:311–4.

62. Roush JK, McLaughlin RM, Radlinsky MA. Understanding the pathophysiology of osteoarthritis. Vet Med 2002;97:108–12.

63. Kerwin SC. Osteoarthritis in cats. Top Comp Anim Med 2010;25:218–32.

64. Johnston SA. Osteoarthritis. Joint anatomy, physiology and pathobiology. Vet Clin North Am Sm Anim Pract 1997;27(4):699–723.

65. Goranov NV. Serum markers of lipid peroxidation, antioxidant enzymatic defense, and collagen degradation in an experimental (Pond-Nuki) canine model of osteoarthritis. Vet Clin Pathol 2007;36:192–5.

66. Maccoux LJ, Salway F, Day PJR, et al. Expression profiling of select cytokines in canine osteoarthritis tissues. Vet Immunol Immunopathol 2007;118:59–67.

67. Foye PM, Stitik TP, Chen B, et al. Osteoarthritis and body weight. Nutr Res 2000;20:899–903.

68. Kealy RD, Lawler DF, Ballam JM, et al. Effects of diet restriction on life span and age-related changes in dogs. J Am Vet Med Assoc 2002;220:1315–20.

69. Marshall WG, Bockstahler BA, Hulse DA, et al. A review of osteoarthritis and obesity: current understanding of the relationship and benefit of obesity treatment and prevention in the dog. Vet Comp Orthop Traumatol 2009;22:339–45.

70. Scarlett JM, Donoghue S. Associations between body condition and disease in cats. J Am Vet Med Assoc 1998;212:1725–31.

71. Rai MF, Sandell L. Inflammatory mediators: tracing links between obesity and osteoarthritis. Crit Rev Eukaryot Gene Exp 2011;21:131–42.

72. Fernandez-Sanchez A, Madrigal-Santillan E, Bautista M, et al. Inflammation, oxidative stress and obesity. Int J Mol Sci 2011;12:3117–32.

73. Marshall WG, Hazewinkel HAW, Mullen D, et al. The effect of weight loss on lameness in obese dogs with osteoarthritis. Vet Res Commun 2010;34:241–53.

74. Impellizeri JA, Tetrick MA, Muir P. Effect of weight reduction on clinical signs of lameness in dogs with hip osteoarthritis. J Am Vet Med Assoc 2000;216:1089–91.

75. Millis DL, Weigel JP, Moyers T, et al. The effect of deracoxib, a new COX-2 inhibitor, on the prevention of lameness induced by chemical synovitis in dogs. Vet Ther 2002;3:7–18.

76. Dionne RA, Khan AA, Gordon SM. Analgesia and COX-2 inhibition. Clin Exp Rheumatol 2001;19(Suppl 25):S63–70.

77. Holtzsinger RN, Parker RB, Beale BS, et al. The therapeutic effect of carprofen (Rimadyl) in 209 clinical cases of canine degenerative joint disease. Vet Comp Orthop Traumatol 1992;5:140–4.

78. Trumble TN, Billinghurst RC, McIlwraith CW. Correlation of prostaglandin E2 concentrations in synovial fluid with ground reaction forces and clinical variables for pain or inflammation in dogs with osteoarthritis induced by transection of the cranial cruciate ligament. Am J Vet Res 2004;65:1269–75.

79. Burnett BP, Bitto A, Altavilla D, et al. Flavocoxid inhibits phospholipase A2, peroxidase moieties of the cyclooxygenases (COX) and 5-lipoxygenase, modifies COX-2 gene expression, and acts as an antioxidant. Mediators Inflamm 2011;2011:385780.

80. Laufer S. Role of eicosanoids in structural degradation in osteoarthritis. Curr Opin Rheumatol 2003;15:623–7.

81. Drevon CA. Marine oils and their effects. Nutr Rev 1992;50:38–45.

82. Schoenherr WD, Jewell DE. Nutritional modulation of inflammatory diseases. Semin Vet Med Surg (Sm Anim) 1997;12:212–22.

83. LeBlanc CJ, Horohov DW, Bauer JE, et al. Effects of dietary supplementation with fish oil on in vivo production of inflammatory mediators in clinically normal dogs. Am J Vet Res 2008;69:486–93.

84. Curtis CL, Rees SG, Little CG, et al. Pathologic indicators of degradation and inflammation in human osteoarthritic cartilage are abrogated by exposure to n3 fatty acids. Arthritis Rheum 2002;46:1544–53.

85. Richardson DC, Schoenherr WD, Zicker SC. Nutritional management of osteoarthritis. Vet Clin N Am Small Anim Pract 1997;27:883–911.

86. Hurst S, Zainal Z, Caterson B, et al. Dietary fatty acids and arthritis. Prostaglandins Leukot Essent Fatty Acids 2010;82:315–8.

87. Miller WH, Scott DW, Wellington JR. Treatment of dogs with hip arthritis with a fatty acid supplement. Canine Pract 1992;17:6–8.

88. Hansen RA, Harris MA, Pluhar E, et al. Fish oil decreases matrix metalloproteinases in knee synovial of dogs with inflammatory joint disease. J Nutr Biochem 2008;19: 101–8.

89. Fritsch DA, Allen TA, Dodd CE, et al. A multicenter study of the effect of dietary supplementation with fish oil omega-3 fatty acids on carprofen dosage in dogs with osteoarthritis. J Am Vet Med Assoc 2010;236:535–9.

90. Roush JK, Cross AR, Renberg WC, et al. Evaluation of the effects of dietary supplementation with fish oil omega-3 fatty acids on weight bearing in dogs with osteoarthritis. J Am Vet Med Assoc 2010;236:67–73.

91. Moreau M, Troncy E, del Castillo JRE, et al. Feeding a high omega-3 fatty acids diet improves the pain-related disability in dogs with naturally occurring osteoarthritis. J Sm Anim Pract 2012, in press.

92. Lascelles BDX, DePuy V, Hansen TB, et al. Evaluation of a therapeutic diet for feline digestive joint disease. J Vet Intern Med 2010;24:487–95.

93. Sierra S, Lara-Villoslada F, Comalada M, et al. Dietary eicosapentaenoic acid and docosahexaenoic acid equally incorporate as decosahexaenoic acid but differ in inflammatory effects. Nutrition 2008;24:245–54.

94. Bauer JE. Responses of dogs to dietary omega-3 fatty acids. J Am Vet Med Assoc 2007;231:1657–60.

95. Talahalli RR, Vallikannan B, Sambaiah K, et al. Lower efficacy in the utilization of dietary ALA as compared to preformed DPA + DHA on long chain n3 PUFA levels in rats. Lipids 2010;45:799–808.

96. Anderson MA. Oral chondroprotective agents. Part I. Common compounds. Compendium 1999;21:601–9.

97. Richy F, Bruyere O, Ethgen O, et al. Structural and symptomatic efficacy of glucosamine and chondroitin in knee osteoarthritis. Arch Intern Med 2003;163:1514–22.

98. Jerosch J. Effects of glucosamine and chondroitin sulfate on cartilage metabolism in OA: outlook on other nutrient partners especially omega-3 fatty acids. Int J Rheumatol 2011;2011:969012.

99. Bucsi L, Poor G. Efficacy and tolerability of oral chondroitin sulfate as a symptomatic slow-acting drug for osteoarthritis (SYSADOA) in the treatment of knee osteoarthritis. Osteoarthritis Cartilage 1998;6(3):31–6.

100. Michel B, Stucki G, Frey D, et al. Condroitins 4 and 6 sulphate in osteoarthritis of the knee: a randomized, controlled trial. Arthritis Rheum 2005;52:779–86.

101. Iovu M, Dumais G, duSouich P. Anti-inflammatory activity of chondroitin sulfate. Osteoarthritis Cartilage 2008;16(Suppl 3):S14–8.

102. Aragon CL, Hofmeister EH, Budsbuerg SC. Systematic review of clinical trials of treatments for osteoarthritis in dogs. J Am Vet Med Assoc 2007;230:514–21.
103. McCarthy G, O'Donovan J, Jones B, et al. Randomised double-blind, positive-controlled trial to assess the efficacy of glucosamine/chondroitin sulfate for the treatment of dogs with osteoarthritis. Vet J 2007;174:54–61.
104. Gupta RC, Canerdy TD, Lindley J, et al. Comparative therapeutic efficacy and safety of type-II collagen (uc-II), glucosamine and chondroitin in arthritic dogs: pain evaluation by ground force plate. J Anim Physiol Anim Nutr 2011. DOI: 10.1111/j.1439-0396.2011.01166.x.
105. Moreau M, Dupuis J, Bonneau NH, et al. Clinical evaluation of a powder of quality elk velvet antler for the treatment of osteoarthrosis in dogs. Can Vet J 2004;45:133–9.
106. Bierer TL, Bui LM. Improvement of arthritic signs in dogs fed green-lipped mussel (Perna canaliculus). J Nutr 2002;132:S1634–6.
107. Hielm-Bjorkman A, Tulamo RM, Salonen H, et al. Evaluating complementary therapies for canine osteoarthritis. Part I: green lipped mussel (Perna canaliculus). Evid Based Complement Alternat Med 2009;6(3):365–73.
108. Dobenecker B, Beetz Y, Kienzle E. A placebo-controlled double-blinded study on the effect of nutraceuticals (chondroitin sulfate and mussel extract) in dogs with joint diseases as perceived by their owners. J Nutr 2002;132:1690S–1S.
109. Maheu E, Mazières B, Valat JP, et al. Symptomatic efficacy of avocado/soybean unsaponifiables in the treatment of osteoarthritis of the knee and hip. Arthritis Rheum 1998;41:81–91.
110. Lippiello L, Nardo JV, Harlan R, et al. Metabolic effects of avocado/soy unsaponifiables on articular chondrocytes. Evid Based Complement Altern Med 2008;5:191–7.
111. Boileau C, Martel-Pelletier J, Caron J, et al. Protective effects of total fraction of avocado/soybean unsaponifiables on the structural changes in experimental dog osteoarthritis: inhibition of nitric oxide synthase and matrix metalloproteinase-13. Arthritis Res Ther 2009;11:R41.
112. Pavelka K, Coste P, Géher P, et al. Efficacy and safety of piascledine 300 versus chondroitin sulfate in a 6 months treatment plus 2 months observation in patients with osteoarthritis of the knee. Clin Rheumatol 2010;29:659–70.
113. Altinel L, Saritas ZK, Kose KC, et al. Treatment with usaponifiable extracts of avocado and soybean increases TGF-β_1 and TGF-β_2 levels in canine joint fluid. Tohoku J Exp Med 2007;211:181–6.
114. Henrotin YE, Bruckner P, Pujol JPL. The role of reactive oxygen species in homeostasis and degradation of cartilage. Osteoarthritis Cartilage 2003;11:747–55.
115. Yudoh K, van Trieu N, Nakamura H, et al. Potential involvement of oxidative stress in cartilage senescence and development of osteoarthritis: oxidative stress induces chondrocyte telomere instability and downregulation of chondrocyte function. Arthritis Res Ther 2005;7:R380–91.
116. Kurz B, Jost B, Schanke M. Dietary vitamins and selenium diminish the development of mechanically induced osteoarthritis and increase the expression of antioxidative enzymes in the knee joint of STR/1N mice. Osteoarthritis Cartilage 2002;10:119–26.
117. Canter PH, Wider B, Ernst E. The antioxidant vitamins A, C, E and selenium in the treatment of arthritis: a systemic review of randomized clinical trials. Rheumatology 2007;46:1223–33.
118. Firuzi O, Miri R, Tavakkoli M, et al. Antioxidant therapy: current status and future prospects. Curr Med Chem 2011;18:3871–88.

119. Peregoy J, Wilder FV. The effects of vitamin C supplementation on incident and progressive knee osteoarthritis: a longitudinal study. Public Health Nutr 2011;14: 709–15.

120. Pelletier J, Jovanovic D, Fernandes JC, et al. Reduction in the structural changes of experimental osteoarthritis by a nitric oxide inhibitor. Osteoarthritis Cartilage 1999; 7:416–8.

121. Calamia V, Ruiz-Romero C, Rocha B, et al. Pharmacoproteomic study of the effects of chondroitin and glucosamine sulfate on human articular chondrocytes. Arthritis Res Ther 2010;12:R138.

122. Li ZH, Zhao WH, Zhou QL. Experimental study of velvet antler polypeptides against oxidative damage of osteoarthritis cartilage cells. Zhongguo Gu Shang 2011;24: 245–8.

123. Kremer JM, Bigaouette J. Nutrient intake of patients with rheumatoid arthritis is deficient in pyridoxine, zinc, copper, and magnesium. J Rheumatol 1996;23(6): 990–4.

124. Stone J, Doube A, Dudson D, et al. Inadequate calcium, folic acid, vitamin E, zinc, and selenium intake in rheumatoid arthritis patients: results of a dietary survey. Semin Arthritis Rheum 1998;27:180–5.

125. McGreevy PD, Thomson PC, Price C, et al. Prevalence of obesity in dogs examined by Australian veterinary practices and the risk factors involved. Vet Rec 2005;156: 695–702.

126. Colliard L, Ancel J, Benet JJ, et al. Risk factors for obesity in dogs in France. 2006;136:1951S–4S.

127. Colliard L, Paragon BM, Lemuet B, et al. Prevalence and risk factors of obesity in an urban population of healthy cats. J Fel Med Surg 2009;11:135–40.

128. Courcier EA, O'Higgins R, Mellor DJ, et al. Prevalence and risk factors for feline obesity in a first opinion practice in Glasgow, Scotland. J Fel Med Surg 2010;12: 746–53.

129. Courcier EA, Thomson RM, Mellor DJ, et al. An epidemiological study of environmental factors associated with canine obesity. J Sm Anim Pract 2010;51:362–7.

130. German AJ. The growing problem of obesity in dogs and cats. J Nutr 2006;136: 1940S–6S.

131. Montoya JA, Morris PJ, Bautista I, et al. Hypertension: a risk factor associated with weight status in dogs. J Nutr 2006;136:2011S–3S.

132. Back JF, Rozanski EA, Bedenice D, et al. Association of expiratory airway dysfunction with marked obesity in healthy adult dogs. Am J Vet Res 2007;68:670–5.

133. Lawler DF, Larson BT, Ballam JM, et al. Diet restriction and aging in the dog: major observations over two decades. Br J Nutr 2008;99:793–805.

134. Bouthegourd JC, Kelly M, Clety N, et al. Effects of weight loss on heart rate normalization and increase in spontaneous activity in moderately exercised overweight dogs. Intern J Appl Res Vet Med 2009;7:153–64.

135. Gayet C, Leray V, Saito M, et al. The effects of obesity-associated insulin resistance on mRNA expression of peroxisome proliferator-activated receptor-γ target genes, in dogs. Br J Nutr 2007;98:497–503.

136. Eirmann LA, Freeman LM, Laflamme DP, et al. Comparison of adipokine concentrations and markers of inflammation in obese versus lean dogs. Intern J Appl Res Vet Med 2009;7:196–205.

137. German AJ, Hervera M, Hunter L, et al. Improvement in insulin resistance and reduction in plasma inflammatory adipokines after weight loss in obese dogs. Dom Anim Endocrinol 2009;37:214–26.

138. Radin MJ, Sharkey LC, Holycross BJ. Adipokines: a review of biological and analytical principles and an update in dogs, cats and horses. Vet Clin Pathol 2009;38:136–56.

139. Wakshlag JJ, Struble AM, Levine CB, et al. The effects of weight loss on adipokines and markers of inflammation in dogs. Br J Nutr 2011;106:11–4S.

140. Root MV, Johnston SD, Olson PN. Effect of prepuberal and postpuberal gonadectomy on heat production measured by indirect calorimetry in male and female domestic cats. Am J Vet Res 1996;57:371–4.

141. Nguyen PG, Dumon HJ, Siliart BS, et al. Effects of dietary fat and energy on body weight and composition after gonadectomy in cats. Am J Vet Res 2004;65:1708–13.

142. Backus RC, Cave NJ, Keisler DH. Gonadectomy and high fat diet but not high dietary carbohydrate induce gains in body weight and fat of domestic cats. Br J Nutr 2007;98:641–50.

143. Belsito KR, Vester BM, Keel T, et al. Impact of ovariohysterectomy and food intake on body composition, physical activity, and adipose gene expression in cats. J Anim Sci 2009;87:594–602.

144. Heuberger R, Wakshlag JJ. The relationship of feeding pattern and obesity in dogs. J Anim Physiol Anim Nutr (Berl) 2011;95(1):98–105.

145. Bjornvad CR, Nielsen DH, Armstrong PJ, et al. Evaluation of a nine-point body condition scoring system in physically inactive pet cats. Am J Vet Res 2011;72:433–7.

146. German AJ, Morgan LE. How often do veterinarians assess the bodyweight and body condition of dogs? Vet Rec 2008;163:503–5.

147. Laflamme DP, Kuhlman G, Lawler DF. Evaluation of weight loss protocols for dogs. J Am Anim Hosp Assoc 1997:33:253–9.

148. Wakshlag JJ, Struble AM, Warren B, et al. Physical activity and body size influence weight loss during a weight reduction protocol. J Am Vet Med Assoc 2011, in press.

149. Laflamme DP, Kuhlman G. The effect of weight loss regimen on subsequent weight maintenance in dogs. Nutr Res 1995;15:1019–28.

150. Rosenbaum M, Hirsch J, Gallagher DA, et al. Long-term persistence of adaptive thermogenesis in subjects who have maintained a reduced body weight. Am J Clin Nutr 2008;88:906–12.

151. Villaverde C, Ramsey JJ, Green AS, et al. Energy restriction results in mass-adjusted decrease in energy expenditure in cats that is maintained after weight regain. J Nutr 2008;138:856–60.

152. Bosy-Westphal A, Kossel E, Goele K, et al. Contribution of individual organ mass loss to weight loss-associated decline in resting energy expenditure. Am J Clin Nutr 2009;90:993–1001.

153. Diez M, Nguyen P, Jeusette I, et al. Weight loss in obese dogs: evaluation of a high-protein, low-carbohydrate diet. J Nutr 2002;132:1685–7S.

154. Bierer TL, Bui LM. High-protein low-carbohydrate diets enhance weight loss in dogs. J Nutr 2004;134:2087S–9S.

155. Laflamme DP, Hannah SS. Increased dietary protein promotes fat loss and reduces loss of lean body mass during weight loss in cats. Int J Appl Res Vet Med 2005;3:62–8.

156. Paddon-Jones D, Westman E, Mattes RD, et al. Protein, weight management, and satiety. Am J Clin Nutr 2008;87:1558S–61S.

157. Vasconcellos RS, Borges NC, Goncalves KNV, et al. Protein intake during weight loss influences the energy required for weight loss and maintenance in cats. J Nutr 2009;139:855–60.

158. Wei A, Fascetti AJ, Liu KJ, et al. Influence of a high-protein diet on energy balance in obese cats allowed ad libitum access to food. J Anim Physiol Anim Nutr (Berl) 2011;95(3):359–67.

159. Jackson JR, Laflamme DP, Owens SF. Effects of dietary fiber content on satiety in dogs. Vet Clin Nutr 1997;4:130–4.

160. Jewell DE, Toll PW, Novotny BJ. Satiety reduced adiposity in dogs. Vet Ther 2000;1:17–23.

161. Bosch G, Verbrugghe A, Hesta M, et al. The effects of dietary fibre type on satiety-related hormones and voluntary food intake in dogs. Br J Nutr 2009;102: 318–25.

162. Weber M, Bissot T, Servet E, et al. A high-protein, high-fiber diet designed for weight loss improves satiety in dogs. J Vet Intern Med 2007;21:1203–8.

163. Morris PJ, Calvert EL, Holmes KL, et al. Energy intake in cats as affected by alterations in diet energy density. J Nutr 2006;136:2072S–4S.

164. Pan Y. Use of soy isoflavones for weight management in spayed/neutered dogs. FASEB J 2006 20:A854–5.

165. Cave NJ, Backus RC, Marks SL, et al. Oestradiol, but not genistein, inhibits the rise in food intake following gonadectomy in cats, but genistein is associated with an increase in lean body mass. J Anim Physiol Anim Nutr 2007;91L400–10.

166. Pan Y, Tavazzi I, Oberson JM, et al. Effect of isoflavones, conjugated linoleic acid, and L-carnitine on weight loss and oxidative stress in overweight dogs. Comp Cont Educ Vet 2008;30(3A):69.

167. Center SA, Harte J, Watrous D, et al. The clinical and metabolic effects of rapid weight loss in obese pet cats and the influence of supplemental oral L-carnitine. J Vet Intern Med 2000;14:598–608.

168. Umeda T, Bauer JE, Otsuji K. Weight loss effect of dietary diacylglycerol in obese dogs. J Anim Physiol Anim Nutr 2006;90:208–15.

169. Bauer JE, Nagaoka D, Porterpan B, et al. Postprandial lipolytic activities, lipids, and carbohydrate metabolism are altered in dogs fed diacylglycerol meals containing high- and low-glycemic index starches. J Nutr 2006;136:1955S–7S.

170. Dyck DJ. Dietary fat intake, supplements, and weight loss. Can J Appl Physiol 2000;25:495–523.

171. Brandsch C, Eder K. Effect of L-carnitine on weight loss and body composition of rats fed a hypocaloric diet. Ann Nutr Metab 2002;46:205–10.

172. Melton SA, Keenan MJ, Stanciu CE, et al. L-carnitine supplementation does not promote weight loss in ovariectomized rats despite endurance exercise. Int J Vitam Nutr Res 2005;75:156–60.

173. Yaissle JE, Holloway C, Buffington CAT. Evaluation of owner education as a component of obesity treatment programs for dogs. J Am Vet Med Assoc 2004; 224:1932–5.

174. German AJ, Holden SL, Bissot T, et al. Dietary energy restriction and successful weight loss in obese client-owned dogs. J Vet Intern Med 2007;21:1174–80.

175. Wadden TA, West DS, Neiberg R, et al. One-year weight losses in the look AHEAD study: factors associated with success. Obesity 2009;17:713–22.

176. Garaulet M, Perez de Heredia F. Behavioural therapy in the treatment of obesity (I): new directions for clinical practice. Nutr Hosp 2009;24:629–39.

177. Rohlf VI, Toukhsati S, Coleman GJ, et al. Dog obesity: can dog caregivers' (owners') feeding and exercise intentions and behaviours be predicted from attitudes? J Appl Anim Welf Sci 2010;13(3):213–36.

178. Jackson M, Ballam JM, Laflamme DP. Client perceptions and canine weight loss. Comp Cont Educ Pract Vet 2001;23(9a):90.

179. Bland IM, Guthrie-Jones A, Taylor RD, et al. Dog obesity: veterinary practices' and owners' opinions on cause and management. Prev Vet Med 2010;94:310–5.
180. German AJ, Holden SL, Mason SL, et al. Imprecision when using measuring cups to weigh out extruded dry kibbled food. J Anim Physiol Anim Nutr (Berl) 2011;95(3): 368–73.
181. Stoa Luedtke E, Schmidt C, Laflamme D. The effect of food bowl size on the amount of food fed to cats. Proc Am Assoc Vet Nutr Annual Symposium 2011. June 15. St Charles (MO): Royal Canin; 2011. p. 8.
182. Murphy M, Lusby AL, Bartges JW, et al. Size of food bowl and scoop affects amount of food owners feed their dogs. J Anim Physiol Anim Nutr (Berl) 2012;96(2):237–41.
183. Gossellin J, McKelvie J, Sherington J, et al. An evaluation of dirlotapide to reduce body weight of client-owned dogs in two placebo-controlled clinical studies in Europe. J Vet Pharmacol Ther 2007;30(Suppl 1):73–80.
184. Wren JA, Ramudo AA, Campbell SL, et al. Efficacy and safety of dirlotapide in the management of obese dogs evaluated in two placebo-controlled, masked clinical studies in North America. J Vet Pharmacol Ther 2007;30(Suppl 1):81–9.
185. Dobenecker B, De Bock M, Engelen M, et al. Effect of mitratapide on body composition, body measurements and glucose tolerance in obese beagles. Vet Res Commun 2009;33(8):839–47.

Veterinary Dentistry in Senior Canines and Felines

Steven E. Holmstrom, DVM

KEYWORDS

- Dentistry • Senior canines • Senior felines • Anesthesia free dentistry
- Oral tumors • Neoplasia

KEY POINTS

When you have completed this article, you will be able to:

- Understand grade patients with periodontal disease and prescribe proper treatment for them.
- Describe the AVDC Stages of Tooth resorption and the treatment.
- Describe the not clinically aggressive and aggressive oral tumors.
- Be knowledgeable of the American Animal Hospital Association Guidelines on Veterinary Dental Procedures and how to obtain them.
- Understand the disadvantage of Non-Professional Dental Scaling (NPDS) and why it should not be performed.

As with many other systems in the "senior" pet, the oral cavity undergoes aging changes that need to be addressed for the comfort of the patient. In their Senior Care Guidelines, the American Animal Hospital Association states that there should be focused attention to client education for the increased veterinary attention to dental/oral care and to home dental prophylaxis.[1] In reality, this dental care should start at an early age to prevent or manage problems when the pet is older.[2] This article will discuss findings that may be discovered by complete oral exam. Typical conditions that can occur in senior dogs and cats include undiagnosed orthodontic disease, periodontal disease, tooth resorption, and oral tumors.

DENTAL WEAR

Attresion is wear of a tooth against another tooth. It may take many years for attresion caused by orthodontic malocclusion to become clinical. For example, a patient with a prognathic mandible may have chronic wear of the maxillary lateral incisors against

The author has nothing to disclose.
Animal Dental Clinic, 987 Laurel Street, San Carlos, CA 94070, USA
E-mail address: steve@toothvet.info

Vet Clin Small Anim 42 (2012) 793–808
http://dx.doi.org/10.1016/j.cvsm.2012.04.001
0195-5616/12/$ – see front matter © 2012 Elsevier Inc. All rights reserved.

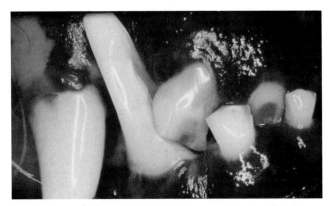

Fig. 1. Attrition Class 3 occlusion. This patient has an occlusion that has resulted in the maxillary incisor chronically wearing into the mandibular canine.

the mandibular canine teeth (**Fig. 1**). This wear may become so severe that the canine teeth may spontaneously fracture, exposing the pulp chamber. The simple prevention at an earlier age would have been to extract the maxillary lateral incisors. Another example for this same orthodontic condition would be chronic trauma between the maxillary and mandibular incisors. The incisors may become lose due to the chronic stretching of the periodontal ligament. These cases are often misdiagnosed as "periodontal disease" when the teeth become loose.

Chronic chewing from skin disease can cause wear of the tooth against an external source known as abrasion. In this case, the teeth may become so worn down that the pulp chambers may become exposed or the wear can cause recession of the gum tissue. As these conditions progress they may become painful and reduce the quality of life.

STAGING PERIODONTAL DISEASE

The American Veterinary Dental College (AVDC) has staged periodontal disease in 4 stages. The AVDC system is a radiographic system and not a clinical grading system.

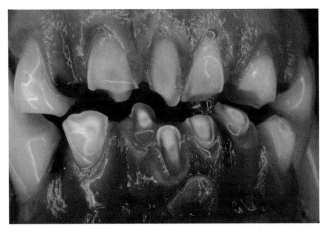

Fig. 2. Abrasion—skin chewing. This patient has been chronically chewing its skin. As a result, labial walls of the incisors are worn.

To use this system, you must have radiographs to evaluate state of periodontal health with the AVDC system. Staging is performed only after the radiographs. The degree of severity of periodontal disease relates to a single tooth; a patient may have teeth that have different stages of periodontal disease (**Fig. 2**).

- *Normal* **(PD 0):** Clinically normal—no gingival inflammation or periodontitis clinically evident.
- *Stage 1* **(PD 1):** Gingivitis only without attachment loss. The height and architecture of the alveolar margin are normal.
- *Stage 2* **(PD 2):** Early periodontitis—less than 25% of attachment loss or, at most, there is a stage 1 furcation involvement in multirooted teeth. There are early radiologic signs of periodontitis. The loss of periodontal attachment is less than 25% as measured either by probing of the clinical attachment level, or radiographic determination of the distance of the alveolar margin from the cemento-enamel junction relative to the length of the root.
- *Stage 3* **(PD 3):** Moderate periodontitis—25% to 50% of attachment loss as measured by probing of the clinical attachment level or radiographic determination of the distance of the alveolar margin from the cemento-enamel junction relative to the length of the root, or there is a stage 2 furcation involvement in multirooted teeth.
- *Stage 4* **(PD 4):** Advanced periodontitis—more than 50% of attachment loss as measured by probing of the clinical attachment level or radiographic determination of the distance of the alveolar margin from the cemento-enamel junction relative to the length of the root or there is a stage 3 furcation involvement in multirooted teeth.

Because many senior pets have not had adequate dental care throughout their life, they may be showing advanced signs of periodontal disease, yet this may not be the case for all. Treatment for PD 0 would be home care. Treatment recommendations for PD 1 would be a thorough prophylaxis followed by home care. Treatment for PD 2 patients would be periodontal therapy, which includes subgingival scaling with a curette or ultrasonic scaler with ultrasonic tips. PD3 patients will require deeper scaling and possibly the use of a medication such as Doxirobe (Pfizer Animal Health, Exton, PA, USA) or Arestin (Oropharma, Warminster, PA, USA). Unfortunately, the damage through years of neglect may already have been done and most with PD4 will require extraction. Bone augmentation procedures can be attempted but are seldom effective in the long term as the same conditions exist after the surgery that existed before the surgery (**Figs. 3** and **4**).

TOOTH RESORPTION

Tooth resorption (TR) is very common in the cat and, with more veterinarians taking whole mouth intraoral radiographs, is very often seen in the dog. TR was formerly called feline odontoclastic lesion (FORL). While TR can occur in any age, for the most part, it is seen in senior pets.

AVDC STAGES

The AVDC has created a system of classifying TR by stages. There is some controversy in this system as it is not known whether the disease progresses in stages. Also, staging assumes one cause, which may not necessarily be so.

- **Stage 1 (TR 1)**: Mild dental hard tissue loss (cementum or cementum and enamel) (**Fig. 5**)
- **Stage 2 (TR 2)**: Moderate dental hard tissue loss (cementum or cementum and enamel with loss of dentin that does not extend to the pulp cavity) (**Fig. 6**)

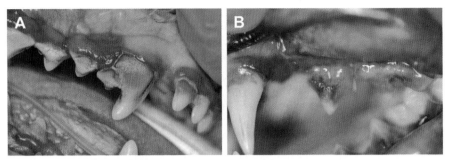

Fig. 3. (A) Photograph of PD4 dog. (B) Photograph of PD4 cat. These patients show signs of advanced periodontal disease. While there is a large amount of calculus present, more concerning is the amount and depth of gingival inflammation.

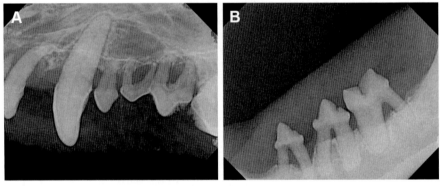

Fig. 4. (A) Radiograph of PD4 dog. (B) Radiograph of PD4 cat. Canine (A) and feline (B) radiographs showing advanced bone loss with exposure of the furcation (area between the roots).

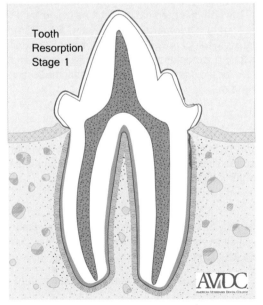

Fig. 5. TR1 drawing. Stage 1 has mild loss of cementum or cementum and enamel as shown by the circle.

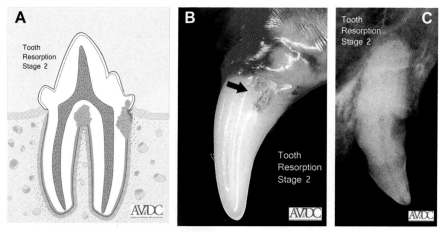

Fig. 6. (*A*) TR2 drawing. (*B*) TR2 photograph. (*C*) TR2 radiograph.

- **Stage 3 (TR 3)**: Deep dental hard tissue loss (cementum or cementum and enamel with loss of dentin that extends to the pulp cavity); most of the tooth retains its integrity (**Fig. 7**)
- **Stage 4 (TR 4)**: Extensive dental hard tissue loss (cementum or cementum and enamel with loss of dentin that extends to the pulp cavity); most of the tooth has lost its integrity.
- *TR4a* Crown and root are equally affected (**Fig. 8**)
- *TR4b* Crown is more severely affected than the root (**Fig. 9**)
- *TR4c* Root is more severely affected than the crown (**Fig. 10**)
- **Stage 5 (TR 5)**: Remnants of dental hard tissue are visible only as irregular radiopacities, and gingival covering is complete (**Fig. 11**).

TREATMENT OF TR

The treatment of TR is radiographic evaluation, followed by extraction of teeth with Stage 2 to 4 lesions. Stage 1 lesions usually do not cause pain, and stage 5 lesions, unless there is gingival inflammation, do not require treatment.

ORAL TUMORS
Not Clinically Aggressive

Oral neoplasia
While they may grow locally and in rare instances convert to malignant tumors, non–clinically aggressive tumors generally do not spread deep into tissue or metastasize to lymph nodes or lungs. Generally, they respond well to surgical removal. If not completely removed, however, they may return to the same or an adjacent location.

Granulomas
Benign granulomas are common, usually incidental findings and are caused by periodontal disease or other irritation. They respond well to local excision and removal of the originating cause. While they can occur at any age, they tend to occur more in senior pets (**Fig. 12**).

Gingival hyperplasia
Gingival hyperplasia, the proliferation of gingival cells, is common among some breeds, particularly the collie, boxer, and cocker spaniel. Pocket formation and

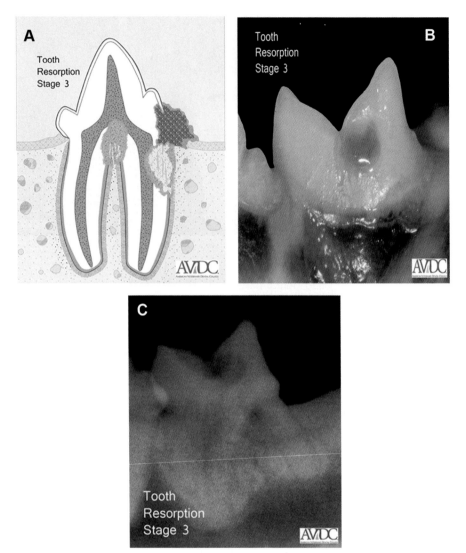

Fig. 7. (*A*) TR3 drawing. (*B*) TR3 photograph. (*C*) TR3 radiograph.

periodontal disease may result from this hyperplastic tissue. Certain medicines such as cyclosporine, calcium channel blockers, and phenytoin can cause gingival hyperplasia (**Fig. 13**).

Peripheral odontogenic fibroma
Peripheral odontogenic fibroma, also known as fibromatous epulides, are characterized by the presence of a tumor in the tissues of the gingiva, containing primarily fibrous tissues. Generally, the peripheral odontogenic fibromas respond well to excision; however, they may return if the excision is incomplete.

An ossifying epulis resembles a fibromatous epulis but also contains large amounts of bone material, which give it a bony quality apparent during excision.

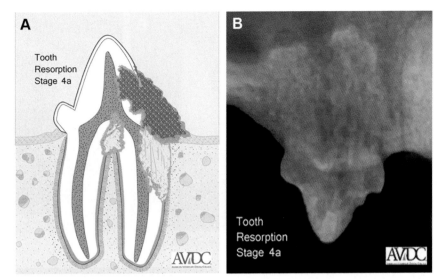

Fig. 8. (*A*) TR 4A drawing. (*B*) TR 4A radiograph.

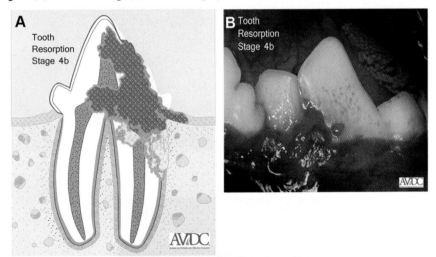

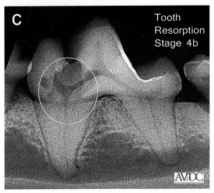

Fig. 9. (*A*) TR 4B drawing. (*B*) TR 4B photograph. (*C*) TR 4B radiograph.

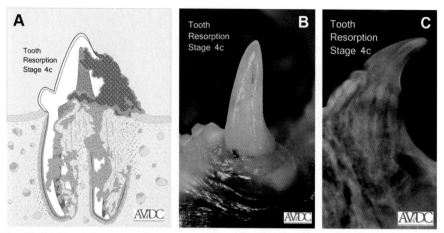

Fig. 10. (*A*) TR 4C drawing. (*B*) TR 4C photograph. (*C*) TR 4C radiograph.

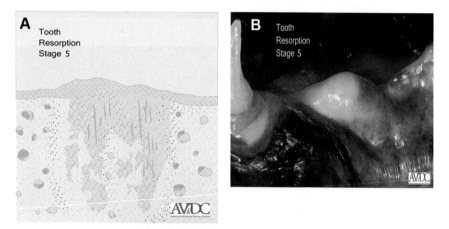

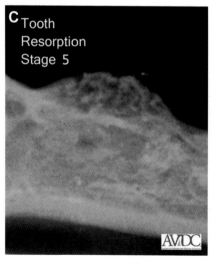

Fig. 11. (*A*) TR 5 drawing. (*B*) TR 5 photograph. (*C*) TR 5 radiograph.

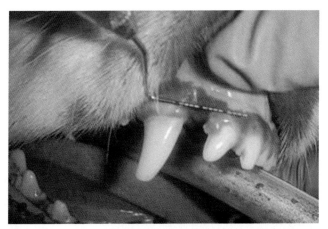

Fig. 12. Gingival granuloma. This benign gingival granuloma will respond well to surgical excision.

Because of the depth of the bone, these tumors sometimes are difficult to remove (**Fig. 14**).

Clinically Aggressive Tumors

Acanthomatous ameloblastoma

The acanthomatous epulis is primarily composed of proliferating epithelial cells of dental origin associated with the tissue. While they are classified as benign, these epulides tend to invade bone, which makes dental radiographic evaluation and aggressive surgery important (**Fig. 15**).

Malignant melanoma

Malignant melanomas occur on any site in the oral cavity: gingiva, buccal mucosa, hard and soft palates, and tongue. They are locally invasive and highly metastatic to

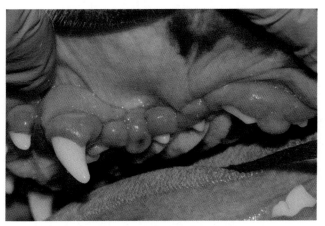

Fig. 13. Gingival hyperplasia of the left maxilla. The first premolar (1P, 205) and supernumary first premolar (1Ps, 205N) are completely covered with hyperplastic tissue.

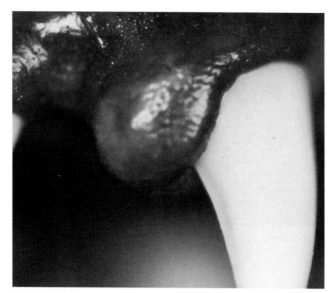

Fig. 14. Peripheral odontogenic fibroma ossifying epulis.

the lungs, regional lymph nodes, and bone. As with many malignancies, clients may first notice a minor change, such as bad breath. Clients also sometimes report oral bleeding. Malignant tumors may appear darkly pigmented or nonpigmented. Loose teeth, caused by bone involvement, is another symptom. The prognosis is poor because reoccurrence is common. They are the most common oral neoplasia in the dog[3] (**Fig. 16**).

Fibrosarcoma

Fibrosarcomas occur in the mandible or maxilla. They may create fleshy, protruding, firm masses that sometimes are friable. As the masses grow, they can become ulcerated and infected. They are locally aggressive but slow to metastasize[4] (**Fig. 17**).

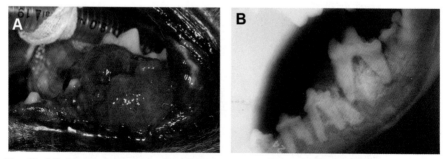

Fig. 15. (*A*) Acanthomatous epulis. (*B*) Acantomatous epulis radiograph. Acanthomatous ameloblastoma that has formed in the region of the mandibular fourth premolar (4P, 308) and first molar (1M, 309).

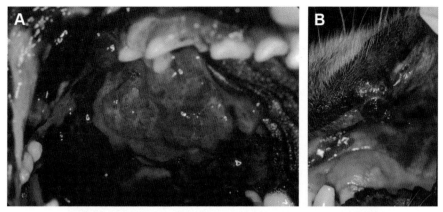

Fig. 16. (*A*) Malignant melanoma in the maxilla. (*B*) Malignant melanoma in the lip.

Squamous cell carcinoma

Squamous cell carcinomas arise in a variety of locations in the mouth. Their cell type is from the epithelium. They can occur in tonsillar crypts and the gingiva. Their appearance varies, but generally they are nodular, gray to pink, irregular masses that invade the bone and cause tooth mobility. Generally, the farther away from tonsils or the floor of the mouth, the better is the prognosis. Typically the only clinical sign of the presence of this tumor is tooth mobility. Teeth are often extracted without biopsy and radiograph. Only when the wound does not heal is the problem investigated. They are the most common neoplasia in cats and are associated with osteolysis.[5] Any lesion that looks clinically or radiographically abnormal must undergo biopsy (**Figs. 18** and **19**).

PROCEDURE CONSIDERATIONS

Properly performed anesthesia as a low rate of mortality.[6–8] The reader is encouraged to read the article by Nora Matthews on anesthesia elsewhere in this issue. The protocol commonly used by the author is noted in the later case report.

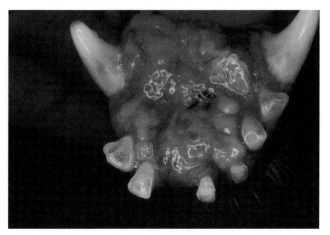

Fig. 17. Fibrosarcoma on the rostral portion of the mandible in a dog.

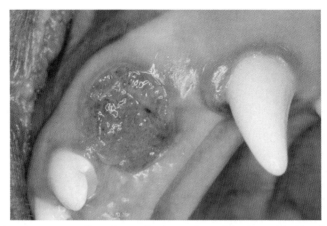

Fig. 18. Canine squamous cell carcinoma in the region of the lateral incisor that had been extracted because it was mobile.

TREATMENT CONSIDERATIONS

The American Animal Hospital Association has published "Dental Care Guidelines for Dogs and Cats"[9] (the reader is encouraged to download).

Among the guidelines is the necessity to perform dental procedures for the best benefit of the patient. This includes a preoperative oral examination on the conscious patient, taking intraoral radiographs using film or digital systems while the patient is under anesthesia, scaling the teeth with hand or powered devices, polishing the teeth, applying antiplaque substances, probing and recording pocket depths, performing periodontal therapy as necessary, administering perioperative antibiotics when indicated, performing periodontal surgery when indicated, extracting teeth when indicated, taking a biopsy sample of all abnormal masses that have been visualized either grossly or radiographically, taking postoperative radiographs to evaluate and document treatment as necessary, and, finally, recommending referral to a specialist if the practitioner does not feel capable of completely treating the patient.

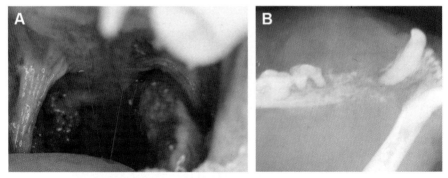

Fig. 19. (*A*) Squamous cell carcinoma of the right tonsil of a cat. (*B*) Advanced squamous cell carcinoma in radiograph of a cat's mandible. The prognosis in both cases is poor.

"ANESTHESIA-FREE DENTISTRY"

There has been an increase in individuals "selling" dental cleaning without anesthesia to both the public and veterinarians. In most states, this is the practice of veterinary medicine and it is illegal to perform outside the direct supervision of a veterinarian. Unfortunately, some veterinarians have accepted this procedure into their practice. The AVDC has a position statement on this procedure (see **Appendix**). It is providing less than the standard of care and is doing harm to patients due to neglect. The following case report is provided as an example of years of negligent practice resulting in chronic dental disease with nonsalvageable teeth.

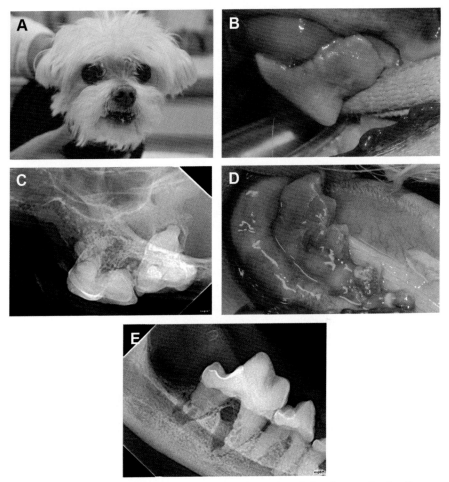

Fig. 20. (A) Ricky has had numerous "anesthesia-free" dental cleanings and pulse therapy. (B) Left maxillary fourth premolar showing gingival inflammation, calculus, and plaque. (C) Left maxillary fourth premolar radiograph showing bone loss and root resorption of the left maxillary fourth premolar and bone loss of the palatal root first molar. (D) Right mandibular third, fourth premolars, and first molar showing gingival inflammation, plaque, calculus, and pus; pockets were noted on periodontal probing. (E) Radiograph of right maxillary first molar showing bone loss and tooth resorption.

Abbreviated Case Report—"Ricky"

"Ricky" is a 13-year-old neutered male Maltese canine weighing 4 kg. Previous history includes placement of an amyloid constrictor for a hepatic portal shunt. Other than his teeth, "Ricky" had received excellent veterinary care. The client had relied on nonanesthesia dental cleanings at a local groomer and pulse antibiotic therapy (clindamycin) prescribed by the referring veterinarian. A conscious oral exam revealed heavy amounts of plaque, calculus, and pus and moderate to severe gingival inflammation. The patient would allow examination on the left side but was more tender on the right. Blood values were all within normal limits.

"Rickey" was premedicated with 0.5 mg butorphanol subcutaneous (0.125 mg/kg) (Butorphanol tartarate, Intra Vet Inc, Millsboro, DE, USA) and 0.1 mg atropine intramuscular (0.025 mg/kg) (Atropine sulfate, Med-Pharmex, Pomona, CA, USA). An intravenous catheter was placed, and 80 mg ampicillin intravenous (20 mg/kg) was administered. Propofol 25 mg (Abbott Animal Health, North Chicago, IL, USA) was administered (to effect). The patient was intubated and sevoflurane 3% to 4%/oxygen was administered. Continuous monitoring of blood pressure, electrocardiography, pulse oximetry, temperature, and respirations was performed during the procedure. Intraoral radiographs were taken, which showed bone loss tooth resorption as the result of chronic periodontal dental disease of all the remaining teeth. Exodontia was performed; the alveolus was debrided and gingiva was sutured with 4-0 MONOCRYL (Ethicon, Guaynabo, PR, USA). As the infection was deemed to have overwhelmed the tissues, Clavamox 62.5 mg (Pfizer Animal Health, New York, NY, USA) every 12 hours was dispensed for 5 days. Tramadol 10 mg (Anneal Pharmaceutical, Glasgow, KY, USA) every 8 to 12 hours was dispensed for 3 to 5 days (**Fig. 20**).

Most dental disease is of chronic nature and is best to be dealt with before it becomes severe. The quality of life of the senior pet can be enhanced by proper care at all times in the patient's life.

APPENDIX
AVDC Position Paper Dental Scaling Without Anesthesia

In the United States and Canada, only licensed veterinarians can practice veterinary medicine. Veterinary medicine includes veterinary surgery, medicine, and dentistry. Anyone providing dental services other than a licensed veterinarian, or a supervised and trained veterinary technician, is practicing veterinary medicine without a license and is subject to criminal charges.

This page addresses dental scaling procedures performed on pets without anesthesia, often by individuals untrained in veterinary dental techniques. Although the term Anesthesia-Free Dentistry has been used in this context, AVDC prefers to use the more accurate term Non-Professional Dental Scaling (NPDS) to describe this combination.

Owners of pets naturally are concerned when anesthesia is required for their pet. However, performing NPDS on an unanesthetized pet is inappropriate for the following reasons:

1. Dental tartar is firmly adhered to the surface of the teeth. Scaling to remove tartar is accomplished using ultrasonic and sonic power scalers, plus hand instruments that must have a sharp working edge to be used effectively. Even slight head movement by the patient could result in injury to the oral tissues of the patient, and the operator may be bitten when the patient reacts.

2. Professional dental scaling includes scaling the surfaces of the teeth both above and below the gingival margin (gum line), followed by dental polishing. The most critical part of a dental scaling procedure is scaling the tooth surfaces that are within the gingival pocket (the subgingival space between the gum and the root), where periodontal disease is active. Because the patient cooperates, dental scaling of human teeth performed by a professional trained in the procedures can be completed successfully without anesthesia. However, access to the subgingival area of every tooth is impossible in an unanesthetized canine or feline patient. Removal of dental tartar on the visible surfaces of the teeth has little effect on a pet's health, and provides a false sense of accomplishment. The effect is purely cosmetic.

3. Inhalation anesthesia using a cuffed endotracheal tube provides three important advantages . . . the cooperation of the patient with a procedure it does not understand, elimination of pain resulting from examination and treatment of affected dental tissues during the procedure, and protection of the airway and lungs from accidental aspiration.

4. A complete oral examination, which is an important part of a professional dental scaling procedure, is not possible in an unanesthetized patient. The surfaces of the teeth facing the tongue cannot be examined, and areas of disease and discomfort are likely to be missed.

Safe use of an anesthetic or sedative in a dog or cat requires evaluation of the general health and size of the patient to determine the appropriate drug and dose, and continual monitoring of the patient.

Veterinarians are trained in all of these procedures. Prescribing or administering anesthetic or sedative drugs by a non-veterinarian can be very dangerous, and is illegal. Although anesthesia will never be 100% risk-free, modern anesthetic and patient evaluation techniques used in veterinary hospitals minimize the risks, and millions of dental scaling procedures are safely performed each year in veterinary hospitals.

To minimize the need for professional dental scaling procedures and to maintain optimal oral health, AVDC recommends daily dental home care from an early age in dogs and cats. This should include brushing or use of other effective techniques to retard accumulation of dental plaque, such as dental diets and chew materials. This, combined with periodic examination of the patient by a veterinarian and with dental scaling under anesthesia when indicated, will optimize life-long oral health for dogs and cats.

For information on effective oral hygiene products for dogs and cats, visit the Veterinary Oral Health Council web site (www.VOHC.org).

For general information on performance of dental procedures on veterinary patients, read the AVDC Position Statement on Veterinary Dental Healthcare Providers (http://www.avdc.org/healthproinfo.html).

Reprinted with permission from American Veterinary Dental College.

REFERENCES

1. Epstein M, Kuehn NF, Landsberg G, et al; Senior Care Guidelines Task Force, AAHA. AAHA senior care guidelines for dogs and cats. J Am Anim Hosp Assoc 2005;41:81–91.
2. Boss N, Holmstrom S, Carlos S, et al; American Animal Hospital Association-American Veterinary Medical Association Preventive Healthcare Guidelines Task Force. Development of new canine and feline preventive healthcare guidelines designed to improve pet health. J Am Anim Hosp Assoc 2011;47:306–11.

3. Bergman PJ. Canine oral melanoma. Clin Tech Small Anim Pract 2007;22:55–60.
4. Coyle VJ, Garrett LD. Finding and treating oral melanoma, squamous cell carcinoma and fibrosarcoma in dogs. Vet Med 2009;104:292–305.
5. Martin CK, Tannehill-Gregg SH, Wolfe TD, et al. Bone-invasive oral squamous cell carcinoma in cats: pathology and expression of parathyroid hormone-related protein. Vet Pathol 2011;48:302–12.
6. Brodbelt DC. Perioperative mortality in small animal anaesthesia. Vet J 2009;182: 152–61.
7. Brodbelt DC, Pfeiffer DU, Young LE, et al. Results of the confidential enquiry into perioperative small animal fatalities regarding risk factors for anesthetic-related death in dogs. J Am Vet Med Assoc 2008;233:1096–104.
8. Brodbelt DC. Feline anesthetic deaths in veterinary practice, Top Comp Anim Med 2010;25:189–94.
9. Holmstrom S, Bellows J, Colmery B, et al. AAHA dental care guidelines for dogs and cats. J Am Anim Hosp Assoc 2005;41:277-83. Available at: https://www.aahanet.org/Library/DentalCare.aspx.

Alternative Medicines for the Geriatric Veterinary Patient

J. Randy Kidd, DVM, PhD

KEYWORDS

- Holistic health • Geriatric • Alternative medicine
- Complementary and alternative medicine • Integrative medicine

KEY POINTS

- There are many medical modalities that are considered "alternative" or "complementary"—in this article, the methods with which the author is most familiar will be discussed: acupuncture, chiropractic, herbs, flower essences (Bach flowers), and aromatherapy.
- Each alternative medicine (as does any medicine) has its advantages and disadvantages, and these are discussed.
- While they are somewhat controversial, alternative medicines are being used by more and more pet owners to treat their pets for a variety of diseases. So, while individual practitioners may or may not choose to offer them for their own patients, a working knowledge of how the various alternative medicines work is almost mandatory in today's world of veterinary health care.
- Although scientific evidence for the effectiveness of many of the alternative medicines is not always well defined, evidence of effectiveness is accumulating. And, while all medicines are capable of producing some adverse side effects, as a general rule, alternative medicines are extremely safe to use.
- With most alternative medicines, emphasis is placed on a holistic approach, involving the body, mind, emotions, and spirit of the patient. And in the case of alternative veterinary medicines, the human–animal bond, as well as the veterinary–animal–patient triad, is also considered important.

INTRODUCTION

The author discusses how holistic practitioners might use some of today's more popular "alternative" medicines as they apply to the geriatric pet. Many practitioners are currently using one or more of the alternative medicines (other terms have been used to describe these medicines, including complimentary, integrative, holistic, and complementary and alternative medicine [CAM]), but they are not without controversy.

The author has nothing to disclose.
Coyote Consulting LLD, 16879 46th Street, McLouth, KS 66054, USA
E-mail address: drrkidd@gmail.com

Vet Clin Small Anim 42 (2012) 809–822
http://dx.doi.org/10.1016/j.cvsm.2012.04.009   vetsmall.theclinics.com

ARGUMENTS AGAINST THE ALTERNATIVE MEDICINES

Until recently, there were few valid scientific studies that used conventional, unbiased methods to evaluate results. While alternative medicines are being taught in approximately two thirds of all medical schools in this country,[1] only a few veterinary schools are actively involved[2]—thus the complaint that "if it wasn't taught in vet school, it can't be valid."

Alternative methods use different ways of diagnosing, evaluating symptoms, prescribing, and evaluating results—methods that are often not easily understood by conventional practitioners. Some of the alternatives are so different from conventional practices that because they violate some basic premises about "our" conventional medicine, it does not seem possible that they could work.

ARGUMENTS IN FAVOR OF USING ALTERNATIVE MEDICINES, ESPECIALLY FOR THE GERIATRIC PATIENT

While alternative treatments are not totally without adverse side effects, as a general rule, they are nontoxic and well tolerated by an older body and its organ systems that are functionally in decline. Typically, alternative medicines approach wellness and healing from the perspective that the patient's body, mind, and spirit are all involved—creating a much more profound and longer-term, whole-body healing.

- Alternative medicines also rely on the assumption that the body, given the chance, can take care of itself. Rather than confronting disease, this assumption places the practitioner's focus on helping to recreate and prolong the animal's innate ability to heal itself and to maintain homeostasis. Alternative medicines are individualized for the patient, with each patient treated as an individual with its own needs for overall health. The human–animal bond is an important part of a holistic approach, making owner compliance in treatment regimens more likely. Beneficial results, observed by the practitioner and owner alike, are often so dramatic that they do not require a large body of supportive research data for validation.

Many of the alternative medicines use a hands-on approach, and there is some evidence that simply putting one's hands on a patient greatly enhances healing.[3]

Finally (and perhaps the most persuasive argument): Today's consumer is dictating that practitioners be at least aware of the alternative medicines and how they might be used in a total wellness program. According to a recent report from the National Center for Complementary and Alternative Medicine, approximately 38% of adults in the United States are using some form of CAM, and this number has continued to rise over the past several years.[4]

Please note that it is the author's conviction that in order to authentically criticize (either positively or negatively) any "alternative" modality, the practitioner must have tried it in a clinical environment and/or for personal use. This, of course, presupposes that the practitioner has versed him/herself in the modality with sufficient study to apply it in an appropriate manner.

In light of this personal "bias," the author briefly discusses the following alternative methods: acupuncture, chiropractic, herbal, flower essences (Bach flowers), and homeopathy. The author has personal experience with each of these methods as a practitioner and as a consumer but realizes that this list is not a complete sampling of all the many alternative methods that are currently being used by various practitioners.

Box 1
Intake form/protocol

Intake Form

Patient Information:

Referring veterinarian:

Entering Complaint:

Temp ____ H/R___ Resp___ Weight____ O N U ____ Ideal=____

Symptoms:

Diagnoses:

Current Medications:

Family and Lifestyle:

Current Diet/Supplements:

Daily Exercise and Play:

****

Objectives: 1,2,3 +

Treatment Protocol:

Treatments:Rx:

Recommendations:

Reevaluate

Box 1 presents an intake and treatment format that represents what might be a typical protocol for a holistic practitioner using alternative medicines. This is the form (slightly modified for this publication) the author used in his holistic practice.

Note that the beginning of the form—patient information, entering complaint, body temperature, heart rate, respiration evaluation—is the same or similar to that used by Western practitioners.

With obesity as a critical factor in the health/disease status of pet animals (and especially geriatric pets), the more ways we can discuss the importance of maintaining a healthy, normal body weight, the better it is for the holistic health of that animal. The opening part of the intake form allows the opportunity to discuss the animal's weight: U = underweight; N = normal weight; O = overweight; and then there is a space to list what the animal's ideal weight should be (one of the treatment goals).

Symptoms

While a holistic practitioner is interested in the normal listings of symptoms such as diarrhea or vomiting, many of the alternative modalities have different ways of evaluating and/or describing symptoms. Traditional acupuncturists, for example, might describe a condition as a "blockage of chi," whereas a Western medicine practitioner might refer to this condition as arthritis of the joint. Chiropractic evaluations involve physically palpating the functional mobility of the spine and other joints, realizing that the symptoms the animal shows (leg limp, poor posture, etc) may or may not directly relate to the actual problem area found on palpation. Physical symptoms are only a part of a homeopath's interest; mental and emotional symptoms are thought of as equally important.

Diagnoses

A Western medicine diagnosis may help a holistic practitioner devise his or her ultimate treatment protocol, but alternative medicines often have very different terminologies and evaluation tools.

Current Medications

In this day and age where over-the-counter medications and nutritional supplements are common and everyone has access to Internet experts waiting to sell their own special treatments, it is critical to know **ALL** the medications the animal is currently taking—including Western medicines, herbs, supplements, and anything else they have obtained from other sources.

Family and Lifestyle

Open-ended questions here can often reveal the extent of the human–animal bond and how involved the entire family (of pets and people) is in using health and wellness methods. This section also gives the practitioner a chance to offer suggestions for healthier lifestyle choices (nutrition, exercise, etc).

Current Diet/Supplements

This gives the practitioner a chance to understand the possibility that the patient's disease symptoms may be diet related and offers another chance to emphasize the importance of a good-quality, high-protein, low-carbohydrate diet for all geriatric animals.

Daily Exercise and Play

What would a normal week of play and exercise look like for this pet? Has this changed recently? Can the owner explain why?

Note: These last 3 items—family and lifestyle, current diet/supplements, and daily exercise and play—could be referred to the "coax and cajole" portion of the form. Spurring people to act holistically is more about coaxing and cajoling than convincing. The remaining portion of the protocol is where the team of owner, patient, holistic veterinarian, and other health care members will be convinced (or not), through observation, that the therapies being used are beneficial.

An example here is to recognize the poor overall results that have accrued trying to convince people (through a multitude of scientific facts and figures) that obesity is indeed harmful to health. But, if we can coax and cajole one individual to take small steps (take the pet on a walk around the block twice a day, for example), we can achieve tremendously beneficial, long-range results. Furthermore, when even small action steps are taken toward achieving better health for the pet, caretakers also benefit.[5,6] Actions, no matter how small, are the key here.

Objectives: 1, 2, 3+

Clients who seek alternative medicines often have different expectations from those who use Western medicines. It is therefore important that the practitioner ensures (ie, does not assume) that caretaker, patient, and practitioner are all on the same page. When caretakers articulate their objectives for therapies and when these objectives are written down, it provides everyone with a one-time log entry for continuing dialogue throughout the treatment regimen. Since many holistic treatments will be given over the course of several visits, each visit offers a good time to reevaluate the caregiver's objectives to make sure these have not changed.

Treatments/Rx

This is the section where the veterinarian's alternative treatments are described. Prescribed medications from holistic practitioners are most often in the form of herbs, homeopathic remedies, nutritional supplements, Bach flowers, aromatherapy, or similar items. Most of these are readily available from health food stores; some holistic veterinarians carry their own inventory; and even some drug stores, pet stores, and groceries are now carrying many of the alternatives.

A typical holistic practitioner will resort to Western medicine drugs such as antibiotics or steroids only as a very last result. In fact, this section might be used more typically to define how the patient can, if appropriate, be gradually withdrawn from the Western drug. On the other hand, some cases will ultimately need (or continue to need) conventional drugs, and this section would be used to prescribe the more appropriate ones.

Recommendations

This section offers a last attempt to get everyone on the pet's treatment team on board and heading in the same direction. Specific dietary and exercise recommendations can be spelled out—perhaps in a step-by-step or one-small-step-at-a-time format.

Reevaluate and expectations

This is the date when the practitioner thinks a reevaluation will be indicated. By establishing a set date, you know everyone is on the same page. As an example, most acupuncturists think that at least 3 to 6 treatments are indicated in order to give the method a fair trial, especially when treating a chronic condition.

ACUPUNCTURE
History

The practice of acupuncture has been used for at least 3000 years in various areas of the Near and Far East. Acupuncture—the insertion of fine needles in specific points of the patient's body—is actually only a portion of traditional Chinese (or Oriental) medicine (TCM), which also incorporates lifestyle recommendations, nutrition, and herbal remedies as additional parts of the overall, holistic approach to health and healing.

It has been estimated that there are several million acupuncture practitioners in the world and that, of these, more than 100,000 are veterinarians and paraveterinary assistants. There are several schools that teach the complex of acupuncture and TCM to veterinarians. The International Veterinary Acupuncture Society is the worldwide professional society for veterinary acupuncturists, and the American Academy of Veterinary Acupuncture was formed to meet the specific needs of American veterinary acupuncturists.

Acupuncture Application

Very fine, filament-like needles are inserted at specific predefined acupoints. Stimulated acupoints have an effect on neurologic, immunologic, and endocrine systems, relieving pain, stimulating leukocyte production, enhancing endocrine function, and, in the words of TCM practitioners, releasing and redirecting blocked energy (*Qi* or *chi*) while treating imbalances between the two polarities of *Qi*, *yin* (–) and *yang* (+). Practitioners may insert needles alone, or they may add electrical stimulation (electroacupuncture) or warmth and herbal stimulation (moxibustion). Substances such as vitamin B12 or gold beads may be inserted at the acupoints to enhance treatment effects and to make them last longer.

In 1997, the National Institutes of Health released a consensus report indicating that promising results were seen when using acupuncture for a variety of (human) conditions such as postoperative and chemotherapy nausea, and postoperative pain. Additional conditions where acupuncture could be considered as an acceptable alternative treatment by the NIH included joint pain, osteoarthritis, lower back pain, and asthma. In the interim since 1997, several studies appeared that indicate acupuncture's efficacy in many more conditions, including incontinence, pain of dysplasia, and cardiovascular disorders.

Compiling information from several sources,[7–9] general conditions in the veterinary geriatric patient that often respond well to acupuncture include musculoskeletal problems, such as arthritis or vertebral disc pathology; chronic respiratory problems, such as asthma; and gastrointestinal problems, such as diarrhea. Other conditions that have been successfully treated with acupuncture include otitis, cardiovascular disorders, dermatologic disorders, immune-mediated disorders, and neurologic disorders.

There are several theories for how acupuncture works, and many of these involve neurophysiologic ways of modulating one or more of the pain pathways or mechanisms via (1) endorphin and enkephalin release working on neurotransmitter receptors, (2) bioelectric stimulation that induces local and distant neuroendocrine responses, (3) stimulation of internal organs via an autonomic response generated by needling the acupoints, and (4) local vasodilation, which stimulates the immune-inflammatory systems.

Acupuncture is a very safe procedure, with only rare adverse side effects reported. Infections can occur at the needling sites (needles should be sterile and not reused); needles can puncture the lungs if inserted improperly; and needles can break off, but the fragments are usually nonreactive and do not cause problems.

Conclusion

Acupuncture is now routinely used by holistic practitioners to combat the pain of arthritis in all ages, and many practitioners have found it useful for a variety of other conditions associated with aging.

CHIROPRACTIC
Introduction

Chiropractic is a health care discipline that emphasizes the inherent recuperative power of the body to heal itself without the use of drugs or surgery. The practice of chiropractic focuses on the relationship between structure (primarily the spine) and function (as coordinated by the nervous system) and on how that relationship affects the preservation and restoration of health.

Modern day chiropractic dates back to 1895 when D.D. Palmer began using spinal adjustments to treat many conditions he saw in his clinic. The modern practice of animal chiropractic began in 1988 when Sharon Willoughby, DVM, DC, founded Options for Animals, a school that teaches veterinarians and chiropractors the art, science, and philosophy of animal chiropractic. Now there are several other schools in the United States and worldwide that teach animal chiropractic techniques. The American Veterinary Chiropractic Association is a professional organization that acts as the certifying agency for animal chiropractic schools and graduates of those schools, and it is a policing agency for the profession.

Animal chiropractic is widely employed by several thousand practitioners worldwide. Practitioners find that it is especially beneficial for helping the athletic animal achieve maximum performance, and chiropractic adjustments also help create a better quality of life for the geriatric patient.

Note: Chiropractic (for humans) is the most commonly used form of provider-delivered complementary health care, with 11% of American adults seeking care annually. Currently, more than 30% of patients with low back pain seek chiropractic care, and 17% of chiropractic patients are over age 65. Most often, especially among the elderly, patients will use chiropractic care for health conditions that other medical providers do not address. Well over 90% of chiropractic patients' chief complaints are musculoskeletal, usually spine-related back pain, neck pain, and headache, with osteoarthritis one of the more common conditions seen by doctors of chiropractic. The patients who received chiropractic care in addition to traditional medical services in the long-term care setting had fewer hospitalizations and used fewer medications than patients receiving medical care only.[10] While these are statistics based on human patients (numbers for pet patients are lacking), it can be assumed that similar numbers would occur in geriatric pet populations.

Applying Chiropractic

The practice of chiropractic focuses on the relationship between structure (primarily the spine) and function (as coordinated by the nervous system) and how that relationship affects the preservation and restoration of health. More specifically, chiropractic focuses particular attention on the vertebral subluxation complex (VSC). A VSC is an aberrant relationship between 2 adjacent articular structures that may have functional or pathology consequence, causing an alteration in the biomechanical and/or neurophysiologic reflections of these articular structures, their proximal structures, and/or body systems that may be directly or indirectly affected by them.

There are many types of chiropractic, some of which rely on a "thrusting" adjustment that uses a very specific short-lever, high-velocity, controlled thrust, by hand or instrument, that is directed at specific articulations. Other methods use low-impact or light-touch techniques to achieve results.

A chiropractic examination includes posture and gait analysis, static and motion palpation of the spine and extremities, short leg analysis, and orthopedic and neurologic evaluations.

In recent years there has been much interest in the potential for chiropractic care to help geriatric patients. From the human literature, clinical trial data found that chiropractic geriatric patients are "less likely to have been hospitalized, more likely to report a better health status, more likely to exercise vigorously, and more likely to be mobile in the community."[11] Of patients who were asked for their reaction to their own chiropractic care, 95.8% claimed that it was either "considerably" or "extremely" valuable. The longer they were in chiropractic care, the fewer nonprescription drugs they used, and there was a reduction in contacts with a physician.[12]

A review of the published chiropractic literature regarding older patients from 2001 through 2010 cites 188 retrievable articles and has 232 listed references.[13]

In the conclusion section of the 2004 White House Conference on Aging, the American Chiropractic Association, it is stated that, relative to musculoskeletal care in elderly patients, chiropractic adjustments (spinal manipulative treatment) are recommended by the Agency for Health Care Policy and Research for the care of acute low back pain and the American Geriatric Panel guidelines for the management of chronic pain state that nonpharmaceutical interventions such as chiropractic may be appropriate.[10]

Safety

Chiropractic is in general a very safe procedure, with a small percentage of (human) patients complaining of pain that exists for a short period after adjustments. However, there has been some recent concern about its potential for causing adverse events, especially when adjusting the cervical area (and especially when using high-velocity low-amplitude techniques, or "thrusting"). While numbers have not been collected from animal patients, several (human) articles have addressed this potential problem. And while the statistical data vary somewhat from study to study, the overall conclusion is that although minor side effects following cervical spine manipulation do occur, the risk of a serious adverse event, immediately or up to 7 days after treatment, was low to very low.[14–16]

Additional concern comes from treating the geriatric population where chronic arthritic conditions may exist or where bone density may be diminished. While high-velocity low-amplitude methods have not yet been shown to be more harmful for geriatric animal patients, trained animal chiropractors are aware of the low-impact, light-touch methods that may alternatively be used for these patients. Furthermore, some practitioners believe that older (human) patients may not actually experience more injuries from adjustments, but rather fewer.[17]

HERBAL MEDICINES
Introduction

Herbal medicine is the oldest form of health care known to mankind. Herbs have been used by all cultures throughout history—herbs were found in the personal effects of Otzi the Iceman whose body was frozen in the Otzal Alps for more than 5300 years. Researchers have identified 122 compounds used in mainstream medicine that were derived from traditional ethnomedical plant sources.[18]

The recently formed Veterinary Botanical Medicine Association[19] is a group of more than 100 veterinarians and herbalists dedicated to developing responsible herbal practice by encouraging research and education, strengthening industry relations, keeping herbal tradition alive as a valid information source, and increasing professional acceptance of herbal medicine for animals.

Herbal medicines may be one of the easiest of the alternatives for the Western practitioner to understand because they rely on biochemically active substances derived from plants to affect organ systems in a healthy manner. However, there are some distinct factors about herbal medicines that an herbal practitioner needs to understand.

Each medicinal plant may contain several dozen bioactive ingredients. Thus, the biochemicals from that one plant (or one plant species) may affect many of the patient's biochemical pathways and organ systems.

The plethora of bioactive ingredients within an herbal remedy may create (1) a synergistic effect where the sum of all the ingredients reacts in a stronger fashion than would be expected from the sum of the ingredients, taken separately, and (2) bidirectionality where one of the plant's substances works in one direction in the body; another in the opposite direction—in many cases, the body has the ability to select the ingredient it needs. (Examples of bidirectionality include *Ginseng,* which has 2 fractions—Rb ginsenosides and Rg ginsenosides—which have opposing actions on blood pressure, and *Echinacea,* which has biochemical constituents that are capable of sending either of 2 signals to the body: producing white cell counts in patients with low white cell counts and decelerating the production of white cells in patients with an excess.).

The biochemistry of a medicinal plant depends on many factors: what part(s) of the plant are used (flowers, leaves, roots), weather and soil conditions during the growing

---

Box 2
Examples of herbs with tonic or specific activities for the listed organ systems or conditions

Adaptogens (whole body systems): Asian and Siberian ginseng, *Panax* spp and *Eleutherococcus senticosis;* astragalus, *Astragalus* spp

Immune system: Echinacea, *Echinacea* spp; Asian and Siberian ginseng; licorice root, *Glycyrrhiza* spp; gotu kola, *Centella asiatica;* schisandra, *Schisandra chinensis;* astragalus

Kidney/urinary tract: Astragalus, dandelion root, *Taraxacum officinale,* marshmallow, *Althaea officinalis,* thyme, *Thymus vulgaris*

Cardiovascular: Hawthorn, *Crataegus oxyancantha,* motherwort, *Leonurus cardiaca,* Asian ginseng

Liver: Milk thistle, *Silybum marianum,* dandelion, turmeric, *Curcuma* spp, artichoke, *Cynara scolymus;* Oregon grape, *Mahonia aquifolium;* yellow dock or curly dock, *Rumex crispus*

Adrenal glands: Licorice root

Cognition: Ginkgo, *Ginkgo biloba;* gotu kola

Nervous system: Oats, *Avena sativa;* St John's wort, *Hypericum perforatum;* skullcap, *Scutellaria lateriflora;* valerian, *Valeriana officinalis;* gingko, hops, *Humulus lupulus;* chamomile, *Matricaria recutita* related to *Anthemis nobilis;* cat nip, *Nepeta cataria;* lemon balm, *Melissa officinalis*

Digestive system: Ginger, *Zingiber officinale;* slippery elm, *Ulmus rubra;* meadowsweet, *Filipendula ulmaria;* goldenseal, *Hydrastis Canadensis;* chamomile, milk thistle, artichoke, turmeric, several of the mints have intestinal soothing activities.

Musculoskeletal system: Devil's claw, *Harpagophytum procumbens;* capsicum, *Capsicum annuum;* boswellia, *Boswellia serrata;* yucca, *Yucca achidigera;* yarrow, *Achillea millefolium;* wild yam, *Dioscorea villosa;* sarsaparilla, *Smilax* spp; burdock, *Arctium lappa;* meadowsweet, turmeric, licorice root

***Qi* tonic:** Astragulus

Analgesics: Corydalis, *Corydalis* spp; California poppy, *Eschscholzia californica;* St John's wort; wild yam

Anti-inflammatory: Willow, *Salix alba;* devil's claw; boswellia; ginger; meadowsweet

Data from Refs.[21–26]

---

season, when the plant was picked, what methods were used for harvesting and transporting to the packaging plant, etc.

There are 2 ways to standardize herbs: (1) by selecting 1 (or more) of the bioactive ingredients and standardizing the final product to the percentage contents of this ingredient or (2) by standardizing to ensure that the product contains the plant that is listed on the label. Both of these methods have their advantages and disadvantages.

Many herbs affect multiple organ systems. Tonic herbs create homeostasis or balance with the biochemical and physiologic events that comprise body systems. Adaptogen is a term coined by herbalists to refer to any of many rejuvenating herbs used to normalize and regulate the systems of the body (**Box 2**).

As a general rule, only small amounts of bioactive ingredients are found in the whole plant. One or more of these ingredients may be concentrated by various methods of extraction, including (1) hot water (teas and tisanes), (2) alcohol (tinctures), and (3) glycerol (and other nonalcoholic extractions). Note that any method of extraction will (1) diminish the potential of synergistic effects and (2) increase the potential for a "concentrated" ingredient to reach a toxic level.

> **Box 3**
> **Veterinary homeopathic resources**
>
> - The Academy of Veterinary Homeopathy: www.theavh.org.
> - Day C. Homeopathic Treatment of Small Animals. Cambridge (UK): CW Daniel; 1990.
> - Hamilton D. Homeopathic Care for Cats and Dogs. Berkeley (CA): North Atlantic Books, 1999.
> - Llewellyn G. Homeopathic Remedies for Dogs. Mail Neptune (NJ): TFH, 1998.
> - Macleod G. Cats: Homeopathic Remedies and Dogs: Homeopathic Remedies. Cambridge (UK): CW Daniel; 1990, 1991.
> - Pitcairn RH. Dr. Pitcairn's Complete Guide to Natural Health for Dogs and Cats. 3rd edition. Emmaus (PA): Rodale; 2005.

While dosage levels may be important for some herbs for certain conditions, many herbalists claim that very small amounts of whole herbs often yield excellent results.

Advantages of Herbal Remedies for the Geriatric Patient

- As a general rule, their actions on organ systems are mild.
- The small amounts of active ingredients they contain (especially when using whole herbs) will not tax the geriatric animal's compromised organ system's ability to eliminate them.
- Their synergistic effects may make even small amounts of active ingredients effective.
- Many herbs have beneficial effects on multiple organ systems, and some affect almost all systems.
- Herbal remedies are available that have proven activity for all organ systems and for many of the biochemical pathways of the body, thus making it easy to provide for each patient's individual needs.
- In addition to their medicinal qualities, herbal plants have nutritional value as well, including vitamins, minerals, fiber, and proteins.
- Many herbs/plants are very high in antioxidant content (helping delay the aging process and activating many of the beneficial healing pathways); many more have a diuretic effect (helping to eliminate toxins).

Disadvantages

- Some herbs may be toxic (and toxicities may be species specific); some may interfere with the activity of conventional drugs or with normal biochemical pathways (have an anticoagulant effect, for example); and some plants may even be poisonous (for more information on both safety/efficacy and potential harmful side effects of individual/specific herbs see Refs.[20–26])
- Palatability may be a problem, especially with some herbs and more especially when using alcoholic tinctures.
- Their mild activity may not be what is needed in all situations. (Or as one herbalist said, "If you've just been hit by a car, you probably don't want to call for an herbalist.")

Box 3 lists some herbs that have tonic or specific activity for the listed organ systems or condition.

HOMEOPATHY
Introduction

Homeopathy was developed in the early 1800s by the German physician Samuel Hahnemann. Its methodology assumes that "like treats like." Homeopathic remedies are developed by first observing symptoms in patients given dosages of various substances and then treating them with highly diluted preparations of the same substance.

Founded in 1995, the Academy of Veterinary Homeopathy is comprised of veterinarians who share the common desire to restore true health to their patients through the use of homeopathic treatment.

Homeopathy is probably the most controversial of the alternative medicines. Critics complain that (1) it has very few scientifically validated trials to validate its claims; (2) it does not seem possible that it could work, given the fact that its remedies are so highly diluted; c) contrary to Western concepts, as a remedy is diluted more and more, it becomes ever more potent; (4) it seems to rely on the "energetics" of the remedies rather than their chemical composition—a concept alien to Western science; and (5) diagnosis and treatment are based on combining the patient's body/mind/spirit into one inseparable whole, rather than focusing on the physical aspects commonly relied on in Western medicine.

However, dedicated practitioners and millions of satisfied users (human and animal) would testify to its safety and efficacy, and there are many recent studies that attest to this.[27] Furthermore, since homeopathic remedies have no chemical composition to be eliminated and/or dealt with by the patient's body, it could be the ideal medicine for treating the geriatric patient with compromised organ system function.

Using Classic Homeopathy

When classic homeopathy is used to treat any of the chronic diseases especially prevalent in geriatric patients, the remedies are individualized to the specific patient's totality of symptoms (physical, mental, and emotional), not to the disease. This means that 2 different patients with the same Western-diagnosed disease might be prescribed 2 entirely different homeopathic remedies. Thus, it is almost impossible to make up a list of diseases, geriatric or otherwise, and their appropriate homeopathic cures (**see Box 3**).

FLOWER ESSENCES/BACH FLOWERS
Introduction

Systems of healing with flower essences use similar principles to homeopathy, although individual flower essence remedies have not been potentized as have homeopathic remedies.

The modern therapeutic system based on flower essences was developed by the British physician, Edward Bach, in the mid-1930s. Flower essence remedies are made from individual plant flowers, each containing a specific vibrational imprint that responds in a balancing, repairing, and rebuilding manner to imbalances in patients on their physical, emotional, mental, and spiritual or universal levels.[28]

Bach identified 38 flower essences, each with a natural affinity to certain mental states, and based on their resonance with normal body rhythms, Bach showed that these healing remedies have the ability to restore healthy states of mind. Since Bach's days, many more flower remedies, developed by various practitioners, also have been shown to be effective.

Table 1 shows some selected flower remedies that might be helpful for the geriatric patient.[28]

Table 1
Selected flower essence remedies

Essence	Remedies	Restores	Keynote
Agrimony	Concealed distress	Inner peace	Subtle signs of distress: panting, rapid heart rate
Aspen	Fear of unknown things	Courage	Apprehension
Clematis	Absentmindedness	Alertness	Absentmindedness
Gentian	Discouragement	Perseverance	Setback
Gorse	Hopelessness	Endurance	Despair
Hornbeam	Weakness	Vitality	Unresponsiveness
Larch	Hesitancy, loss of confidence	Confidence	Loss of confidence
Mustard	Depression	Serenity	Gloominess
Oak	Lack of resilience in normally strong animals	Resilience	Persistence in spite of adversity
Olive	Mental and physical exhaustion	Strength	Fatigue and exhaustion
Scleranthus	Imbalance, uncertainty	Stability, balance	Imbalance
Sweet chestnut	Extreme mental and physical distress	Endurance	Intense pain and distress
Wild rose	Resignation	The will to live	Apathy

Data from Graham H, Vlamis G. Bach flower remedies for animals. Forres (Scotland): Findhorn Press Ltd.; 1999. p. 94–6.

SUMMARY

During the past 20+ years of the author's veterinary career, before recent retirement from active practice, the author operated a wholly holistic practice. Most of the patients were geriatric or end-of-life dogs and cats. The greatest majority of the patients received acupuncture along with chiropractic adjustments and herbal and nutritional supplement prescriptions. The author would always discuss (coax and cajole) the topics of nutrition and exercise and the importance of the human–animal bond, and for those patients where it seemed appropriate, other therapies such as massage, flower essences, Reiki, etc, were recommended.

In the author's hands, this combination for treating arthritis in the geriatric patient has been almost always beneficial, consistently alleviating pain and often returning the animal to nearly normal musculoskeletal function. Further, this combination was used to treat immune-mediated diseases, skin conditions, urinary incontinence, and a host of other diseases—most of which were also responsive.

To be honest, though, conditions such as epilepsy, diabetes, thyroid imbalance, and other organ-specific dysfunctions would sometimes have seemingly miraculous responses; other times not much change was noticed, although some other practitioners have better results.

The author's experience with homeopathy is that a small percentage of clients were adamant that it be used as the primary therapy, and that was obliged. Homeopathic remedies (and the flower essences) were not as consistently effective as was acupuncture, but when they did work, the response was often dramatic and oftentimes seemingly miraculous.

Finally, in addition to the good results seen using the alternative medicines, the real reason the author kept his practice entirely holistic was purely selfish. The author became a veterinarian (many years ago) because he loved animals, not because he loved the science behind treating animal diseases. Using alternative medicines gave an opportunity to get hands on the animals (a chiropractic treatment is an intimate way to go skin-to-skin and heart-to-heart with your patient); to watch as animals actually enjoyed the treatments (most of the acupuncture patients would fall asleep during the treatment); and to spend some quality time with the patients and their owners, helping them and the clinic healing team come up with ways to provide the animal patient with a better quality of life for his or her end-of-life phase.

Admittedly, in the end, these factors—hands-on therapy, treatments that relaxed rather than confronted, and quality, compassionate time spent with patient and owner—may have been the biggest contributors to the successes of the author's treatments.

REFERENCES

1. Barzansky B, Jonas HS, Etzel SI. Educational programs in US medical schools, 1999-2000. JAMA 2000;284(9):1114–20.
2. Schoen A. Results of a survey on educational and research programs in complementary and alternative veterinary medicine at veterinary medical schools in the United States. J Am Vet Med Assoc 2000;216(4):502–9.
3. Benor DJ. Healing research: volume I, spiritual validation of a healing revolution. Bellmawr (NJ): Wholistic Healing Publications; 2007. Available at: www.Wholistic HealingResearch.com. Accessed April 10, 2012.
4. US Department of Health and Human Services; National Institutes of Health; National Center for Complementary and Alternative Medicine. The use of complementary and alternative medicine in the United States. December 2008. Available at: www.nccam. nih.gov/news/camstats/2007/camsurvey_fs1.htm. Accessed April 10, 2012.
5. Owen CG, Nightingale CM, Rudnicka AR, et al. Family dog ownership and levels of physical activity in childhood: findings from the child heart and health study in England. Am J Public Health 2010;100(9):1669.
6. Reeves MJ, Rafferty AP, Miller, CE, et.al. The impact of dog walking on leisure-time physical activity: results from a population-based survey of Michigan adults. J Phys Activity Health 2011;8(3):436–44.
7. International Veterinary Acupuncture Society. Available at: www.IVAS.org. Accessed April 10, 2012.
8. Durkes TE. Gold bead implants. Probl Vet Med 1992;4(1):207–11.
9. Gulanber EG. The clinical effectiveness and application of veterinary acupuncture. American Journal of Traditional Chinese Veterinary Medicine 2008;3(1):9–22.
10. McClelland GB. Chiropractic and geriatrics: care for the aging. White House Conference on Aging, American Chiropractic Association, September 10, 2004. p. 4.
11. Coulter ID, Hurwitz E, Aronow H, et al. Chiropractic patients in a comprehensive home-based geriatric assessment. Top Clin Chiro 1996;3(2):46–55.
12. Rupert RL, Manello D, Sandefur R. Maintenance care: health promotion services to US chiropractic patients aged 65 and over. J Manipulat Physiol Ther 2003;23(1):10–9.
13. Gleberzon BJ. A narrative review of the published chiropractic literature regarding older patients from 2001–2010. J Can Chiropract Assoc 2011;55(2):76–95.
14. Cassiday JD, Boyle E, Cote P, et al. Risk of vertebrobasilar stroke and chiropractic care. Spine 2008;33(4 Suppl):S176–83.
15. Thiel HW, Bolton JE, Docherty S, et al. Safety of chiropractic manipulation of the cervical spine: a prospective national survey. Spine 2007;32(21):2375–8.

16. Gouveia LO, Castanho P, Ferreira JJ. Safety of chiropractic interventions: a systematic review. Spine 2009;34(11):E405–13.

17. Cooperstein R., Killinger LZ. Chiropractic techniques in the care of the geriatric patient. In: Gleberzon BJ, editor. Chiropractic care of the older patient. Oxford (UK): Butterworth-Heinemann; 2001. p. 359–83.

18. Fabricant DS, Farnsworth NR. Value of plants used in traditional medicine for drug discovery. Environ Health Perspect 2001;109(Suppl 1):69–75.

19. Veterinary Botanical Medicine Association. Available at: www.vmba.org. Accessed April 10, 2012.

20. Mills S, Bone K. The essential guide to herbal safety. Amsterdam: Elsevier Churchill Livingstone; 2005.

21. Fougere BJ. Approaches in veterinary herbal medicine prescribing. In: Wynn SG, Fougere BJ, editors. Veterinary herbal medicine. St Louis (MO): Mosby; 2007. p. 275–90. Chapter 19.

22. Materia medica. In: Wynn SG, Fougere BJ, editors. Veterinary herbal medicine. St Louis (MO): Mosby; 2007. p. 459–684. Chapter 24.

23. Mowery DB. Herbal tonic therapies. Chicago (IL): McGraw Hill publishers; 1996.

24. Medical Economics. PDR for Herbal Medicines (Physician's Desk Reference for Herbal Medicines). North Olmsted (OH): Thomson Healthcare, Advanstar Communications; 1998.

25. Kidd JR. Dr. Kidd's guide to herbal dog care. North Adams (MA): Storey Publishing; 2000.

26. Kidd JR. Dr. Kidd's guide to herbal cat care. North Adams (MA): Storey Publishing; 2000.

27. Ullman D. Homeopathic family medicine: evidence based homeopathy. Available at: www.homeopathic.com. Accessed April 10, 2012.

28. Graham H, Vlamis G. Bach flower remedies for animals. Forres (Scotland): Findhorn Press Ltd.; 1999.

Implementing a Successful Senior/ Geriatric Health Care Program for Veterinarians, Veterinary Technicians, and Office Managers

William D. Fortney, DVM

KEYWORDS

- Geriatric • Aging • Senior • Health care

KEY POINTS

- A successful, comprehensive senior health care program can significantly increase the quality of life and longevity of all older dog and cats.
- Regularly scheduling a senior wellness examination is one of the most important steps pet owners can take to keep their older pets healthy.
- Since each organ ages at a different biological rate, the assessment of a patient's overall health status should be based on a screening of each organ function.
- Early benchmark changes of aging are commonly identified on "routine" senior profiling, further validating the value of routine screening testing protocols of healthy older patients.
- A senior health care program implies both a preventative wellness strategy and a comprehensive therapeutic approach to the management of acute and chronic conditions in aging dogs and cats.

INTRODUCTION

Senior health care, geriatric health care, senior wellness, geriatric wellness, and senior care are all terms for specific health care programs that are designed to improve the routine veterinary health care of older dogs and cats. While the veterinary profession may not agree on what to call the program, what age to start the program, what diagnostics evaluations to include in the program, or even how often per year the patient should be evaluated, we are all in agreement that the program should significantly increase the older patient's quality of life and their longevity.

In the early 1990s, the concept of a geriatric wellness and geriatric health care program was being considered in veterinary teaching hospitals. Veterinarians were

The author has nothing to disclose.
Department of Pathobiology and Diagnostic Medicine, Kansas State University College of Veterinary Medicine, Manhattan, KS 66506, USA
E-mail address: wfortney@vet.k-state.edu

doing a good job of managing age-related diseases once they were made aware of the patient's problem(s). However, in general neither the veterinarians nor the owners were aggressively "looking" for subclinical or early problems.

"Senior Care" exploded in the mid 1990s when Pfizer Animal Health implemented the national marketing concept of Senior Care. In essence, their Senior Care model was the newly emerging geriatric health care program but was also a set of marketing tools and education client brochures that dovetailed with their new senior-specific line of products. In the past 2 decades, senior/geriatric health care programs evolved as the recognized platform for healthy old pet evaluations, preanesthetic protocols, and approach to testing clinically ill animals and chronic drug monitoring protocols.

AGING

It is difficult to totally understand older dog and cat health programs without at least having some understanding of how animals age.

An animal's life can be divided into 4 stages; pediatric, adult, senior (mature, middle age), and the traditional geriatric (senior/super senior). The senior/middle age years represent the transition period between the relatively "healthy" adult years and the traditional "geriatric" age period where serious age-related diseases are significantly more prevalent. The senior (transition) period signals the patient's initial decline in physical condition, organ function, sensory function, mental function, and immune responses.[1] During this period of progressive decline, it would be appropriate on all veterinarians to take an age-specific history of the senior patient, perform complete age-related physical examinations, recommend selected diagnostic screening testing, advocate a premium senior diet, and provide weight consultations, plus increasing the caregiver's awareness and educate him/her on age-related disease symptoms.

Although the exact time of each life stage could be argued for each breed, it is generally agreed that cats live longer than dogs; smaller breed dogs live longer than larger breed dogs; and each life stage has a corresponding chronologic difference. In the early 1980s, Dr Richard T. Goldston took a more scientific approach to this premise.[2] The result was various versions of the popular human/pet age analogy charts.

The current human/pet age analogy chart (**Fig. 1**) helps clarify the longevity versus size concept for both clients and hospital staff. These relative age charts also emphasize the concept of comparable "time compression" differences between humans and animals. The take home message being that animals require shorter intervals between routine wellness testing than humans, in pets, all chronic diseases progress much faster than similar conditions in people and the need for repeated drug monitoring intervals to be undertaken more often in older dogs and cats. Hanging an age analogy chart in each exam room is a useful and inexpensive marketing strategy.

DECLINING PHYSIOLOGIC RESERVES HELPS DEFINING AGING

Aging is the sum of the deleterious effects of time on the cellular function, microanatomy, and physiology of each body system. Aging is not a specific disease but rather a complex process of genetic, biological, nutritional, and environmental factors all contributing to the progressive regression called aging. These factors affect varying rates of progressive and irreversible degenerative changes of all body tissues and organ systems. The rate of the physiologic decline and lack of reserves varies between species, breeds, and even littermates. Individuals at equal chronologic ages may experience different alterations. For some organs, the level of decline may be rapid and dramatic, while for others organs, the changes are much less significant.

Human/Pet Age Analogy

Adult Size in Pounds

Pet Age	Feline	Canine 0-20	21-50	51-120	>120	Human Equivalent Age
3 years	28	28	29	31	39	
4 years	32	33	34	38	49	
5 years	36	38	39	45	59	
6 years	40	42	44	52	69	
7 years	44	46	49	59	79	
8 years	48	50	54	66	89	
9 years	52	54	59	73	99	
10 years	56	58	64	80		
11 years	60	62	69	87		
12 years	64	66	74	94		
13 years	68	70	79			
14 years	72	74	84			
15 years	76	78	89			
16 years	80	82	94			
17 years	84	86				
18 years	88	90				
19 years	92	94				
20 years	96					

Age Analogy Chart: W. Fortney, R. Goldston

☐ Adult
▨ Senior
■ Geriatric

Fig. 1. The current human/pet age analogy chart.

Long-term physiologic declines of the major organ systems lead to an altered patient response to stressors, infections, and various drugs. Therefore, it is the declining physiologic reserves that tailor our medical approach to the geriatric patient. These biological aging changes manifest in progressive deteriorations in physical condition, organ function, mental function, and immune response, but not necessarily correlating with the patient's birth date. The actual age of an organism is referred to as "chronologic" aging and should be distinguished from "biologic" aging, which is the relative functional age of each of an individual's diverse organ systems.

Using the patient's age as a point of reference for their collective decline is appropriate. However, because each organ has a different rate of biologic aging, any critical assessment of a patient's overall health status should be based on a complete health screening of each specific organ function if possible. It is not uncommon in practice to see a 20-year-old cat with the kidneys of an adult or, conversely, a 6-year-old cat with geriatric kidneys. This is the basis for advocating a senior laboratory and diagnostic evaluation in apparently healthy pets starting at 7 years of age.

At some critical stage in the progressive decline, the physiologic "tipping point" for that organ is reached.[3] All of that particular organ's physiologic reserves are exhausted, resulting in overt changes in diagnostic tests; biochemical parameter(s), and/or the onset of clinical symptoms.

These measurable points are referred to as "benchmarks" of organ aging. Usually, these slowly progressive benchmarks are often subtle, undetected, or misinterpreted by the owner until the patient is stressed by an unrelated illness, boarding, medications, or general anesthesia. Increasingly, those early benchmark changes are identified on "routine" senior profiling, further validating the value of routine screening testing protocols of healthy patients.

INTRODUCTION TO SENIOR/GERIATRIC HEALTH CARE PROGRAMS

Senior pets represent 30% to 40% of patients, and this number will most likely increase as technology and education progress.[4] This movement in pet population demographics is due to several interconnected factors involving owners, animals, and the veterinary profession. As a result, senior medicine will continue to be an increasing profit center for practices.

The evolving positive attitudes most owners have toward their pets (the "human–animal" bond) has significantly contributed to increases in their pet's life expectancy. Today, a large group of animal caregivers consider their pets as being "family members." They are more willing to invest the time, the resources, and the commitment necessary to appropriately prevent and manage the chronic infirmities often associated with aging.

In parallel with the rise of the "human-animal bond," the veterinary profession, along with the pharmaceutical industry, has responded with significant developments in comprehensive health care options, diagnostics, and therapies. Enhanced senior diets, improved dental care, superior diagnostic techniques, new drugs, safer anesthetic protocols, newer surgery techniques, advances in cancer chemotherapy, pain management strategies, and the use of multimodal management strategies are changing the senior health care landscape. Advances in procedures, diagnostics, and equipment once reserved for referral centers are now accessible to the primary care veterinarians to provide their older patients the high quality care that even the "average" pet owner is now expecting and is also willing to pay for.

Every senior/geriatric care health program is based on 2 premises: first, there are fundamental differences in the specific diseases, behavior problems, and the nutritional needs of the older pet; and, second, prevention and/or early detection of age-related problems can have a very positive impact on the patient's quality of life and longevity. The purposes of clinical screening of healthy pets are to establish a baseline assessment for future comparison and to detect subclinical abnormalities at a time when preventive and therapeutic intervention may have the most benefit. Armed with the knowledge gleaned from the health screening, the progressive veterinarian is better positioned to prevent and/or manage problems in the earliest stages, thereby increasing the available options and improving the overall outcome.

In many respects, senior/geriatric care health programs have changed the traditional *reactive* veterinary sick animal "fix it shop" approach to a more *proactive* wellness health care tactic. Long-term health and patient well-being for older pets are the emphasized points of this platform. The strategy supports routine screening (history, physical examination, and diagnostics) of patients for early signs of disease, when the patient has the most options and the best opportunity for success.

WHY BUILD A SENIOR CARE PROGRAM IN YOUR PRACTICE?

Scheduling regular wellness examinations is one of the most important steps pet owners can take to keep their pets healthy. Since the risk factors for developing age-related diseases increase with aging, senior wellness examinations are more important than ever. Early detection of any health problem, especially age-related diseases, is paramount to long-term management success. The earlier the detection of any health or behavioral problem, the more options that are available to either cure the condition or slow the progression of the problem. By advocating more comprehensive histories, performing more complete physical examinations, and recommending more diagnostic testing of older pets, the clinician is providing higher-quality veterinary medicine for his/her senior patients.

A great deal of professional satisfaction for the veterinarian and staff comes from helping those long-established senior patients live longer, healthier lives; also, managing most age-related disease in the early phases is far more professionally rewarding than the "end stage."

Finally, while the veterinary profession has been very successful at providing comprehensive pediatric health care programs for decades, there are almost 2.25 times as many senior pets as puppies and kittens.[5] Dogs are puppies for 1 year but are seniors for 4 to 10 years.

A senior/geriatric health care program implies both a preventative wellness strategy and a comprehensive therapeutic approach to the management of acute and chronic conditions in aging dogs and cats. The program emphasizes prevention, early detection, and timely medical intervention, combined with client education.

Senior Care Program Essential Components

Four essential components of any Senior Care program should include:

1. Preventative health programs
2. A comprehensive patient health assessment (discovery)
   - Age-specific history
   - Complete age-related physical examination
   - Laboratory evaluation
   - Additional diagnostics
3. A formal review period where all the findings are communicated to the owner
4. Formulating specific short- and long-term action plans and scheduling a follow-up.

Just like there is no perfect veterinary hospital, there is no perfect blueprint for a senior/geriatric health care program that fits all practice scenarios. Instead, each practice must develop and tweak a program specifically catered to the client's wants, the practice's ability to provide appropriate services, and the associated financial issues.

When implementing a senior/geriatric health care program, the first critical decision each hospital must make is establishing the minimum database "boundaries" of the recommended health assessment. For example, exactly how detailed should the age-related history be? Which diagnostic screening tests should be included in the health assessment? The ultimate decisions for such a program are based on several interrelated factors including patient age, presence or absence of disease, current conditions and medications, and owner's interests and resources. Most hospitals initially use a basic (simple) screening strategy. However, over time, many expand the program to more extensive comprehensive health evaluations.

1. Routine preventive health program

A senior/geriatric health program must start with a comprehensive preventive health program, appropriate risk assessment of vaccine recommendations, endo and ecto parasite control, proper dental care, nutritional advice, weight counseling, and exercise guidance. Since the patient is already scheduled for annual evaluations, it is logical that preventive care be an integral part of the entire program.

2. Comprehensive health assessment

The primary purpose is discovery—to identify early disease conditions, recognize behavior problems, and establish a database for successive evaluations. To be comprehensive, the health assessment must include an age-specific history, complete age-related physical exam, and more appropriate laboratory and diagnostic evaluation.

An **age-specific history** using a medical, behavioral, and dietary history is the starting point of a complete health assessment. Pet owners can be invaluable sources of information on the overall health of their pets. Observant and well-trained owners can detect subtle changes in their pet's activity levels, elimination patterns, and behavior. Often this vital information is unapparent to the veterinarian and veterinary technician in an examination room setting.

Owner's observations, medication skills, and monitoring abilities are paramount to the overall success in managing certain chronic diseases. Therefore, the goal must be to convince each owner to become a much more active partner in the health care of their aging pet including their observation skills. Using a hardcopy history questionnaire greatly expedites time utilization if done in the waiting room, ensures that all the standard questions are asked, and educates the caregiver on those critical pain, disease, and behavior warning signs.

A complete age-related **physical examination** is the second part of the comprehensive health assessment. While a regular physical exam is part of any good health care evaluation, the senior/geriatric patient requires a more extensive examination. In addition to a standard physical, the additional examinations should include a weight assessment and gentle palpation of each skeletal joint for indications of osteoarthritis. Digital rectal examinations of the prostate and the presence of masses are worth the time and effort. Extra time should be taken for an extensive dental/oral examination, as well as diligent palpation of the mammary glands for skin and subcutaneous masses. Each tumor identified should be accurately measured and mapped in the medical record. Unless you are sure it is benign, a fine needle aspiration and cytology is appropriate. Some practitioners believe a Schirmer tear test in their older dogs is prudent.

An **appropriate laboratory evaluation** is the third portion of the comprehensive health evaluation. There is no arguing that the minimum laboratory database will result in early detection of age-related diseases that definitely benefit older pets. Routine testing of the clinicopathologic database is a critical component in the management of mature, senior, and geriatric patients because blood and urine testing allows one to detect subclinical abnormalities at a time when preventive and therapeutic intervention may have the most benefit.[6]

Precise comparisons of the laboratory values (normal and abnormal) changes seen in serial/sequential tests over 2 or more occasions (referred to as trending) is a helpful diagnostic and prognostic tool. Trending may help in recommending future baseline testing intervals.[7] The larger the data trends between samples, the shorter the testing interval should be.

Advantages of baseline testing in senior patients include (1) helping to establish a diagnosis in a patient with a known illness, (2) assessing and monitoring potential adverse drug reactions, (3) providing assessment of the patient's anesthetic risks, (4) perhaps uncovering subclinical/undetectable disease in apparently healthy patients, and (5) establishing a "normal" laboratory baseline for direct comparison at a later date when the patient has an obvious illness.

In addition, senior profiling allows veterinarians to select safer sedation/anesthesia protocols. However, the debate remains regarding what screening tests are appropriate for an apparently "healthy" senior/geriatric dog or cat. That argument will not be solved in this article.

The laboratory profiling and additional diagnostics, part of a simple program, a complex program, or something in-between, is a choice the practice decision maker will make early on. As stated earlier, what constitutes a minimum laboratory and diagnostic database is complicated and not easy to determine. While it would be nice to run all of the tests available, it is not practical or affordable for most clients. Fortunately, some compromise will be found based in the overall practice philosophy and the logistics of providing the testing, combined with the average client's level of financial interest.

A reasonable starting minimum database for the "healthy" older patient should include a complete blood count, biochemical profile with electrolytes, complete urinalysis (specific gravity, urine testing sticks, and urine cytology), fecal flotation, and heartworm and tick-borne disease testing in appropriate patients.[8] The minimum senior feline database includes a complete blood count, biochemical profile with electrolytes, complete urinalysis (specific gravity, urine testing sticks, and urine cytology), fecal flotation, a total thyroxine, and feline leukemia/feline immunodeficiency virus testing in appropriate feline patients.[9,10] Based on the incidence of Cushing disease and hypothyroidism in dogs, some practices routinely incorporate thyroid and adrenal screening in their senior/geriatric health care programs.[8]

Additional diagnostic testing is the final portion of the comprehensive health examination. While arguably not part of a minimum database of the healthy older pet, various additional diagnostics are commonly incorporated into many successful health care programs. Those supplementary diagnostic tests include an electrocardiogram, thoracic radiographs assessing the cardiac silhouette and the presence of a mass(s), abdominal imaging (radiography or ultrasound) for any organ abnormalities, blood pressure measurement in cats, and ocular tonometry in dogs. For a list of additional tests, access the latest AAHA Senior Care Guidelines.[8]

3. Review period

Once the comprehensive health assessment is complete and the results finalized, it is time to inform the caregiver of the findings followed but any short- and long-term action plans and timelines.

A formal review period is the time where all the normal and abnormal findings are communicated to the owner in person or via phone, mail, e-mail, or some combination. Obviously that choice is a practice one. Given a choice, I have always promoted a "face-to-face" conversation. However, good news is very easy to convey with any method, while bad news in not. One of the advantages of pet-side laboratory testing is the rapid results turnaround requiring just a little extra time in the waiting area before receiving the review. In addition to a phone call, my family physician mails me a copy of my laboratory test results, a common practice in human medicine screening programs. The author suggests at least considering sending a copy of the laboratory results home with the owner. This value-added document can be shared with others in the home and the report often becomes part of the patient's private medical record. Obviously sending the report alone will invoke additional questions and time, so sending a corresponding piece, "Understanding Your Pet's Blood Work," minimizes the questions and increases the perceived value of the tests.[11] Good examples of this great continuing education tool can be found online.

Regardless of how your practice elects to manage the review period, the author suggests that you provide a written evaluation (a health "report card") of the pet's summary health report for the owner to take home to share with any other caregivers and a copy for your medical records.

It is commonplace to send home any appropriate client education materials used to help reinforce any health issues at home and distributed to the other home caregivers. To be optimally effective, this step must occur in a timely fashion and not several days later.

Two common errors caregivers of older pets make are (1) failure to observe subtle changes in their pet's activity or patterns and (2) assumption that nothing can be done about old age diseases. Regardless of the cause, the owner's failure to inform the veterinarian of the early symptoms often results in a missed opportunity to help the pet when it could actually help the most.

As the pet ages, each owner must assume an increasing responsibility for the overall health care of their pets. Our task as a health professional is to help our clients fulfill that role. One of the most important steps pet owners can take to keep their pets healthy is to become a better observer and reporter. By using educational tools including brochures and the practice's website, and combining education with some training, most clients can be become an important member of their pet's health care team. Their awareness of any change in their pet can be invaluable . . . only if they know what to look for. Recognition of even mild changes in a pet's habits, activity patterns, behavior, weight, eating, or elimination patterns may be a signal that something serious is developing.

While many other owners do observe many of those subtle symptoms and changes in behaviors in their older pet, sadly those observations are often misinterpreted as just part of "normal aging" and that "nothing can be done about the condition." The owners failure to inform their veterinarian of the early symptoms usually results in a missed opportunity to manage the early condition when it could actually help the most. As a result, their pet continues to suffer from the lack of medical attention and care. Tragically after weeks, months, or years of suffering, the pet is finally presented to the veterinarian for euthanasia.

Some examples of commonly assumed "just old age" conditions include inactivity (chronic pain, arthritis, or a systemic illness), bad breath (dental disease), decreased appetite (chronic pain, dental disease, or a systemic disease) decreased vision (cataracts), periods of disorientation or confusion (cognitive dysfunction syndrome), and early-morning stiffness (arthritis). The slowly progressive symptoms of osteoarthritis are commonly misinterpreted by the owner. They assume the dog or cat is just slowing down and not wanting to play as much due to an old age–related lack of energy. Even minimal education could alter many of these outcomes.

The most common serious problems in older dogs include cancer, heart disease, kidney disease, liver disease, osteoarthritis, and cognitive dysfunction syndrome. In cats, cancer, kidney disease, heart disease, diabetes, and thyroid disease top the list. It is important for owners to observe the early warning signs of the most common life-shortening diseases in elderly pets. Equally important is that they report them to their veterinarian as soon as possible. Waiting for the next annual examination may be too late.

A partial list of warning signs that owners should look for includes:

- Changes in weight, especially weight loss
- Decreased appetite or inappetance
- Increased water consumption
- Changes in elimination patterns (urine or stool)
- New lumps or bumps or swellings, or changes in existing ones
- Persistent cough
- Difficulty breathing or breathing heavily or rapidly at rest
- Sudden collapse or bout of weakness
- Difficulty climbing stairs or jumping
- Foul mouth odor or drooling
- Seizure, convulsion, or fit
- Pain.

4. Short- and long-term action plans and a follow-up

During the review period, the clinician and the client need to formulate specific short and long-term action plans for each new problem identified. If no problem(s) are found, then continue the annual or bi-annual evaluations as scheduled. Either way, specific recommendations for diet, exercise, and dental care should be explicitly communicated. Dietary recommendations should be based on the health needs of the patient and not on cost alone. Those factors influencing the diet selection includes quality of ingredients, specific antioxidants shown to modify the aging process, and a research-based formulation. Any dental procedures, medication, therapies, re-testing, or additional testing should be discussed and scheduled.

Timely follow-up telephone calls and written reminders are essential components and critical in the overall success of any senior/geriatric health care program. A critical part of any follow-up is scheduling the next appointment prior to leaving the hospital if for a healthy patient. Setting a routine appointment time even if it is 6 months or 1 year later reinforces the program timetable.

A standard practice policy of a phone call-back within 72 hours of the examination to discuss questions, concerns, medication issues, dietary needs, etc; it also sends an honest message of caring to the owner.

Senior/geriatric health care reminders should not be vaccine and parasite related but rather focused on wellness and the advantages of health evaluations. While infectious disease preventatives are important, the emphasis is shifted to that of wellness and age-related disease prevention program and strategies.

MAKING THE PROGRAM SUCCESSFUL

Obviously the professional rewards are proportional to the success of the program. And while success is never guaranteed, the 10 steps listed later may help you reach your program's ultimate goals.

A successful program requires a large tool box. Tools for client education, health data gathering and health reporting tools, patient diagnostic and management charts, plus program implementation tips are currently available for successfully implementing a senior/geriatric health care program in your practice. Reinventing the wheel is time consuming and can be frustrating. Veterinary articles and seminars are good sources of ideas and suggestions. One course of information is the earlier mentioned AAHA Senior Care Guidelines.[8]

Other sources of support are marketing tools, the products, and services various industries have available for old dog and cat health care. For example, IDEXX (Westbrook, ME, USA) can provide practices with advanced age-related in-house diagnostics and referral laboratory diagnostic services. In addition, they can also include some marketing and implementation tools necessary to make your program more successful.

TEN STEPS TO MAKE A SENIOR/GERIATRIC HEALTH CARE PROGRAM SUCCESSFUL

1. The practice decision maker must be convinced that a senior/geriatric health care will become a significant asset to the practice before investing the time, energy, training, and resources necessary in developing and maintaining the program. However, because of the commitment necessary for success and growth, this program is not for every practice and—depending on the level of interest and finances—may not appeal to every client. Unfortunately, this is not a "build it and they will come" plan.

2. Convince the entire staff of the significant health benefits the program offers the senior pet. Critical to the success or failure of a senior/geriatric health care program is the involvement and buy-in of your staff. In fact, ownership of the program by every staff member is essential. Staff incentive programs will also help the senior/geriatric health care program patient base grow and maintain the program's momentum.

3. Create a very specific and detailed program including age of onset, frequency of visits, scheduling periods, fee structure, educational materials, and marketing strategies. Decide exactly which tests are to be included in the program. Finally, ensure every member of the staff is "program proficient" and can sufficiently understand the particulars.

4. Convince the owners of the significant health benefits the program offers their aging pet. A percentage of your practice (ie, the "A-list caregivers") will readily accept the program, but the rest will need repeated convincing. Increased client knowledge usually equates to increased client acceptance and compliance. Early and persistent owner education is a long-term investment in a senior/geriatric health care program.

5. A well-designed market strategy correlates with success. Use newsletters, reminder cards, invoices, telephone directory ads, Web pages, and social media to educate your current and prospective clients on age-related problems and solutions. Client marketing efforts should emphasize all the advances in veterinary medicine including newer diagnostic testing, improved anesthetics and anesthetic monitoring equipment, behavioral drugs, newer arthritis therapy options, leading edge cancer chemotherapy, more effective cardiac medications, dental care, and nutritional advancements that are available.

6. Bundle the fee structure to include a senior pet discount. Discount the fee for all the services and also consider a cost reduction in the senior diets for any patients already on the program.

7. Start slow and be patient and the program will grow. A senior/geriatric health care program is a long- term hospital investment. It is much easier to add a test and expand the program than take one away because the cost was considered

excessive for the average owner. Unfortunately, an overzealous program coupled with underdelivery of value is commonplace. The seeds of program success and client subscription actually begin when outlining a life-long preventive health care program the first time a new owner visits the practice, even for puppies or kittens.[5,12]

8. Since a comprehensive health examination will require more time in the exam room, try to schedule these appointments during slow days or during periods of the day when you can devote the time necessary for a complete evaluation.

9. An attractive 3-color trifold brochure for your practice's program is an easy and time-saving marketing tool. The brochure should be uniquely branded to your practice. Highlight the specifics of your program (age of onset, visits per year, etc), but keep the piece simple for an easy read. Emphasize the advantages of the health program to the older pets and the early warning disease signs to watch for.

10. Periodic program review by your clients and staff is essential in maintaining the consistently high standard of care you have established for your senior patients. Do not be afraid to modify the program to meet the emerging minimum database protocols.

SUMMARY

A senior/geriatric care health program is a more inclusive wellness program than those recommended for all healthy "adult" pets. Older dogs and cats have a different set of needs and challenges than when they were younger. Aging in animals is similar to aging in people except at an accelerated rate. To offset this faster aging process and increased "time compression" and to detect potentially serious conditions at the earliest stages, most progressive small animal practices are now recommending examinations every 6 months even with healthy senior/geriatric dogs and cats. Initially, the program starting at around 7 years of age for both species is commonplace.

Comprehensive health evaluations, including senior profiling, allow veterinarians to more successfully diagnose and manage an early condition. The detection of underlying diseases also impacts pharmaceutical selections and chronic drug monitoring. In addition, the routine laboratory evaluation supports safer sedation/anesthesia protocols.

REFERENCES

1. Mosier JE. Effect of aging on body systems of the dog. Vet Clin North Am Small Anim Pract 1989;19(1):1–13.
2. Goldston RT, Hoskins JD. Geriatrics and gerontology of the dog and cat. Philadelphia: WB Saunders; 1995.
3. Fortney WD. Declining physiological reserves: defining aging. Nestle Purina Companion Animal Nutrition Summit Proceedings, March 2010. Available at: http://breedingbetterdogs.com/pdfFiles/articles/CAN2010_updated.pdf. Accessed April 10, 2012.
4. Metzger FL. Senior and geriatric care programs for veterinarians. Vet Clin North Am Small Anim Pract 2005;35(3):743–53.
5. Hoskins JD, McCurnin DM. Geriatric care in the late 1990s. Vet Clin North Am Small Anim Pract 1997;27(6):1273–84.
6. Epstein M, Kuehn NF, Landsberg G, et al. AAHA senior care guidelines for dogs and cats. J Am Anim Hosp Assoc 2005;41:81–91. Available at: https://www.aahanet.org/PublicDocuments/SeniorCareGuidelines.pdf. Accessed April 10, 2012.
7. Fortney WD. Interpretation of baseline testing in senior patients. DVM InFocus, Sept 2007.

8. AAHA senior care guidelines for dogs and cats. Available at: https://www.aahanet. org/Library/SeniorCare.aspx. Accessed April 10, 2012.

9. Rebar A, Metzger F. The veterinary CE advisor: interpreting hemograms in cats and dogs. Vet Med 2001;96(Suppl 12):1–12.

10. American Association of Feline Practitioners/Academy of Feline Medicine. Panel report on feline senior care. Available at: http://www.aafponline.org/about_guidelines.htm. Accessed April 10, 2012.

11. Purdue University College of Veterinary Medicine, Small Animal Clinic. Understanding your pet's blood work. Available at: http://www.vet.purdue.edu/vth/SACP/documents/ understandingyourpetsbloodwork.pdf. Accessed April 10, 2012.

12. Rucinsky R. Implementing a geriatric wellness program. Proceedings of The Central Veterinary Conference; Baltimore (MD), April 2009. Lenexa (KS): Advanstar; 2009.

Index

Note: Page numbers of article titles are in **boldface** type.

A

Vet Clin Small Anim 42 (2012) 835–851
http://dx.doi.org/10.1016/S0195-5616(12)00086-1
0195-5616/12/$ – see front matter © 2012 Elsevier Inc. All rights reserved.

vetsmall.theclinics.com

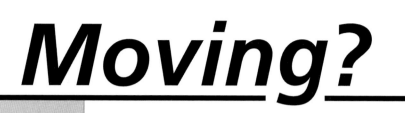